Praise for
And Still We Rise

"If you put no other book on your summer reading list, you should definitely share Corwin's journey through the lives of these students in *And Still We Rise*."

—Los Angeles Times

"An impressive, important work of narrative journalism. . . . A more gifted reporter can barely be imagined."

—San Francisco Chronicle

"Compelling and beautifully constructed. . . . In *And Still We Rise* . . . all the complexities of a carefully chronicled reality coalesce into art."

—Newsday

"Corwin is a thoughtful chronicler . . . giving this book layered meanings."

—St. Louis Post-Dispatch

"Miles Corwin's *And Still We Rise* is a book that both lifts the heart and afflicts the soul. It is an account of dreams fulfilled, of children from shattered families in a murderous neighborhood who will themselves into a program for gifted students and ultimately into college and the American mainstream. It is also an account of dreams endangered—by a society that thinks the SAT is the sole measure of merit, by a ghetto culture that glorifies self-destruction and academic failure, and even by a pair of teachers whose brilliance is undermined by their own bitter feud."

—Samuel G. Freedman, author of Small Victories

"Whether following the travails facing the vividly characterized students or those facing the class instructor, Toni Little, Corwin kept his own journalistic focus throughout a project that presented professional and ethical challenges of the most exasperating sort. He details the subsequent defeats and triumphs of will and discipline and keeps the story gritty and gripping."

—*Kirkus Reviews* (starred)

"Corwin gives added meaning to my grandmother's inspiring words to me as I struggled in poverty on our Alabama tenant farm in the 1940s. 'It doesn't take much yeast to make the bread rise,' she said. Heroic, creative, and productive people don't all come from fine prep schools and successful parents. Corwin reminds us that, given a chance, the spark of genius can be ignited in the most unlikely students from the meanest places in our country."

—Morris Dees, Southern Poverty Law Center

"This is a book as penetrating as it is brilliantly told. Miles Corwin has recorded, like a camera moving through a series of rooms, the human meaning of the lives he observed. What a stunning accomplishment."

—Leon Bing, author of *Do or Die*

PRAISE FOR MILES CORWIN'S
The Killing Season

"Moral, humane, and ultimately uplifting. . . . Rarely has the genre been worked to better effect. . . . He could scarcely have invented a better cast and story."

—*New York Times Book Review*

"Compelling." —*The New Yorker*

"A grab-you-by-the-throat page-turner. . . . Miles Corwin's intelligent, empathetic, and in-depth observations . . . offer rare insights."

—*Los Angeles Times Book Review*

And Still We Rise

AND STILL

WE RISE

WE RISE

The Trials and Triumphs of Twelve Gifted Inner-City Students

Miles Corwin

Perennial

An Imprint of HarperCollinsPublishers

Excerpt from "Mosely Had Charted the Territory Ahead" by Eric Shephard, *Los Angeles Times*, February 22, 1997, © 1997 Los Angeles Times. Reprinted by permission.

Excerpts from *Inherit the Wind* by Jerome Lawrence and Robert E. Lee.
Copyright © 1955 by Jerome Lawrence and Robert E. Lee.
Used by permission of Random House, Inc.

A hardcover edition of this book was published in 2000 by William Morrow and Company, an imprint of HarperCollins Publishers.

HarperCollins books may be purchased for educational, business, or sales promotional use. For information please write: Special Markets Department, HarperCollins Publishers Inc., 10 East 53rd Street, New York, NY 10022.

First Perennial edition published 2001.

Designed by Kellan Peck

The Library of Congress has catalogued the hardcover edition of their book as follows:

Corwin, Miles.
And still we rise : the trials and triumphs of twelve gifted inner-city high school students.
Miles Corwin.—1st ed.
p.cm.
1. Gifted children—Education (Secondary)—United States—Case studies. 2. Socially handicapped children—Education (Secondary)—United States—Case studies. 3. Education, Urban—United States—Case studies. 4. Crenshaw High School (Los Angeles, Calif.). I. Title.
LC3993.9.C678 2000
371.95'09794'94—dc21   99-046775

ISBN 0-380-79829-8 (pbk.)

01 02 03 04 05 JT/RRD 10 9 8 7 6 5 4 3 2 1

In memory of Moritz, Lili,
and Ingrid Wolff

Hope deferred maketh the heart sick;
but when the desire cometh, it is a tree of life.

PROVERBS 13:12

CONTENTS

CONTENTS

PART THREE
SECOND SEMESTER

PART FOUR
SPRING

INTRODUCTION

He was yet another victim of a drive-by shooting, a teenage boy splayed out on a South-Central Los Angeles street corner, with several gunshot wounds to the chest. He died before the paramedics arrived. The two homicide detectives could find no wallet and no identification on the boy, so the coroner's investigator called him John Doe Number 27.

The detectives assumed he was just another gangbanger caught in the wrong neighborhood, on the wrong street, on the wrong night, by the wrong gang. But a closer inspection of the body revealed an exam on the French Revolution neatly folded in his back pocket.

"Damn," a detective muttered in amazement. "Look at that printing."

It was clear to the detectives that the boy had taken the test very seriously. His printing was meticulous, each letter precise and carefully drawn. The test looked as if it had been scripted by a draftsman. And every one of the boy's answers on the exam was reasoned, thoughtful, and well written. At the top of the paper the teacher had written a large A.

"This doesn't look like your typical dipshit," a detective said, as he showed his partner the A. "This looks like a smart kid who was going somewhere."

I was researching a story about homicide in South-Central at the time and was with the two homicide detectives that night. We later discovered that John Doe Number 27 was a fifteen-year-old boy who was enrolled in a junior high school program for gifted students. He had just spent the afternoon at the Boys Club, and was walking home, when a group of gang members in a van asked him where he was from, the traditional gang challenge. He answered: "You don't know me." One of the boys in the van then pulled out a pistol and shot him.

As a reporter for the *Los Angeles Times,* I had written many stories about gangbangers, the kind of boys who were in the van that night. But after seeing the exam, the careful printing, the A, and learning a bit about the boy's life, I decided I wanted to find a way to write about the *other* children of South-Central, the students who avoid the temptations of the street, who strive for success, who, against all odds, in one of America's most impoverished, crime-ridden neighborhoods, manage to endure, to prevail, to succeed.

This idea seemed so consequential because the national debate about affirmative action was intensifying at the time. I wanted to show how truly slanted the playing field remains, how inequality is built into a system touted as a meritocracy, how students from places such as South-Central face such great obstacles that they still need the step up from affirmative action, and how it is not only they—but the universities as well—who benefit from the inclusion of those who excel despite impediments that derail students of lesser character and fortitude.

This idea continued to germinate until 1996, when an antiaffirmative-action initiative qualified for the ballot in California. At the time, affirmative action faced elimination in a number of other states as well and was a heated topic of debate across the country. I now had the topical context in which to frame a book that I had contemplated writing for several years.

To write about those students who would be most affected by the end of affirmative action, I needed to find an inner-city school where the students were bright and accomplished enough to have a chance for acceptance at top universities, but who needed the edge that affirmative action traditionally provides.

There are two high schools for gifted students in Los Angeles. One is in the San Fernando Valley, and the student body is almost 90 percent white and Asian and less than 1 percent black. The other program is located at Crenshaw High School, in the 'hood, and the vast majority of gifted students are drawn from inner-city neighborhoods throughout South-Central and Watts. All the students in the Crenshaw program—who are classified gifted as a result of IQ or standardized test scores—are minorities, most of whom are black. It is one of the few all-minority, gifted public high school programs in the nation.

In his novel, *The Bonfire of the Vanities,* Tom Wolfe, with a mixture of condescension and elitist sarcasm, proffers a stereotypical view of an inner-city high school.

A tabloid reporter calls an English teacher at an all-minority high school in the Bronx and asks if a boy is an "outstanding student."

At the school, the teacher explains, "we use comparative terms, but *outstanding* isn't one of them. The range runs more from cooperative to life-threatening."

The reporter then asks if the boy is a "good student."

"*Good* doesn't work too well . . . either," the teacher replies. "It's more 'Does he attend class or doesn't he?' "

"Let me ask you this," the reporter says. "How does he do on his written work?"

The teacher "lets out a whoop. *Written* work? There hasn't been any written work . . . for fifteen years . . . You're thinking about 'honor student' and 'higher achievers' and all that . . ." But, the teacher explains, at this high school, "an honor student is somebody who attends class, isn't disruptive, tries to learn and does all right at reading and arithmetic."

At Crenshaw's gifted program, however, I found many students who truly are outstanding; students who not only turn in written work, but, in some cases, write essays and poems that are dazzling; students, who, by any measure, are true honor students.

*   *   *

The gifted program is a high school within a high school, separate and autonomous. The gifted students share the hallways with the other Crenshaw students—including the gangbangers and the troublemakers—but they have different classes and teachers, and more demanding assignments. On a recent standardized exam, the tenth graders at Crenshaw's gifted program had the fifth-highest score in mathematics out of 106 high school programs in the school district—including a number of schools in affluent areas—and the sixth highest in reading.

At many inner-city schools, the peer pressure to fail is oppressive. Students who are articulate, who excel in class, are accused of "acting white," of "selling out." Many of the students I write about have endured this type of hazing in the school lunchroom, at the bus stops, in their neighborhoods, on the playgrounds. But in the gifted program, they are safe. In their classes all the students are bright; all the students have the potential to be achievers. And all the students know that, ultimately, they can do more for themselves, their families, and their neighborhoods by earning good grades, winning scholarships, and going on to college.

Ninety-eight percent of the students in the gifted program *do* go on to college. About a third of them attend University of California campuses, which accepts the top eighth of the state's high school graduates. Some of these students do not need affirmative action to qualify for prestigious universities. But many do.

South-Central is a sprawling, multiethnic ghetto with about a half-million residents, about a third of whom subsist below the national poverty level. The area was once virtually all black; now it is more than half Latino. While the rest of South-Central has been transformed by immigration, the neighborhood surrounding Crenshaw—and the composition of the school—has remained largely black. Many nonblack students could attend the gifted program because magnet schools are open to students from throughout the city, but they eschew Crenshaw. Some prefer to attend a school with more members of their own race; others seek a suburban setting or are frightened by the school's reputation for gang violence.

While gender politics and the call for diversity have influenced the debate, affirmative action was created in the 1960s to benefit blacks, whose history of enslavement, legally imposed segregation, and virulent discrimination is unprecedented in America. That is another reason why I thought a predominantly black school such as Crenshaw would be an ideal place to set this book.

The debate on affirmative action always comes back to the issues of "fairness" and "merit." But what if the criteria for university admission are not inherently equitable?

Many parents in suburban neighborhoods hire private Scholastic Aptitude Test tutors or pay for preparation courses for their children. Some of these students spend years preparing for the exam.

Almost every Crenshaw student I followed walked into the SAT test cold, with no preparation whatsoever. They had neither the money nor the time for SAT preparation. Most of the students had jobs ranging from part- to full-time, and when they returned home at night, after a day of school, and a swing shift at a fast food restaurant or clothing store or cleaners or convalescent hospital or taxi-dancing club, they barely had time to squeeze in some homework before dozing off. Preparing for the SATs was a luxury they could not afford.

Also, many schools use weighted grading systems that award extra points for Advanced Placement or honors courses. Students can fill their schedules with these courses and inflate their grade point averages. Most prep schools and high schools in affluent school districts offer many more of these courses than do inner-city schools such as Crenshaw. As a result, when the students apply for college and their grade point averages are analyzed, they have yet another advantage over Crenshaw students.

Sometimes the disadvantages of Crenshaw students are subtle but nonetheless significant. Some of the seniors at Crenshaw's gifted program, for example, enroll in Advanced Placement U.S. Government and Politics. At the end of the year, they take a standardized AP exam and compete against students from across the country, students whose parents subscribe to *Time* or *Newsweek,* who read the newspaper every morning, who discuss current events every night at dinner. Current events are an important variable of the exam, but parents of only two of the Crenshaw students subscribed to a newspaper.

For many of the students I followed, academic disadvantages are the least of their difficulties. I write about A students who live in foster and group homes because they have been abandoned or abused by their parents. I write about academic achievers whose only source of family income is the welfare check, students with fathers or brothers in prison, students who were raised in crumbling housing projects, students who were once members of the city's most violent street gangs. I write about students who are the sons and daughters of maids and crack addicts, street sweepers and street people, who work forty hours a week because they have to put food on the table and pay for rent and clothing.

I wanted to observe on a daily basis the many obstacles and pitfalls these students face during a school year. So I decided to follow the seniors at Crenshaw's gifted magnet—the class of 1997—from their first day of class, during their final year of high school, to graduation.

Advanced Placement English Literature and Composition seemed to be the best class to learn about these students. More gifted seniors take AP English than any other class. And students express themselves freely in AP English—both in classroom discussions and in writing assignments—so this would provide an intimate forum to glean insights into the students' academic and personal lives. I planned to follow other classes as well, but AP English, I decided, would be the book's unifying thread.

I had one major hesitation, however. There have been many books and movies about a year at a clichéd inner-city high school, with unruly, delinquent, menacing minority students, and wide-eyed—but inspirational—school teachers who ultimately lead the unfortunate ghetto youths to academic enlightenment. I wanted *And Still We Rise* to be different on a number of levels. First of all, this book is not the inspirational tale of a messianic schoolteacher. In this book, the students are the heroes and heroines, the ones with the inspirational stories. In this book, the students value education, sacrifice much to further their educations, and overcome many obstacles—including sometimes even their teachers—in order to obtain their educations. This book is not about a group of unerring students who, uniformly, withstand the temptations of their neighborhood. Although many do succeed, some break the law, or drop out, or lose interest in school. This book is not about hallowed students and sainted teachers; this book is not hagiography. This is journalism, and I attempt to present what I observed in a fair, unflinching manner.

The teacher of the AP English class, Toni Little, was an interesting character because of what she was not. She was not a do-gooder with unwavering dedication who decided to teach in the inner city because of her strong social conscience. She simply enjoyed teaching gifted students. Little is forty-one, white, and had taught gifted children at a suburban high school in the San Fernando Valley. She briefly left teaching, and when she returned she accepted the job at Crenshaw because she wanted to teach gifted students again. Her students' race and residence are irrelevant to her.

She is a controversial figure at the school because of her tempestuous personality and her countless battles with administrators, other teachers, and, sometimes, students. While Little is clearly a talented teacher, her volatility and her vexations frequently sidetrack her.

Little, another Crenshaw teacher said, is like the cow who gives a bucket of milk. And then kicks it over.

For much of the year in Little's class, I was a silent observer—Emerson's "transparent eyeball"—a role I have always assumed as a reporter. But there were times when I was forced to take an active role, to become a character in the unfolding drama. This was not a role I sought, or felt comfortable with; it was a role that, at times, was thrust upon me and, at other times, I chose to assume because the students' needs outweighed my desire to maintain the traditional journalistic reserve.

I also closely followed another gifted class at Crenshaw, junior English, taught by Anita "Mama" Moultrie, who was a compelling counterimage to Little. Moultrie has strong views on affirmative action and many other issues pertinent to the black community. And she does not hesitate to discuss them in class.

Moultrie, who also is forty-one, is black, lives in the neighborhood, and has devoted her career to inner-city students. Her manner of teaching English, her views on how to teach the classics, and her commitment to incorporating black writers and black themes into the curriculum were diametrically opposed to Little's. Yet the two teachers are inextricably entwined because Moultrie's juniors eventually became Little's seniors, and during the year I was at Crenshaw, the two teachers frequently clashed.

Two months after the school year began, Californians voted to end affirmative action in the state, which means that the state's public universities and state colleges no longer take race into account in order to increase minority admissions. Moultrie's juniors will be among the first students affected by the end of affirmative action.

Little's seniors, however, had a reprieve. They were among the last group of California seniors to benefit from race-based preferences. But they know that in four years, when they apply to law schools, medical schools, or other graduate programs, the end of affirmative action in the state will have a profound impact on their futures.

Shortly before the school year, I knew that the Crenshaw gifted magnet program had been a serendipitous choice. Because it was then I recalled the fifteen-year-old junior high school student whose murder several years earlier had impelled me to write about accomplished minority students. I realized that, had he not been killed, he would have enrolled at Crenshaw's gifted program the next year.

He would have graduated in 1997, along with the seniors whose stories I tell.

OLIVIA

I DON'T WANT HER

During the years of beatings by her mother, years of being whipped with an extension cord, smacked in the mouth with a telephone, pounded against a wall, punched in the lip, dragged by the hair through the hallway, tossed in the shower, and scalded with hot water, school was Olivia's salvation. The only kind words she heard, the only love she felt, the only compliments she received, were from her teachers. At home, no matter how she was tormented, no matter how long she cried, when the beatings were over, she always read her assignments, and prepared for her tests.

Olivia had always excelled in school and was always one of the brightest students in her class. And the As she strived for and always received enabled her to find a glimmer of happiness and hope during an abysmal childhood.

But when Olivia began the seventh grade, even the diversions and distractions of school were no longer enough. The beatings were now a daily torment. Each evening, when her mother returned from her job as a hotel maid, she always found a reason to beat Olivia. If Olivia's face was bruised, or her lip was split, her mother would tell her to say at school that she fell off a bicycle.

Olivia's stomach churned as she waited for her mother to walk through the door. She was terrified by the image that she knew would confront her: her mother's eyes wild, mouth wide open in a rictus of rage, shouting, "I hate you!" or "I wish you were never born!" and then spitting at her and dragging her around the house until carpet burns covered her body. Olivia could never understand why her mother seemed to detest her; she could never figure out exactly what she did to warrant yet another beating. When Olivia was a little girl she was convinced her mother was possessed by the devil. Her only respite from her anguish, her only reprieve from the beatings, she decided, was suicide. At school, she daydreamed about hanging herself, or swallowing an overdose of pills, or slashing her wrists.

But one afternoon after school, when her mother left for work, Olivia decided to run away instead. She ripped out of the Yellow Pages the shelter listings for abused children and battered women. She stuffed them in her back pocket and filled a duffle bag with clothes. Then, as an afterthought, she grabbed her mother's black leather jacket. Olivia had always been cowed into absolute obedience, and this was a final act of absolute defiance that meant to Olivia that she was never coming back, that, at twelve years old, she was forever severing the bond with her mother.

It was a windy March afternoon, and when Olivia stepped outside, she zipped up the jacket and ran until she was exhausted. At a busy intersection, she spotted a phone booth. She pulled out the list of shelters from her pocket and called a few, until she found one that agreed to pick her up. At dusk, she sat in the phone booth, cross-legged, and watched the light fade from the sky. Finally, two men in a van showed up and asked Olivia her name.

"I can't give you my name," she cried. "You'll just take me back to my mother. She'll kill me! Please don't make me give you my name." Olivia burst into tears. The men assured her that she was safe and drove her to a downtown shelter. That first night she shared a room with another girl and felt both relieved and frightened. Relieved that no one had called her mother. Frightened that someone might call her mother the next day and she would be sent home.

She spent ten days at the shelter before a social worker arranged a meeting with Olivia and her mother. Olivia recounted the beatings and the abuse. Her mother interrupted her and shouted, "She's making it all up! She's a liar!" Then she lunged at Olivia, and several shelter staff members had to restrain her.

A few months later a court hearing was held to determine Olivia's fate. She felt as if she were in a fog as the judge and social workers discussed her case. She remembers only the end of the hearing, when the judge told her mother that if she wanted the opportunity to regain custody of her daughter, she would have to undergo psychological testing, individual counseling, and family counseling. Olivia's mother told the judge, "She's the crazy one. Not me." The last words Olivia remembers her mother saying were, "I don't want her!"

Olivia was made a ward of the county. Her social worker told her she would be placed with a foster family, but there were no openings, so she was sent to a group home where six other girls were living. During the next few years, Olivia was shuttled between a series of Dickensian group homes and foster homes in South-Central Los Angeles. (A group home is an independent business with a hired staff; a foster home is a private house headed by a foster parent who lives there.)

At one group home, a supervisor only let the girls take showers every three days. At a foster home, during the heat of the summer, the foster mother locked the girls in their rooms all day. At another, the girls had to purchase their own food. At a group home, the girls kept stealing Olivia's clothes, and one wild-eyed girl chased her around the house with a hot iron. By the time she was sixteen, she had lived in ten different group or foster homes.

Olivia always felt she was an outsider. Her father, half black, half Cuban, barely played a role in her life. Her mother is Mexican. But Olivia considers herself black, partly because she has spent so many years living with black girls and black foster mothers and attending predominantly black schools. The other girls at the homes, however, never let Olivia forget her mixed heritage. And Olivia was always the only girl who cared about school, who did her homework, who dreamt of attending college. While Olivia was a precocious and articulate child, her housemates often were surly and monosyllabic girls who counted the days until they could drop out of high school, who talked about getting pregnant and living off welfare. Olivia spent more time chatting with the adults at the homes than with the girls.

When Olivia was about to start high school, a rare, compassionate group-home administrator gave her a pamphlet that listed the magnet schools in the Los Angeles school district. These schools were for students who had an interest in a particular field of study, or who had a talent for music or art, or who were classified as gifted because of their high IQ or standardized test scores. Olivia studied the pamphlet and discovered that one of the two high schools in the city for gifted students was located at Crenshaw High School, only a few miles from her South-Central group home.

One afternoon, she took the bus from her junior high school to Crenshaw and talked to several administrators. They told Olivia that her IQ and her standardized test scores—which were in the top 5th percentile of the nation—were well above the minimum requirement. She enrolled in the gifted magnet program in the ninth grade.

Crenshaw is an overcrowded, underfunded South-Central high school where two school district policemen armed with 9mm pistols patrol the grounds and where several neighborhood gangs fight for control. It is a high school where half the students come from families eligible for welfare, where about 90 percent participate in the federal free lunch program, where the dropout rate is almost 50 percent, and where only 4 percent of the seniors score above average on college aptitude tests. Known as "Da Shaw," it is one of the city's most notorious high schools. Crenshaw was the setting for the movie *Boyz N the Hood*, the alma mater of rapper Ice T, and the home base for the Rollin 60s, one of the city's most notorious street gangs.

The gifted magnet program, however, was a refuge for Olivia, and she immediately felt comfortable in the program. She met many other students who, like her, had wretched childhoods, yet had managed to stay focused on school and retain a love of learning. Olivia thrived in the program, and at the end of her first year, she was one of only two ninth graders who received all As in their academic subjects. Her home life remained chaotic, but school, once again, was her escape, her respite from the loneliness of having no family, the rootlessness of having no home. Olivia enjoyed the courses in the gifted program and the challenging class discussions. But most of all she appreciated the interest and concern of her teachers, the camaraderie among her classmates. This, she felt, was the family she never had.

By the tenth grade, however, school was no longer the only priority in Olivia's life. The nerdy bookworm, the girl who had always been teased for her studiousness, was now a pretty teenager who caught the eyes of the boys on campus. And now Olivia felt ashamed because of her shabby clothes. When she started high school, all she owned were three pairs of blue jeans, some hand-me-down tops, a pair of worn sneakers, and a threadbare jacket. The various foster and group homes were supposed to buy her clothes at the beginning of the school year, and to provide her with an allowance. Some gave her $10 a week, some $2.50, and some no money at all. And she rarely received money for clothes.

So now, Olivia had another outlet, besides school, for her intelligence and creativity: She turned her attention to making money. Olivia was a natural entrepreneur who soon realized that with enough chutzpah and savvy she could bend any rule and cut any corner. She became known at Crenshaw as a smooth talker, an operator, who, as one of her classmates said, "could charm a rock off a crackhead."

Each morning before class she stopped by a discount supermarket and purchased boxes of Kit Kats, M&Ms, Butterfingers, Baby Ruths, and Corn Nuts, and sold them for twenty-five cents during lunch and between classes. She cut a distinctive figure in the halls as she lugged her duffel bag bulging with candy, a backpack filled with books, and an oversized purse filled with quarters and dollar bills so she could make change. Olivia was soon netting more than $200 a week. When the principal heard about the unauthorized business and shut down the operation, Olivia began selling fire-safety equipment, including smoke alarms and fire extinguishers, door-to-door. Soon she was able to buy so many stylish outfits that she was considered one of the best-dressed girls on campus. Soon she had enough money to buy her own meals, instead of eating the execrable food at her group home.

The summer before her junior year, Olivia was tired of living in other people's homes, tired of restrictions, tired of dealing with hostile and indolent supervisors. She decided to go AWOL and spent July at a series of friends' houses. When she could not find a place to spend the night, she crawled in the back seat of a friend's car, spread out a blanket, and caught a few hours of fitful sleep. In August, she rented a twenty-dollar-a-night room in a roach-ridden hotel at the fringe of downtown, hard by the tracks of a commuter rail line. The trains rumbled by the old hotel, rattling the rooms with the sound of bells and horns. Bordered by abandoned businesses, the hotel was filled with winos, hookers, and rheumy-eyed pensioners renting rooms by the week.

A few weeks later, she rented a $375-a-month South-Central studio apartment, in a neighborhood of Mexican markets, liquor stores, hot-sheet motels, and empty lots strewn with trash and rusty shopping carts. A week before the first day of school, Olivia was in a panic. She did not know how she was going to juggle a full-time job at a hot-dog stand and her junior year in high school. She decided to stop by Crenshaw and talk to Scott Braxton, who headed the gifted magnet program. Braxton was raised just a few miles from Crenshaw, and, during college, classmates used to yell, jokingly, "Welcome back, Kotter!" when he wandered by because he always talked about returning to South-Central and teaching high school.

Braxton sometimes exasperates the teachers in the program. He is often overwhelmed by the workload of single-handedly running a program for more than 200 students. Some teachers feel he is, at times, disorganized and dilatory. Others feel he is excessively conciliatory when teachers need to be disciplined and not sufficiently decisive when departmental disputes need to be resolved immediately. But among the students such as Olivia, who have no one else to help them, he is venerated. He devotes so much time counseling students that his administrative duties suffer, which angers some of the teachers.

For Olivia, Braxton was her primary academic influence, the father figure she never had. No matter how busy he was, Braxton always found time to listen to Olivia, to help resolve her problems. He often called Olivia's social worker to straighten out disputes, or to find a new place for her to live. He even spent $125 on the fire-safety equipment she was peddling.

She developed a close relationship with Braxton during her first two years in high school because he was one of the few adults she trusted. So when she decided to drop out, the first person she informed was Braxton. She told him she could not afford to quit work and return to school. She had bills to pay, rent that was due. But after a few months of work, she hoped to save enough money so she could return to school for the second semester.

Braxton told Olivia that her plan was a disaster. If she dropped out now, he said, she would never return. She was too bright, he told her, and her potential too great to squander. It was imperative that she return to school. Immediately.

He arranged her courses so she could attend school in the morning and work in the afternoons, a highly unorthodox schedule for a gifted student with honors classes. Braxton's sole concern was her academic future. He did not care if he had to bend the rules a bit; he was determined to keep Olivia in school. Olivia had walked into his office a high school dropout. She walked out of his office a high school junior.

Olivia spent the first six weeks of her junior year living in her apartment, attending class in the morning, and hawking hot dogs in the afternoon and evenings. But then she was laid off. She could not pay her rent and, knowing she had no other alternative, she contacted her social worker. Olivia, unhappily, returned to another group home.

She still needed money, so she decided to find another job, a job, however, with more cachet than the hot-dog stand. Since she had to be eighteen to get the kind of job she wanted, Olivia obtained a fake ID and was hired as a salesclerk at a women's clothing store at a mall near the high school. She attended class in the morning, worked the swing shift at the clothing store, and tried to squeeze in an hour of homework before she collapsed at midnight.

Olivia staggered to her morning classes bleary-eyed, although she usually arrived late. She turned in most of her homework, although she usually turned it in late. And while she was no longer an all-A student, she was still on track for college.

Then, midway through her junior year, she punched a girl whom she suspected had broken open her locked storage box and stolen some of her candy earnings. The foster mother threw her out of the house. Olivia tossed all her belongings in a green plastic garbage bag, the foster child's luggage, sat on the front porch, and cried.

She did not know where to go or what to do. She ended up calling a classmate's family, and they agreed to put her up for a while. Later, the family agreed to apply for foster care certification and let her live with them until she graduated. Olivia felt she had finally found a real home.

The classmate's mother, Lita Herron, had a neighbor who, on a rainy afternoon, spotted a little dog shivering on her front porch, trying to stay dry. The woman gave the dog a home. When Olivia came to Herron's house, asking for a place to stay, Herron thought of that little dog. Herron, too, felt as if she were adopting a stray. And Herron respected Olivia's drive, her indomitable spirit, her determination to take challenging classes in a high-powered academic program.

Olivia lived with the Herrons during the last few months of her junior year. She followed the house rules and respected the family curfew. But in August, a few weeks before Olivia was to begin her senior year, she bought a beat-up, 1977 Volkswagen bug, and Herron soon discovered that Olivia did not have a driver's license, registration, or insurance. Herron and her husband, who were responsible for Olivia, forbade her to drive the car, but Olivia insisted. After a number of heated arguments, she went AWOL. Again.

The Herrons had treated Olivia like a member of the family. But Olivia was so used to living with people who did not care about her, people who only looked after her because they were paid to do it, that after the argument with the Herrons, she simply reverted to form. In the past, whenever she was angry or hurt, whenever she was confronted with what she considered to be an insuperable problem, Olivia knew only one way to respond: run.

Herron worried because she knew Olivia had almost dropped out of school before her junior year. Now she worried that Olivia might not return to Crenshaw for her senior year. This was to be a big year for Olivia, a critical year. She had signed up for a full regimen of demanding classes, including three Advanced Placement classes: Computer Science, U.S. Government and Politics, and English Literature and Composition. If she did well in her AP classes—courses that offer college-level curriculum—and on the SATs, she could count on a college scholarship.

Olivia had been looking forward to the AP literature class, in particular, and seeing the teacher, Toni Little, again. Little had taught Olivia in sophomore English, and it was one of her favorite classes. She was entertained by Little's classroom antics and theatrics, and she enjoyed the books she read. *The Great Gatsby* was her favorite because she identified with Gatsby's humble background, his raffish past, and how he used hustle and guile to achieve great wealth and social standing.

When Olivia sold candy, Little was the only teacher who was a customer. Other teachers ignored Olivia's business, or reported her to the principal. Little, however, was never one to pay scrupulous attention to school rules. She even special-ordered candy from Olivia, who bought Chick-O-Sticks specifically for her.

Little was the one female authority figure in Olivia's life with whom she could identify. Olivia felt a deep kinship because Little, too, was stubborn and rebellious, did things her own way, battled the school authorities. And Little, who lived in a small duplex with her three dogs, also seemed alienated and angry and, ultimately, alone.

As news of Olivia's disappearance spread, her friends and teachers wondered if she would return to Crenshaw for her senior year. Would she fulfill her great promise, graduate with honors, and proceed to college? Or would she end up just another abused teenager who succumbed to the odds, who dropped out of high school, and extinguished the flame of her future? As summer waned, everyone wondered where Olivia would be at 8:00 A.M., Thursday, September 6—the first day of school. When Toni Little called roll that morning, would Olivia be there?

PART ONE

SEPTEMBER

ONE

SADIKIFU

TELL ME WHY

On a warm September morning, at 7:59 A.M., on the first day of school, during Toni Little's first class of the day, she surveys the seniors arrayed before her in the stuffy classroom and her cheeks redden, her eyes narrow, and her mouth tightens. The students who know her exchange nervous glances and whisper among themselves, "Miss Little's mad."

She is mad because there are forty-two seniors in her Advanced Placement English class. Because to properly teach an Advanced Placement class, she believes, she should only have half that many. Because she will now have twice as much homework to read, twice as many exams to grade. Because she dislikes the chairwoman of the English Department and has to take orders from her again this year. Because she believes *she* should be the department chairwoman. And, finally, because just the sight of this overflowing classroom makes her feel fatigued, frazzled, a bit burnt out, and school has not even started yet.

There are only enough desks for half the students. The others stand along the sides of the room, teeter on plastic storage crates, or crowd onto a narrow wooden bench in back. They laugh and chatter about their summers.

Little pounds a fist on her desk and quiets the class. "This class is too damn big. I can't believe they dumped all of you on me. I can't properly teach AP English with so many students." She rolls her eyes and sighs heavily. "I'm going to have to weed some of you out. So I'm going to give you a writing prompt to do." The students groan in unison. "This will make or break you getting into this class."

Little nervously paces in front of the class. She is dressed in black leather boots, black stretch pants, and an oversized, pale green T-shirt. She has red hair, cut short, and vivid blue eyes. When she is amused or engrossed in a lecture, the students are mesmerized by her eyes, which seem to sparkle. But when she is angry, her eyes quickly darken, like a cloud drifting past the sun. Then all her fury, her pent-up irritation are centered in those forbidding eyes, which can impel even the most unruly gangbangers, whom she occasionally confronts in the hall, to back off.

She walks to her desk and picks up a memo—a suggested writing assignment for the first day of class—that the English department chair-woman sent to all the English teachers in the school: "Discuss a film, novel, video, or event that you saw this summer." Little snorts derisively, tosses the memo in a drawer, and spins, theatrically, toward the black-board. She writes: "The British novelist Fay Weldon offers this observation about happy endings: 'The writers, I do believe, who get the best and most lasting response from readers are the writers who offer a happy ending through moral development. By happy endings, I do not mean mere fortunate events—a marriage or a last-minute reprieve from death—but some kind of spiritual assessment or moral reconciliation, even with the self, even at death.' "

Little tells the class, "Now, here's the prompt," and then writes: "Choose a novel or play that has the kind of ending Weldon describes. In a well-written essay, identify the 'spiritual assessment or moral reconcili-ation' evident in the ending and explain its significance in the work as a whole."

"Okay, rock 'n rollers, get started," Little announces. "Also, on a separate sheet of paper, write why you want to be in this class. State your case."

Those students on the bench and the plastic crates pull up cardboard boxes to use as makeshift desks. The students who are standing balance their notebooks with one hand and write with the other. The students are serious, intent, and the only sounds are the occasional whispers: "Who was the preacher in *The Scarlet Letter?*" or "What was the name of the narrator in *The Great Gatsby?*"

In many inner-city high schools, teachers are confronted with rows of bored, insolent students, but Little teaches at Crenshaw High School's program for gifted students. The students, who are from throughout South-Central Los Angeles, have been given a special opportunity to succeed. And the vast majority go on to college. They are used to a more rigorous and disciplined academic environment, so as they write their first essay, the class has a decidedly different ambience than the rest of the school. Outside the classroom, students walk the halls and scrawl graffiti on the walls, and in a few nearby classrooms, students shout and pound their feet while teachers frantically try to establish order. In Little's classroom, however, the students hunch over their papers and scribble furiously until the bell rings.

Little gathers the papers, checks the names against her roll book, and discovers that several students are absent. One of them is Olivia.

Scott Braxton, who heads the Crenshaw Gifted Magnet program, is overwhelmed on the first day of school. He stands up and stretches in his small, sweltering office, the size of a walk-in closet, glances at the jumble on his desk, and ruefully shakes his head. His desk is cluttered with "change of program" forms, "elective course selection" sheets, computer printouts, and stacks of attendance records. Dozens of students and parents line the hallway outside his office, waiting to see him. Students need to drop a class. Or they need to add a class. Or they need to change a class. Parents hope to get their children into the gifted program. Or parents are moving and transferring their children out.

The heat in Braxton's office leaves the secretaries irritable, mopping their brows, but he appears cool and comfortable. Braxton is nattily attired in royal blue slacks, Italian tasseled loafers, royal blue and white silk tie. His white-on-white, long-sleeved dress shirt still is sharply creased and, despite the heat, the top button remains buttoned. The lines outside his office do not subside during the day, but Braxton remains endlessly patient with the students and the occasional teacher who drops by with a complaint.

Despite today's busy schedule, Braxton still attempts to track down Olivia. During the past three years he has probably spent more time with Olivia than with any other student. He has counseled her during countless lunch hours, frequently changed her schedule to accommodate her various jobs, and conferred with her social worker numerous times.

Olivia is different from the other students with tumultuous home lives whom Braxton counsels. They usually try to persuade him to assign them easier, less challenging classes. Olivia, however, always wants the most advanced classes. Most students in the gifted magnet program enroll in one, maybe two Advanced Placement classes during their senior year. Olivia requested three. Braxton, well aware of her arduous work schedule, tried to dissuade her, but she insisted. He respected her tenacity.

He remembers Olivia as a shy, shabbily dressed ninth grader. He watched her grow up during the past three years, watched as she hustled to make money and buy herself clothes, watched as she struggled to stay in school, despite circumstances that prompted other students to drop out. He has been through too much with Olivia to allow her to quit school now. So he calls Lita Herron, whom Olivia lived with before she went AWOL a few weeks ago. Herron says she has not talked to her and has not been able to find out where she is living. Braxton tells her that if she finds Olivia, please ask her to call him.

Braxton removes his glasses and wearily massages the bridge of his nose. "Nine months," he tells me. "I just need nine more months from her." Last year he was worried about Olivia keeping up her grades so she could win a college scholarship. Now he is worried that she will not even enroll for her senior year.

The next morning, at 8:00 A.M., Little calls roll and Olivia is still absent. Little asks a few students if they know where she is. They shake their heads. Little walks over to the windows and jams them open, hoping for a breeze. In Southern California, people often can smell and taste the onset of a hot day before they can feel it. On this morning, the asphalt is starting to bake and the acrid smells of oil stains and exhaust fumes drift into the classroom. The smog already obscures the horizon with a bourbon-colored scrim and fills the air with the metallic taste of pollutants.

When Little finishes taking roll, she discovers that her mission on the first day of class was accomplished. Five students, intimidated by the essay, dropped out. Although the class still has thirty-seven students, Little's irritation has been ameliorated. The principal has authorized extra pay because Little is, in essence, teaching two classes.

She finds a teacher across the hall who can spare a half-dozen desks, and a few of the boys bring them into her classroom. Still, about ten students must sit on plastic milk crates and on the bench in the back and write on cardboard boxes. But at least nobody has to stand.

Today is another abbreviated class—less than an hour—and the end of a short week. Next week the school's regular schedule begins. AP English will be almost two hours, Mondays and Wednesdays, and about fifty minutes on Fridays. Little quickly introduces the first play the class will study—*The Crucible,* by Arthur Miller. She tells them that the root of the word Puritan is purify, discusses the difference between the Puritans and the Pilgrims, talks about the travails of Hester Prynne from *The Scarlet Letter,* which the class read last year, and links it to *The Crucible.*

She is distracted by two girls who are talking, giggling, and ignoring her lecture. The class is so big that they have to sit in chairs in the corner of the room, behind Little. She whirls around and shouts, "You two have been giving me trouble since I started this morning. What's your *problem*? I'm already sick of *both* of you."

The girls, best friends, are wearing tight jeans, tank tops, and their orange lipstick is rimmed dramatically with dark lip liner.

"You were like this in the tenth grade, but I thought you both would have grown up by now. You're still gabbing about your *idiotic* social life." Little looks them up and down, with disdain. "You're still just two little girls with weird lipstick."

One of the girls, clearly hurt, says softly, "That's not right for you to say that in front of the whole class."

"It's not that deep," Little says, walking to the other side of the classroom. She introduces the first act of the play and asks the class what some of the characters are afraid of in the forest?

"Angry black men," one student, with a goatee, shouts, as the class chuckles.

Little talks about a character who is searching for herbs.

"What kind of herbs, homegrown?" a girl with dyed orange hair calls out. The class titters.

Little ignores the quips and then reads from Act 1 of *The Crucible:* "They—the Puritans—believed, in short that they held in their hands the candle that would light the world. We have inherited this belief . . ."

A student in the back row, with the mellifluous first name of Sadikifu—everyone calls him Sadi—raises a hand and interrupts Little.

"We didn't *inherit* it," he says. "It was *forced* on us."

"Okay," Little says. "We were *forced* to believe . . ."

"Not *you*," says Sadi, who has a buzz cut and whose oversized jeans sag to the middle of his hips. "*Us!* Religion was forced on *us*. Black people. We had no choice. Our African religions were taken away from us. We were forced to believe what our slave masters wanted us to believe."

"Amen," a few students shout.

"And if this God that was forced on us in America is so good, why are black people in America on the bottom of the totem pole? Prisons are the number-one industry in California, and who fills them? Black people."

Yesterday, when Little asked students to include in their essay why they wanted to take AP English, Sadi wrote, "I wish to be a writer. So with that goal in mind, it's almost impossible not to sign up for the hardest English class in the school."

A girl with corn rows challenges Sadi. "I understand what you're saying, to an extent. But people have to take responsibility for their actions. Can't just blame it on God or white society. Blacks aren't getting arrested and thrown in jail for standin' still. No one's kickin' blacks out of libraries."

"Black people couldn't even go to libraries fifty years ago," Sadi says. "Yeah, there are certain pitfalls out there—"

Little cuts him off and attempts to guide the discussion to the Puritans' view of God in *The Crucible*. The discussion soon drifts to the students' own views. One student says God is a myth, and Sadi raises his hand.

"God created us parallel to the universe, so our existence can't be random," says Sadi, echoing a sermon he heard at the Muslim mosque he attends with his mother. "There are nine planets and there are nine major organs in the body. There is the sun and there is the brain. The brain gives off light. The light symbolizes knowledge. Without knowledge, we'd be in the dark. Without the sun, the universe would be in the dark."

"*Preach* it," students call out, as if they were in the amen corner in church.

"All *right* now," others say.

"Stand up and *tell* it," a few shout.

Sadi stands up, continues his impromptu sermon, and concludes with the Muslim interpretation of heaven, as students clap their hands, fan themselves with their notebooks, and sway in their desks.

"I don't believe in heaven," shouts a tall student, wearing a black do-rag. He pumps a fist, smiles, and shouts, "My heaven is a *fine,* black woman."

The class erupts into laughter. Little briefly closes her eyes and throws up her hands in frustration. She realizes she has lost control of the class. But she knows it is warm and uncomfortable in the room and the students, who have just had three months off, are not accustomed to sitting and concentrating on literary symbolism and imagery patterns. So she cuts them some slack, draws from her small reserve of patience, and maintains her equanimity.

"Let's get out of church," Little says, tapping a stapler on her desk to focus the students' attention. "Let's get back into literature class."

She tells the class that being in AP English is a privilege, that they will be doing college-level work, that she expects more out of them than any other English class she teaches. She tells them the course culminates in a three-hour exam that they—and students from across the country— will take in May. If they pass with a score of three or better—out of a possible five—they will earn college credit. She tells them they will be competing against students from tony prep schools and wealthy suburbs, and this is their chance to show that kids from South-Central can compete with anyone.

A student named Kurt, who earned a summer scholarship to Stanford two years ago and attended UCLA this past summer, responds, "Everybody used to look at me like I was stupid because I was an African American. Then you do more work than anyone else and get good grades. Everyone shakes their heads in amazement and says, 'How'd you do that?' "

Little nods and then the bell rings. "Everyone better be serious on Monday," she shouts. "No more screwing around."

As the students stuff their books and notebooks into their backpacks, she tells me she is worried about this class. Not only are there almost twice as many students as last year, but last year's group seemed more serious to her, more academically inclined. "I don't know about these kids," she says. "I hope what we saw today was because of the heat and it was just the last throes of summer in them."

When the last student files out, the room suddenly seems smaller and more shabby, a standard, austere high school classroom, painted a pale institutional yellow, with a brown-and-white-flecked linoleum floor and rows of metal and plastic desks. An American flag hangs in one corner, a jumble of books, storage boxes, and files fill another corner, and blackboards cover three walls. Little's chipped, wooden desk faces the class. She has added a few homey touches. There is a Georgia O'Keeffe poster of a large white lily in one corner. A section of the back wall is covered with lavender paper and pictures of women writers.

Although Little's students are drawn from some of South-Central's most impoverished neighborhoods, Crenshaw is not a typical inner-city school. The older, crumbling South-Central high schools were built on major thoroughfares, in blighted commercial districts. But Crenshaw, which opened in 1968, is one of the newest high schools on the Southside and is located in a modest residential neighborhood several blocks from bustling Crenshaw Boulevard, the central artery in Los Angeles' black community. The school, with about 2,800 students, is a weathered, three-story, tan-brick building built around a quadrangle of desiccated grass, where students gather at lunch.

From a distance, the school seems as if it could be in any working-class neighborhood in America. But inside, the graffiti sets the school in the inner city. It is only the second day of class, yet the walls, hallways, and bathrooms are already cloaked with gang graffiti. In the stairwell between the second and third floors, the names of students killed over the summer, T-Gunn, Baby Sextage, and Papa Fuck, are spray-painted beneath: R.I.P.——WE LOVE Y'ALL. On other hallways are scrawled the names of various gangs, including the Rollin 30s, Rollin 40s, and Rollin 60s; EastSide 97th Street Crips, Harlem Crips, and Georgetown Crips; Van Ness Gangster Bloods, Inglewood Family Bloods, and 87th Street Bloods. Almost every square inch of the first floor bathroom—including the walls, windows, ceiling, door, and the paper towel, soap, and toilet paper dispensers—are covered by gang graffiti. Taggers—also known as tagbangers because some are becoming as violent as street gangs—have scrawled the names of their crews in the bathroom, including WestSide Young Thugs, Sex Riders, and Youngstas Gettin High. On every bathroom wall there is also the obligatory: FUCK ALL SLOBS (Bloods), with the *B* crossed out, and KILL ALL CRABS (Crips), with the *C* crossed out.

The busiest man at Crenshaw High School is the school painter. He has the Sisyphean task of forever painting walls, only to see them—sometimes hours later—defaced yet again. The acrid smell of fresh paint is a constant and pervasive presence at Crenshaw.

After Little's AP English class, she walks over to a window, lifts the venetian blinds and surveys the campus. The quadrangle is framed by spindly jacaranda trees that flower in spring. A few lavender blooms still cling to the branches. On a broiling September morning, the shadows are razor sharp, and the lavender rosettes and scarlet blooms of the bottlebrush trees on the edge of campus gleam in the brilliant desert light. The commercial thoroughfares of South-Central, not far from Crenshaw, seem impervious to the light and the seasons. The streets, without a hint of vegetation, are devoid of color, dreary black-and-white cityscapes of liquor stores, check cashing shops, tiny storefront churches, and gutted buildings.

Little turns away from the window and pours herself a cup of coffee from her coffee machine hidden behind a metal file cabinet. She sips the coffee and then grabs from her desk the second memo of the week from the English Department chairwoman, Anita Moultrie. She waves it in the air and shouts, "This is insidious. I won't do it. She doesn't pay my salary. I am a scholar. I should be treated with some deference. I will *not* be ordered around like this."

Moultrie wrote the memo in response to a handbook for the school's English teachers that the principal asked Little to create during the summer. Little, who was paid for the work, compiled the handbook, which includes a sample reading list for ninth to twelfth graders; lists of literary terms; sample homework, essay and exam assignments; and numerous other projects and teaching aids that she has collected during her almost twenty years of teaching.

Moultrie's memo merely asked Little to "please send the handbook to me so that I can look it over . . . I need a copy . . . today for assignment of novels . . . Thanks for your continued assistance and support." Little was angry because she did not like Moultrie giving her what she construed as an order, she did not want her editing the handbook, and, most importantly, Little wanted to make sure *she* received all the credit for the handbook, not Moultrie. Little writes Moultrie a frosty response, ensuring that the cold war between the two teachers will escalate and that, in the future, they will communicate only by memo.

"I hereby withdraw my volunteer services to develop and produce a plan under your leadership . . ." Little writes. "Please place all necessary correspondence to me in my mailbox . . ."

She is interrupted when a few students wander into her classroom. One of them, Julia, is Olivia's best friend.

Little rushes over to Julia and asks, "Where's Olivia?"

Julia shrugs.

"Why isn't she in school?" Little asks.

"She's got no transportation."

"Where's she living?"

"I'm not sure."

"Tell her to call me. I'll get her to school."

"Okay," Julia says, nodding.

Little grabs her by the bicep and fixes her with an intent stare. "Can you save her?" Little asks.

"I'll try," Julia says.

"Save her!" Little urges, squeezing her arm. "She helped you when your parents were getting a divorce. She was there for you when you needed it. Now it's your turn to be there for her."

Little lets go of Julia's arm and says, "Tell her it's important that she gets her butt to school. Tell her I want her in my class."

A few minutes ago, Little was angry, vindictive, and consumed by the minutiae of an interdepartmental dispute. Now she is concerned only with Olivia's welfare. She volunteers to pick Olivia up, if necessary, and drive her to school. Many of Little's colleagues are baffled by her bifurcated personality, her contradictory qualities. The students call her Dr. Jekyll because of her mercurial moods. During one class she might be a consummate professional, lecturing brilliantly and inspiring impassioned class discussion. The next class she might be thoroughly distracted and spend two hours vilifying O.J. Simpson or railing against school administrators. She is caring and kind to some students. She invites them to her home, lets them use her computer to write class papers, sits with them at her kitchen table, and helps them to draft their college applications. Other students irritate her, and she denounces them in class, driving them to tears.

Little teaches tenth and twelfth grade English. She had about half of the AP English students in her class two years ago, including Sadikifu, the student who wants to be a writer and who delivered the impromptu sermon today. She still recalls the comments he made when he was a tenth grader and the class was discussing *The Great Gatsby*. He admitted that he once hated white people, but reading the novel changed his perspective. Like Olivia, Sadi identified with Gatsby. He identified with his love for Daisy, his modest beginnings, his desire for success, his need to be accepted. "Gatsby's feelings are universal," Sadi said during the class discussion. "Gatsby could be anybody. Gatsby could be me." Sadi realized after reading the book, he told the class, that to hate people because of the color of their skin was wrongheaded and intellectually shallow.

Sadi was one of Little's favorite tenth graders. He impressed her because he was so passionate about the literature, because his insights were so penetrating, and because he had transformed himself, in a very short time, from a gangbanger to a scholar.

Sadi's mother, Thelma, who was one week shy of her forty-first birthday when her only child was born, considers her son a gift from Allah. He was unexpected and unplanned. Thelma and Sadi's father, who never married, became Muslims in the 1970s, and they gave their son an Islamic name—Sadikifu—which means "truthful and honest."

When Sadi was five, his father moved out. He later became addicted to crack, ended up homeless, and served a few jail terms. Sadi rarely saw him. Thelma, the child of a single mother, now a single mother herself, moved into a Section 8, federally subsidized apartment complex and began cleaning houses. But Thelma had health problems—she now needs a liver transplant—and she and Sadi soon survived on welfare.

Because Thelma never had been around children, and Sadi was her only child, she talked to him like a peer. That is one reason, she believes, why he is so bright and articulate. In the third grade he was classified as gifted by the school district when he scored in the 95th percentile on a national achievement test. In the fourth grade he won an oratorical contest, sponsored by a local bank, for a speech on homelessness. Thelma still proudly displays the trophy—next to a picture of Elijah Muhammad—in her small, immaculate two-bedroom apartment.

All through elementary school Sadi attended classes for the gifted. In the seventh grade, he was on the verge of winning a full scholarship to an exclusive prep school in Pasadena. Sadi had passed the entrance examination and the oral interview. Thelma was elated. Sadi was not an athlete or a musician. Academics, she knew, would be his way out of the ghetto.

A few weeks later, Sadi's father briefly resurfaced. Thelma told him she was still waiting for the acceptance letter from the prep school, but that she was certain Sadi would get a scholarship. Sadi's father, perhaps out of guilt for his long absence, perhaps out of a need to feel important, perhaps because he truly thought it would help, called the school and demanded to know his son's status. The call was a disaster. On the application Thelma had filled out, she wrote that she, alone, was supporting

Sadi, that she did not know where Sadi's father was. Now school officials wondered why Sadi's father had called. Sadi's application was rejected.

His father disappeared again, and Sadi remained at his South-Central junior high school. He lived in a gang-ridden neighborhood interlaced with dozens of warring gang factions and tagging crews. In the eighth grade he lost interest in school and joined a group of tagbangers called the All Out Kickin' It Gangstas, which was like a minor-league farm team for the Front Hood 60s, a hard-core Crip gang. If the young taggers, most of whom were twelve and thirteen, proved themselves on the street, the Front Hood 60s would jump them in.

Sadi was consumed with anger at his father for leaving and resentment at his mother for her constant lectures about academics. But Thelma was just trying to ensure that her son did not repeat her mistakes and the mistakes of Sadi's father. She had been caught transporting drugs and served time in jail, where another inmate introduced her to Islam. She wanted Sadi to have a different kind of life.

Sadi continued to rebel in school, however, and was on his way to the penitentiary or an early grave. He was suspended from junior high school numerous times, for shooting dice, for throwing gang signs, for fighting with rival gang members. He was constantly in trouble in his gifted classes because he did little work. One morning his mother emptied the trash and discovered several sheets of notebook paper that Sadi had doodled on. The writing style resembled the gang graffiti she had seen around the neighborhood. She took the paper to the security guard at Sadi's junior high school.

The guard scanned the writing and told Thelma, "He's still young enough to change. But he could go either way."

Sadi, unfortunately, went the wrong way. In the ninth grade, he enrolled in Crenshaw's gifted program, but after only two months of high school he was thrown out for instigating a fight between his tagging crew and a rival set. Although his mother was livid, Sadi's expulsion probably saved his life because the next afternoon his best friend was shot to death by a rival tagging crew called Nothin But Trouble. Sadi always spent every day after school with his friend, whose street name was Chaos. Sadi knew if he had not been stuck all afternoon enrolling in his new high school, he would have been walking down Vermont Avenue with Chaos. He probably would have been killed, too.

After Sadi was expelled from Crenshaw, his mother signed him up to be bussed, along with a group of other South-Central students, to a predominantly white high school in the San Fernando Valley. Despite Sadi's test scores, his new counselor refused to assign him to gifted classes. At the school, many of the South-Central students were placed in the remedial program. The counselor did not believe a black child could be classified as gifted.

Thelma still held out hope for Sadi, still prayed that he would regain his enthusiasm for school. She did not know much about Crenshaw's gifted program, but she knew Sadi was getting a better education there than at a standard high school. She wanted him to have the same opportunity at the Valley high school. So every day for a week, she drove an hour to the school and pestered administrators until they finally agreed to enroll him in gifted classes.

On Sadi's first day of school he discovered he was the only black student in his gifted classes. When students passed out work sheets they skipped him. When he asked for the assignments the students invariably said: "I thought you were here for detention."

Although he was now attending a suburban high school far from South-Central, at night and on weekends he was immersed in the gang life. He had graduated from his tagging crew to the Front Hood 60s and was known by his street name—Little Cloudy. And even though he had been arrested several times, three of his homies had recently been killed in drive-bys, and about ten were in jail, he kept gangbanging.

One weekday afternoon, when school was canceled because of an earthquake, he and two other 60s were walking down Western Avenue, on their way to buy some Thunderbird at a liquor store near 69th Street. They spotted a teenager across the street whom they did not recognize. Sadi and his two homies threw up the hand sign for the Front Hood 60s. The gangbanger across the street threw up the sign for the Eight-Tray Gangsters, a bitter rival of the 60s. One of Sadi's homies pulled out a semiautomatic .380-caliber pistol and fired at the Eight-Tray. Then everyone sprinted for cover. Two LAPD officers in a patrol car heard the shots, pulled up, and grabbed Sadi and another 60. The shooter and the Eight-Tray, who had not been hit, escaped.

Sadi and his homie were handcuffed, arrested, and taken to the 77th Street Division station. They were questioned by detectives, who then dabbed their hands with a sticky aluminum tab that tests for gunshot residue. When the test came back negative, and a witness told detectives neither of them was the shooter, they were released. But the incident precipitated an epiphany for Sadi.

Seeing the flash of the gun, just inches away, marked a turning point for him. It inalterably changed the course of his life. In an instant, he realized how transitory life was, how transitory *his* life was. How all his decisions were wrong. How he was destined to die in a drive-by, or languish in prison. He realized that maybe his mother had been right about school. Maybe his intelligence was, as his mother told him, a gift from Allah.

He decided to transform every aspect of his life. He attended the Muslim mosque in South-Central where his mother worshiped. He avoided his old homies. He met with Yvonne Noble, the principal at Crenshaw, told her that he had left the gang scene forever, and implored her to take him back. He told her that the long bus ride to the San Fernando Valley was exhausting, that he wanted to return to the gifted program at Crenshaw, that he felt more comfortable with other bright black students than with condescending suburban kids. Noble told him if his grades were good, he could return. He studied hard during the second semester, and Noble allowed him to enroll in the fall for his sophomore year, but she warned him that she would throw him out for good if he flirted with the gang scene on campus.

His first year back at Crenshaw was difficult for him. Each day after school, when he walked down 71st Street to his apartment, he fought a gauntlet of temptations.

"Come kick it with us," his old homies, who were hanging out on the corner, would call to him.

"Let's blaze," others would shout, lighting up joints.

Sadi would put them off by telling them he had to take care of some business at home. Fortunately, the Front Hood 60s he had been closest to, who could have exerted the most pressure on him, were no longer around. They were either dead or in jail.

His neighborhood, where the sidewalks are streaked with gang graffiti, is less than a mile from the flash point of the 1992 riots. He lives in a three-story apartment complex, filled with many other welfare families, off a depressed section of Western Avenue; an area of storefront churches, hamburger stands, and abandoned businesses. Next door to Sadi's apartment is a boarded-up home covered with gang graffiti and the names of two gangbangers targeted for death. A rival spray-painted LOCO and SPARKY and, beneath it, the number 187—the California Penal Code for murder.

After Sadi returned to Crenshaw in the tenth grade, he felt lonely and isolated. The gifted students did not want to hang out with him because they thought he was a gangbanger. The gangbangers on campus thought he had turned into an Urkle, a nerd.

In the past, when he had classes outside the gifted program, and he had participated in class discussions and tried to articulate his opinions, other students often would mock him or shout: "Stop trying to act white." But in the tenth grade all of his classes were in the gifted program, and most of the students were accustomed to participating enthusiastically in class discussions. They competed against—rather than ridiculed—each other. He no longer felt as if he were a traitor to his race or was contravening his culture if he tried to excel in school.

Still, even within the supportive confines of the gifted program, it is not easy for a young black man. At Crenshaw's gifted program, only about one-third of the students are boys; at the city's other high school program for gifted students—which is largely white and Asian and less than 1 percent black—almost two-thirds of the students are boys.

Given the distractions and disadvantages, it is difficult for all inner-city students to succeed academically. But boys have an added burden. In the ghetto, where teenage machismo is venerated in rap songs and music videos, where athletes and gangbangers gain the most attention in the school hallways, an affinity for academics is something to camouflage, not celebrate. The serious student often is regarded as effete, as a sellout, as someone who has disdained his culture. In Little's AP English class, for example, there are only seven boys.

"I rarely see a girl trying to get out of the gifted program," Braxton says. "But every year a number of boys come by my office, begging to get out. They feel that by going the academic route, they just can't fit in. The pressure gets to them. They just get dragged down by this strong undercurrent in the neighborhood against carrying books, against studying, against striving to succeed in school."

During Sadi's first year back at Crenshaw, he struggled against that current. During lunch and after school, he felt like an outsider. He had no one to hang out with, so he decided to attend the Speech Club meetings. Sadi immediately gravitated to the poetry competitions. Drawing on his years in gangs, his father's crack addiction, his growing awareness of black history, he won a number of poetry contests. He was a natural performer and he read his poems with great feeling and panache. Although a bit rough, his gritty poems were infinitely more dramatic than those of the suburban poets he competed against.

When Sadi was a junior, he won first prize in the original poetry category at the city speech championships. His poem was about his family, his neighborhood, and the plight of black people in America:

Tell me why.
Why my dad and uncle were strung out on crack . . .
That's why I have to grow up strong and black
I can't let nothing hold me back.
Tell me why we were emancipated, but still segregated and hated.
Why we never got a chance to be fully integrated.
Tell me why.
Tell me why, for the average African American
The American dream has become the American nightmare. . . .
To those who are unaware of times of despair and no more welfare . . .
Prepare.
Tell me why . . . my life is full of so much anxiety.
Curiosity almost got me shot . . .
Got me smoking pot . . . nonstop.
Tell me why.
Look at me and tell me what you see

Because my pants sag, I'm perceived to be a G. [gangster]
Tell me why there are more black men in prisons than college. . . .
Tell me why . . .

Teachers at Crenshaw now asked him to recite the poem for their classes and during school assemblies. The gifted students accepted him. Even the gangbangers on campus appreciated the raplike cadence and street-level perspective of the poem. When they saw him walking by they nodded to him and called out, "Hey, there goes the poet."

Last year Sadi won the city championship; this year he has a chance to become the state champion. But his teachers know he is not the most disciplined student. While he is enthusiastic about his poetry and his literature classes, he often coasts in classes that do not capture his interest. His teachers hope that knowing how important this year is, how much is riding on it, he will summon the discipline to keep his grades up. Because with his onerous upbringing and academic transformation—which always impresses college admissions officials—and his writing ability and poetry prizes, he could have a number of college scholarships to choose from by the end of the year.

When Sadi's mother talks about his transformation, she says, "He's come out of the darkness and into the light." Still, she is concerned. She knows that he has to earn a scholarship because she has no money for college. And his teachers know the pitfalls and dangers his neighborhood presents. They hope he can stay focused and survive another year.

TWO

TOYA

I NEVER DREAMED I WOULD SEE SIXTEEN

On a Monday morning, during the second week of school, Toni Little watches the students drift into class, and she checks their names off the roll sheet. Many of the students have names so distinctive and mellifluous that there is a kind of poetry in merely reading the roll. There is Latisha, LaCresha, and Miesha; Nikia and Khaliah; Taaji and Akindeji; Princess and Aphrodite; Tashana, Shana, and Andriana; Naila and Venola; Sabreen and Sadikifu.

After finishing the role, Little decides to do some remedial work, to revisit some basic literary terms. She tells the students that she has read their essays from the first day of class and is *not* impressed. She furiously fills the blackboard with thematic principles such as "conflict," "point of view," "narrative method," "tone," "characterization," "plot," and "setting." Underneath each heading, she writes a brief explanation.

The students scribble pages of notes. This process wastes precious time, but Little has no choice because she has not been able to Xerox her assignments. In order to use the federally funded Xerox machine—provided to Crenshaw because it has so many low-income students—Little has to complete a host of forms and wait several days for her copies. She finds it easier simply to use the blackboard.

She is also frustrated because she feels that to teach this class properly, to prepare them for the AP exam in May, she needs world literature textbooks. But she has been unable to secure funding for the textbooks, so she will have to improvise with the materials she cobbled together over the years.

By the time Little finishes the exercise, her mood has soured. She groans loudly and tells the class, "I shouldn't have to go over all this stuff again. This is AP lit. This should be a three-year program, not a one-year program. You should know this already. I taught all this to you in the tenth grade. Did you forget everything? Where *were* all of you last year?"

Little knows where they were last year. And this exacerbates her irritation. The students had Little's nemesis last year for English—Anita Moultrie, who serves as a lightning rod for Little's various complaints. Little often attributes a wide range of student inadequacies to a single, unambiguous source—Moultrie—although there often are manifold reasons for gaps in the students' knowledge.

Little looks flushed in the warm classroom as streaks of light slice through the venetian blinds. A girl in the front row, with short, copper-colored hair, interrupts Little. In a role reversal, the student, patient and soothing, lectures the teacher, rash and incensed.

"Chill, Miss Little," the student says. "In eleventh grade English we didn't follow the kind of outline you would have liked. Okay. But we *did* get some good teaching. So just calm down and bear with us. Let's just review what you've got on the board and get *on* with it."

The student's comments break Little's mood, and she resumes her lecture. But in a few minutes, a surprise visitor walks through the door.

"Well, well, well," Little says, smiling broadly. "Look who's here."

Olivia has arrived.

Usually when students are late, they are nabbed by a security officer who mans the heavy metal gate by the main entrance. He sends them to the principal's office where they pick up tardy slips before they can attend class. But Olivia the operator simply pulls out a key to the teachers' elevator, which she somehow procured last year, slips into the elevator on the basement level, rides it to the third floor, and walks down the hall to Little's classroom. She sashays through the halls with such authority that the administrators who patrol the halls do not stop her.

Little motions for Olivia to find a desk. The other girls in class are dressed casually in jeans or shorts, sneakers and T-shirts. In contrast, Olivia, who is dressed for her afterschool job at a women's clothing store, is wearing black rayon slacks, a maroon silk blouse, and black patent leather high heels. Her improbably long nails are painted bright red, her hair swirls atop her head in an elaborate creation of dips and curls, and she is wearing heavy makeup and rust-colored lip gloss. She has a gold stud in her nose, a diamond stud in one ear, and large gold hoop earrings. Olivia is seventeen, but she seems older. Only her braces—provided free at a dental school—give her away. She has no backpack, no books, and no notebook. When Little begins discussing *The Crucible,* Olivia pulls a small pad out of her black leather purse and casually jots down a few notes, like a businesswoman taking inventory.

After class, a few students crowd around Olivia. They ask her why she has been absent. She tells them she is living on her own again and is working at the mall to support herself.

"Wow, you got your own place again," a girl says, wide-eyed with admiration. "That's cool."

Olivia flashes the girl a skeptical glance. "It's not cool at all. All I've got in my purse is twenty dollars. When that runs out I don't know what I'll do."

"You still selling fire extinguishers?" the girl asks.

"Naw," Olivia says. "That was a while ago."

"Where you staying at?" another girl asks.

"An apartment."

"Where is it?"

"What is this, Twenty Questions?" Olivia asks, looking irritated. She strides to the front of the class to see Little.

Little hugs Olivia and asks her why she has not been in class. Olivia tells her that she has had to work. Last year, Olivia says, her supervisor let her set her own hours. She had a night job so she could attend school during the day. But her new boss assigned her the day shift last week. Her boss thinks she is nineteen—the company does not hire seventeen-year-olds—and Olivia has a fake ID. She could not tell her boss she needs her mornings off for her high school English class. This week, Olivia says, she finagled a night shift, so she can get to class in the morning.

"Then why were you so late today?" Little asks.

Olivia tells her she bought an old VW bug and it would not start. She had to take two buses to get to school.

Little asks her where she is living. Olivia is evasive. She tells her the apartment is about a dozen miles west of the high school, not too far from Little's Culver City duplex. Little tells her to be at a specific intersection at 7:30 A.M. "I'll swing by, pick you up and get you to class on time," Little says.

"Okay," Olivia replies. "I'll be there."

Before class on Wednesday, a group of students congregate in the hall and discuss the stabbing on campus the day before—the fourth day of school. It was the first gang attack of the year. There is some confusion about the incident, so a few students ask Sadi, a recognized authority on the subject, for clarification. Sadi still has neighborhood friends in the gang scene.

Two Rollin 60s, Sadi explains, attacked a Harlem 30 who was walking across campus and was about to enroll. The Harlem 30 was not even a student yet. He pulled out a knife and slashed his two rivals. They were rushed to the emergency room.

Later that same day, Sadi tells his classmates, he was jumped as he walked across the football field after class. A group of Bloods spotted his blue shirt and blue cords. Crenshaw is in a neighborhood dominated by Crips—who wear blue—but a small pocket of Bloods live behind the school.

"About four of them surrounded me and started shoutin', 'Hey, Blood, where you from?' I told 'em I wasn't into that anymore. I told 'em I'm just tryin' to go to school and get an education. But they wouldn't listen. All they saw was that blue. One dude, who looked like a real ruffian, socked me.'' Sadi lowers his chin and points to a knot under his ear the size of a walnut.

"How'd you survive it?'' a boy asks.

"I did what any intelligent person would do. I ran.''

Little sweeps into the hall with Olivia in tow and breaks up the crowd surrounding Sadi. She shepherds them into her classroom and tells them they will read *The Crucible* out loud. In many high school classrooms, teenage boys read their parts in an inhibited, reluctant monotone. But the boys—and the girls—in Little's class fight over roles and they infuse their parts with great authority and passion, without a hint of self-consciousness.

Little occasionally interrupts and questions the class about what they have just read.

"Why do the Puritans forbid witchcraft?'' she asks.

"Because it's devil's work,'' a student says.

"Is witchcraft bad?'' Little asks.

"Of course it's bad.''

"Is it only bad if you're a Christian?''

The student is baffled for a moment.

Little reminds the students that Tituba, a slave accused of practicing witchcraft, is from Barbados. She is not a Christian, so if she practices witchcraft, can that be construed as evil? A dozen students wave their hands, and for the next half hour they excitedly discuss the play.

Little steers the discussion to another topic by asking, "What role does the devil play in our life today?''

For most of the students religion is a central part of their upbringing, and the traditions of the black Baptist church form their identities and belief systems. To them, the devil is a familiar force, identified and vilified every Sunday morning.

Several students chant in unison a line they learned in church: "The devil is the author of confusion. His role is to build and to destroy.''

Olivia raises her hand. "I don't think God makes you do good, or the devil makes you do evil,'' she says. "In the end, it's up to you.''

"The pitchfork and the horns are all mythology,'' adds Sadi. "People who do evil things use the devil as a copout.''

LaCresha, a devout Christian who twice a week attends the Shackelford

Miracle Temple, Church of God in Christ, asks, "How can you say there's no devil when there's so much evil in this world."

"How do you know there's a God?" Olivia asks.

"Because God is in my heart," LaCresha says, "and he talks to me every day."

The discussion rages, and the students shout out answers, leaf through the play, and quote sections to buttress their points. Little plays the role of the moderator, calling on the students, guiding the discourse, wheedling the quiet ones to participate.

She was distracted during the first few days of class by academic politics, the interdepartmental feuds, the stuffy, overcrowded classroom. But today she has hit her stride. She subtly extracts conclusions and interpretations from the class. She sparks a genuine enthusiasm for the literature. She helps the students see how a play set in seventeenth-century Salem can help them interpret and understand their lives in South-Central Los Angeles.

She is unable, however, to sustain the thoughtful, academic ambience. About three-quarters of the way through the class, Little is distracted by loud voices emanating from the quad. She walks to the window, glances through the blinds, and sees more than a hundred students milling about, talking and laughing. Furious, she stomps over to the phone and calls the administration office. A secretary tells her several science classes are being held in the quad.

"Why can't the noise level be managed? How can I be expected to teach with these distractions?" She faces the class, rolls her eyes, and holds the phone at arm's length, mocking the reply. She jams the phone back into her ear and shouts, "Where is the teacher? . . . Will somebody tell those kids to SHUT UP!" She slams down the phone.

She storms to the front of the class and paces back and forth. "This is *outrageous*," she tells the class. "No one ever does *anything*. It's always Toni Little who has to take care of the problem," she says wearily, flashing the class a look of martyrdom. "This is a public school. Not a *playground*. *Hundreds* of kids are out there, without *any* supervision." She holds out her hands and shakes them violently, as if she is strangling a Rottweiler.

"THE STUPIDITY!" she shouts. "Not *one* teacher is an activist here. I stand *alone*. The conditions for teaching here are becoming *intolerable*."

She snorts in anger, her face convulsed, like an infant ready to burst into tears. The noise in the quad finally subsides, but by the time the class returns to *The Crucible,* the bell rings.

After the stabbing, the lunchtime ambience on the quadrangle where students gather is more like a penitentiary than a high school. Administrators, eager to establish the tone for the year, want to prevent the anticipated retaliatory attacks. In addition to the two school district policemen armed with 9mm pistols who usually patrol Crenshaw, the school district dispatches two more armed officers. And the principal calls the coaches and male teachers to emergency duty. They, too, march up and down the quad, break up fights, grab students who are throwing gang signs, and drag them to the principal's office. Several coaches patrol the school's perimeter to ensure no neighborhood gangbangers try to slip inside and even a score.

Every week school officials conduct random weapons checks in classrooms. Now they step up the frequency. They pull students out of classrooms and run hand-held metal detectors over them, searching for guns and knives. The principal wants to install a high-security metal detector at the school entrance, but the funding is not available.

Braxton, too, is drafted for security duty during lunch. He is forty-one, but still rangy and fit. He played defensive back on his high school football team, and he still runs like an athlete, gliding across the quad to break up a fight.

He does not like having to spend his lunch hour on security duty, but even this obligation does not dampen his mood today. He has been buoyant all morning, ever since Olivia stopped by his office and told him she was returning to school. He does not have long, however, to savor the good news. When the bell rings and he returns to his office, he must turn his attention to Toya, a student who has disappeared just as Olivia has returned.

Braxton is distressed because, like Olivia, Toya has overcome such steep odds. She is a senior, on the verge of making it out of Watts and

on to college. To falter now would be a crushing defeat, not just for
Toya, but also, Braxton feels, for himself. Because he has spent so much
time counseling Toya. Because he cares for her. Because she has experienced so much cruelty in her young life, she deserves a break, she deserves
to succeed.

For years, Toya had prayed for this night. And it was the death threat
that finally did it, finally convinced her mother that her life and her
daughters' lives were truly in danger.

It was a bitterly cold January night in Hinesville, a small south Georgia
town where Toya was raised. Her stepfather, a burly power plant worker
with an unruly Afro, was on another drinking binge, and was arguing again
with Toya's mother. Toya, who was nine, had seen dozens of these arguments. They usually ended with her stepfather pummeling her mother.
Then he would grab an extension cord, or yank a loose board off a wall,
and beat Toya. Sometimes he would just punch her.

But on this night, he threatened to kill Toya's mother, and the set of his
jaw and the narrowing of his eyes made her believe him. When he finally
passed out in a drunken stupor, Toya's mother quietly hustled her two daughters out of the house, and checked into a nearby shelter for battered women.

After about a week, Toya's mother decided to leave the shelter. It was
too far from her job and she could no longer afford the ten dollar a night
fee the shelter charged. So she arranged to stay with a friend. On the morning
of January 29, she told Toya, "I'm going to pack up all our clothes. So when
you get out of school, come straight to the house. We'll get our things and
move out for good."

Toya returned to the house after school at 3:30 P.M. and found her
mother sprawled on the bedroom floor. She thought her mother was
drunk. Toya shook her. Her mother did not move. She shook her again.
Finally, she crouched beside her mother and looked into her eyes. Then
she knew. She ran out of the house screaming, "She's dead! She's dead.
My mommy's dead!"

Toya's stepfather had strangled her.

Toya had never met her biological father, had no idea who he was or
where he lived. So she and her five-year-old sister were sent to live in a

foster home with three other children. At the home, whenever she thought about her mother and started to cry, her little sister would sob, too. Although only a fifth grader, Toya felt she had to be strong for her sister, to present herself as a steadying maternal figure. It was only late at night, when her sister was sleeping soundly, that Toya allowed herself to mourn her mother's death. She tugged the covers over her head and muffled her cries with a pillow.

Later, Toya wrote a poem that chronicled her childhood, her stepfather's cruelty, and her mother's death:

Was I such a bad child
That I deserved to get hit
With boards
And extension cords . . .
He hit me, abused me
Abuse of every kind.
He conquered my hope . . .
You're my mother.
Why must I feel your pain?
Why must I live your grief?
He took you away from me.
He stole my pride.
He left me—no, us—high and dry
I knew, I just knew I was going to die.
I never dreamed I would see . . . sixteen.
I didn't see my life span
Going past the new day.
I didn't have time to think about tomorrow.
I had to survive for today.
Why?
That's all I want to know.
Why?
But I will never find out
Because you left me . . .
So live on mind, spirit, and heart.

Just know that you're my mother and I'm your daughter
And you could have given me a better start.

During these years of abuse, home was a terrifying prison. The cacophony from drunken fights often awoke her at night. Her stepfather beat her repeatedly, for no reason. He sexually molested her several times, the first time when she was three years old.

Toya's elementary school was her only sanctuary. She was a bright child who learned effortlessly, although no one in her family seemed interested in her progress. In the fifth grade, she was one of the few black children placed in the school's gifted classes. Her science teacher, an elderly lady who wore her gray hair in a bouffant, used to tell her, "You're black, so you've got to prove you're as good as everyone else." If Toya did not do well on an exam, her teacher would say, "You're black, so you can't afford to let down." This angered Toya, but it also made her more determined to succeed, to study harder so she could prove she was as smart as her white classmates.

After her mother's murder—and her stepfather's conviction for voluntary manslaughter—Toya and her sister spent about three months in the group foster home. Then her mother's sister agreed to take them in. Toya's aunt lived in Watts, an impoverished neighborhood at the southern edge of South-Central, down the street from the dilapidated Jordan Downs housing projects. Toya was from a small, country town and she was frightened by her new neighborhood, where drug dealing and drive-by shootings and gangbanging were pervasive. She avoided the perils of her neighborhood by leaving the house only to ride the bus to and from school. When she returned home, she stayed inside and did her homework on the kitchen table, where she could hear the occasional staccato of semiautomatic gunfire outside the window. In junior high school she was placed in a gifted program, and in the ninth grade enrolled at Crenshaw's gifted magnet program.

Toya was one of Braxton's favorite students, not just because she had endured so much and not just because she was one of the school's most conscientious students. Braxton appreciated her great enthusiasm for school, how she embraced the challenges of her classes, particularly her honors chemistry and physics classes. While many bright students at Cren-shaw cannot imagine a world outside South-Central, Toya was ambitious. By her junior year she had mapped out her academic goals: Cornell University's summer program for high school students. After high school, Harvard, with a major in chemistry. After Harvard, medical school and then a career as an oncologist.

During the spring of her junior year, Toya had achieved her first goal: Cornell offered her a full scholarship for its summer program. She had only a little more than a year of high school left. Then, Braxton was sure, Toya would win a scholarship and excel in college. But in late March and early April, she missed a few weeks of school. For Toya, this was highly unusual. Her teachers did not know where she was. Her friends had not heard from her. Braxton called her home and left messages on her answering machine, but no one returned his calls.

On a morning in mid-April of her junior year, the mystery surrounding Toya's absence was solved. I was talking to Braxton in his office, when a secretary interrupted us.

"There's something you should see," the secretary told Braxton. We followed her to the conference room.

Toya was sitting there. With her ten-day-old baby.

Braxton collapsed in a chair. He closed his eyes and cradled his head in his hands. During the past few months, Toya had worn increasingly baggy clothes to school. Braxton and all her teachers thought she had just gained weight.

In the conference room, when Braxton spotted Toya's baby, he emitted a long, slow sigh that sounded like a hinge creaking. "I've seen plenty of students have babies," he told her, "but at least I *knew* they were pregnant."

Toya's baby was dressed in a fuzzy, powder blue sleeper and was wearing a matching cap. She smoothed his hair.

When Braxton regained his composure, he asked her, "What are you going to do about school?"

"I want to take home study," she said evenly.

"How about Cornell?" he asked.

"That's out," she said. "But I'm coming back to school in the fall.

I *will* graduate. And I *will* go on to college. A lady helped my aunt raise me and my little sister when we moved out here. She's very strict. So I'll have her take care of the baby next year."

Toya was not cowed as many teenage mothers are who stop by Crenshaw with their babies. "Can you help me get home study?" she asked, lifting her chin and looking him in the eye.

"Of course," he said. "With all of your honors classes it won't be easy. But don't worry about that. Just do your work and get back here next fall."

He walked Toya to the hallway. A teacher spotted her, pointed to the baby, and asked, incredulously, "Is that *yours?*"

"Yes, he is," Toya said, enunciating each word clearly. "This is my little boy."

Toya lugged her baby to the bus stop and boarded the next bus back to Watts. Braxton returned to his office. He shook his head disconsolately and said, "I had *plans* for that girl. That Cornell experience would have been great for her. I can't even tell you how disappointed I am."

He riffled through her file and perused her report cards, which were mostly As, with a few Bs. He studied her teachers' comments, listed below her grades: "Exceptional student." "Outstanding in every respect." "A pleasure to have in class."

During the next week, Braxton called numerous schools, trying to find a home-study program for Toya. This was not his responsibility because Toya had left the gifted program for the year. But he did not care; he just wanted to make sure Toya earned the credits she needed so she could return to Crenshaw in the fall. A few of the home-study programs Braxton called would not enroll new students because it was too late in the year, but he finally found a program that would accept Toya. For the last few months of her junior year, between changing diapers, nursing her baby, and visiting the pediatrician, she completed homework and wrote papers. In June, she assured Braxton she would return to Crenshaw in the fall for her senior year.

But on the first day of class this year, Toya did not show up. Braxton called her aunt. She told him Toya and her baby had moved out and she did not know where they were. Braxton was dejected. Other girls in the gifted program had become pregnant, but stayed in school. Braxton had thought Toya, too, was disciplined and ambitious enough to juggle mother-hood, high school, and, eventually, college. But when she was absent on the first day of school—and did not call—he reconciled himself to the idea that she was gone.

During the second week of school, Toya, who has left her baby with her cousin, stops by Crenshaw. During lunch, she visits Toni Little, who was her English teacher in the tenth grade. Toya is scheduled to take AP English with Little this year.

"Even though I've got way too many students, I'd still love to have you in AP lit," Little says. "You going to make it to class this week?"

"We'll see," Toya says, looking despondent and lost.

Toya then visits Braxton. She explains that last month she moved into a Watts apartment with her cousin, after her aunt threw her out of the house. Her aunt had always told her: "Don't be a mother before you're a wife." Now her aunt was angry. "You're a woman now," Toya's aunt told her. "You have a baby, so it's time for you to go out on your own. The baby's your responsibility, not mine."

Toya tells Braxton she does not know if she can return to Crenshaw. The family friend who was going to watch the baby while she was in school backed out, and she cannot afford an expensive child care center. She tells him she is considering enrolling at a Watts high school, which has a program that includes free child care for teenage mothers. Toya does not want to leave the teachers in the gifted program. She wants to graduate with her friends. And she is accustomed to excelling in honors and Ad-vanced Placement classes. Toya and Braxton both know that the Watts high school will not be much of an academic challenge, will not prepare her for college. Toya dabs at her eyes with a tissue.

"Don't give up yet," Braxton says. "Let me see if I can find some child care around here that you can afford."

"Okay," Toya says, nodding. Then she says, more to herself than to Braxton, "I've been through a lot tougher times than this. If I could survive them, I can get through this."

THREE

OLIVIA

MY ONLY SAFE HAVEN

While Braxton searches for an inexpensive child care center for Toya, he is heartened by the fact that, at least, his other problem student—Olivia—has returned to school. As long as she remains on the lam from the county, however, Braxton knows her future is uncertain. He knows that county authorities can get a court order to apprehend her and contact police. Officers can then track her down, pull her out of school, and toss her in the county's shelter for abused and neglected children.

During Olivia's first few weeks at school, Braxton continually encourages her to return to foster care. She just has to make it until June, he tells her, and then she will walk the stage at graduation, head for Babson College in Massachusetts, where she plans to apply for a scholarship, and finally free herself from county supervision. A few years ago Olivia read a magazine article that rated Babson as the best business college in the nation, and since then she has dreamed of enrolling there. The school offers a major in entrepreneurial studies, which Olivia feels would be perfect for her. She eventually wants to own her own business and make a lot of money, as quickly as possible, because she never wants to be poor again, never wants to rely on another governmental agency for her survival.

Last year, Braxton enrolled in a class on how to run a business from home, and throughout the class he kept thinking about Olivia, how she netted almost $1,000 a month from her shoestring candy operation on campus, how her combination of intelligence and ambition would ideally suit her for the business world. Without a business school curriculum to guide Olivia, however, Braxton fears her proclivity to bend the rules and work the system could get her into trouble. Gifted kids, he knows, do not always use their intelligence in pursuit of academic excellence.

Olivia has written a brief autobiographical essay in preparation for her Babson application:

"Die, you little bitch!" the woman roared as she caught the young girl by her hair. Struggling to escape, the girl was dragged to the bathroom. The girl's tear-drenched face screamed for the woman to stop, as she was thrown into the shower, her head bouncing off the tiled wall. Her skin burned as the hot water soaked through her clothes.

The woman lifted an extension cord. Crack, crack, crack, it resounded, until the girl's yells drowned out its sound . . .

I was that little girl, and the woman, my mother. I wanted to die rather than endure it. Dealing with a situation I did not create, and could not change, became more than I could bear. Society teaches one to honor thy father and mother, for it is morally correct. But what is one to do when they aren't morally correct and being beaten becomes an everyday event?

So one windy March afternoon I ran until my breath escaped me. Later that night, I called a runaway shelter, which began my trek through many group and foster homes.

My life hasn't been an easy one. Group homes are full of teenage pregnancy, high school dropouts, thieves and drugs. The staff only work there. And since caring isn't included in their salary, they don't.

Through it all, school has been my only safe haven. It is my main focus, even though I have allowed the surrounding negativity to sidetrack me at times. I can truly appreciate what an education means, for it is the only *factor that separates me from the hoodlums. It is imperative in order for me to attain the success that I deeply desire in my future.*

Braxton tells Olivia that to ensure her future, to earn a scholarship to Babson, she must keep her grades up this year and stay focused on school until June.

To Olivia, graduation day seems so far in the future that it is an abstraction rather than an inevitability. During the second week of school, she loses her job at the women's clothing store because her sputtering, 1977 Volkswagen bug continues to stall on her and she is late to work several days in a row. She hears about a job as a graveyard-shift dispatcher at an aerospace company. Olivia figures she will be able to do her home-work and catch a few hours of sleep during the quiet early morning hours. When her shift ends, she will have enough time to make it to class in the morning. She tries to schedule an interview for the job as soon as possible because she is down to her last few dollars and is desperate for money. She scans the ads in the newspaper for temporary night work where she can earn some quick cash to tide her over.

Olivia is embarrassed to tell Braxton, or her classmates, but she even-tually takes a job as a taxi dancer. She wears a black, low-cut, spaghetti strap dress, and dances, talks, and plays pool with customers for six dollars an hour and tips. The club is located in a desolate, industrial section of downtown Los Angeles, on the top floor of a grimy brick building, above an electrical supply company and down the street from a printing plant and a cigar factory.

The black awning outside the club advertises: HOSTESS DANCING in large block letters. There is a five dollar cover charge, and a sign by the door: PROSTITUTION & LEWD CONDUCT ARE UNLAWFUL AND IMPERMISSIBLE ACTIVITIES. Inside the dim, smoky club, downtown factory workers and laborers, and a few businessmen in sports coats and ties, ogle the women, who sit on a padded bench, at the edge of the bar. The women, dressed in short skirts, halter tops, and skimpy, low-cut dresses, look bored as they smoke cigarettes, chat, and wait for customers to approach them. In her heavy makeup and thick eyeliner, Olivia looks as if she is in her twenties. Only an occasional girlish gesture or nervous giggle betrays her as a seventeen-year-old high school senior with a fake ID.

In the club's dark recesses, in the padded corner booths, some of the women engage in what is euphemistically called "lap dancing," and afterward obtain "tips" from the men. The empty Trojan wrappers scattered about the floor of the men's bathroom indicate that more goes on in this club than dancing.

Olivia carefully avoids the dark corners of the club. When a man wants to dance or talk with her, he has to line up at a booth by the bar, punch a time card, and pay twenty-one dollars an hour for the privilege. Dancing with the men is distasteful to Olivia, and she tries to persuade them to buy her a Snapple and just sit and talk at a well-lit table near the dance floor. She usually takes home from fifty to seventy dollars a night in tips, but, some nights, she does not return home until 2:00 A.M. She wakes up at 6:30 the next morning, stumbles into class, bleary-eyed and yawning, and fights to stay awake. Other students are penalized for being tardy or for missing class. But most of the teachers cut Olivia some slack. Even though she often is late now for her 8:00 A.M. classes, is occasionally absent, and sometimes turns in her homework late, her teachers know her circumstances are anomalous.

In her AP U.S. Government class, the teacher, Scott Allen, asks students to sign a contract with him, agreeing to obey the class rules regarding homework assignments, attendance, and exams. Allen also asks the students to have a parent sign it. On the day the contract is due, Olivia approaches Allen after class. From a distance, she could pass for a teacher, and Allen, who is thirty-five years old, could pass for a student. He has light brown, shoulder-length hair and wears faded jeans, sneakers, and a T-shirt. Olivia is dressed up again today, in a chocolate brown skirt, matching blazer, stockings, and brown lizard high heels. After school, she is interviewing for the job as the graveyard-shift dispatcher.

"I can't turn the contract in," Olivia tells Allen.

"Why not?" he asks, not looking up from his roll book.

"I don't have any parents to sign it," she says matter-of-factly.

He studies her, now, with genuine concern.

"Are you eighteen?"

"No."

"Well . . ." Allen says, struggling to think of a solution that does not embarrass her. "Just sign it yourself. Don't worry about the rest of it."

She nods and saunters out the classroom, earrings jangling, her high heels clicking on the linoleum, echoing in the hallway.

Olivia's schedule is so hectic now, with school and taxi dancing, that she has little time for homework, so she tries to do most of it during her AP computer science class. While the other students write down the problems and furiously fill pages of paper with their attempts to solve them, Olivia computes the problems in her head. In a moment, she can conceptualize computer or mathematical problems and quickly reach solutions. Her teacher boasts that Olivia is one of the most gifted computer science students she ever taught at Crenshaw and expects her to pass the AP exam this spring with a five—the highest score.

As the other students labor and surreptitiously ask Olivia for help, she quickly whips through her class assignments. She has no computer at home, so despite admonitions from her teacher, she frequently uses her spare class time to write papers and finish homework for other courses.

After a few weeks of taxi dancing four and five nights a week, trying to keep up with her AP courses, and sleeping only a few hours a night, Olivia finally concedes defeat. She cannot sustain this pace until October, much less until June. She does not want to return to a group home, but she has heard about a pilot program for older foster children that provides apartments, stipends, and loose supervision. Olivia decides this could be the solution to her problems.

She decides to cut her computer science class on a September afternoon and visit Ron Johnson, whose firm has a county contract to run the housing program. Johnson knows Olivia because she was a long-time student in a martial-arts class he taught for foster children. And she trusts him, partly because he, too, grew up poor and had a tumultuous childhood; because he, too, was once a bright student with a troubled home life. A former gang member from a Brooklyn housing project, Johnson straightened out his life and graduated from Columbia University.

Olivia pulls out of the high school parking lot and speeds around a corner, grinding her gears, her Volkswagen rattling down the street. On this still, smoggy afternoon, the gauzy haze that encircles Los Angeles seems to compress the horizons and shrink the city. The air is so thick with pollutants, the veiled sun and vaporous shadows create a spectral twilight in the middle of the day.

"If Ron can get me an apartment, all my problems will be solved," Olivia tells me. At a stop sign she puts her hands together, as though praying, and says, "I hope, I hope he can. I'd rather be AWOL than have to deal with another crowded, dirty foster home with another foster mother who doesn't give a damn about anything but her paycheck."

She races down Crenshaw Boulevard and screeches to a halt in front of Johnson's office, housed on the ground floor of a sooty brick building, facing a body shop and down the street from a pawn shop, a hat store, and a strip of boarded-up businesses. She sits on a chair next to his desk. He brings a Coke and she explains her predicament to him, how she is tired of living in foster homes, how his program would be perfect for her.

He shrugs and says, "I understand what you're saying. But as long as you're AWOL, I can't do anything for you. You've got to get back into the system. You've got to let your social worker place you in a home. Once you're placed, I can see about getting you an apartment."

"Why can't I get an apartment right now? I'm turning myself in to you."

"You know that's not the way it works."

The office's front door is open, but there is not much of a breeze, just the rumble of traffic. Olivia cools her forehead with the Coke can. "I can't live like that again," she says. "I can't go back to one of those places."

"Your last placement seemed like a good situation. Why'd you go AWOL?"

"I haven't had a mom since I was twelve. All of a sudden someone wanted to be my mom. It didn't work."

"Part of being an adult is making it work," he says. "It was an impulse decision. You can't make life decisions based on impulses."

"I never respected my mom," Olivia says. "She never deserved respect. And I never respected my foster mothers. They never cared about me.'' Olivia stares off into the distance. ''So I don't care about them.''

''Any problem you've got, you just replay your battle with your mother,'' he says. ''You're angry. You resent authority. You've got to give people some respect.''

''I give people respect who deserve respect,'' she says angrily. ''I respect my teachers. I respect Mr. Braxton. I respect you.''

''Physically, you're okay,'' he says. ''But you've got a lot of emotional problems. Hey, you come from a situation that would make anyone angry and hurt. But you've got to be in the system before I can help you.''

She frowns and twirls an earring. ''If I go back, how long will I have to be there before you can get me in an apartment?''

''One to two months,'' he says. ''That's all I need.''

''I can't handle another two months in one of those homes,'' she says plaintively.

''Olivia!'' he shouts. ''We're talking a few months.'' He pats her shoulder and says softly, ''We're talking about what's best for you, what's best for your future.''

She slinks down in her chair and her eyes begin to tear.

''You're jammed up right now,'' he says. ''But you know you've got to go back. It's your only way out.'' He pauses, grips her by the shoulders, and asks, ''Will you go back?''

''I guess so,'' she says mechanically.

''Okay,'' he says, clapping his hands once. ''We got that straightened out. You still working?''

''Yeah. I got a kind of temporary job now. And I've applied for this night job as a dispatcher. I'm waiting to hear whether I got the job. It's perfect for me—''

He interrupts her. ''When you get back into a foster home, I hope you stop working.''

''I can't.''

''Why not?''

''I can't live poor,'' she says, sounding desperate. ''I gotta buy clothes. I gotta pay for gas.''

''None of that stuff really matters,'' he says. ''Look, you can't play basketball. You're not a musician. But you're bright. School's your ticket out of here. It was my ticket out, too. School should be your priority now, not clothes and your car.''

The teenagers he advises often stare at him sullenly, their eyes opaque with boredom. But Olivia is listening to him now, nodding in assent.

"So first thing you do is call your social worker. Get back into the system. Whatever foster home they send you to—go. Don't get nasty with anyone. Don't give anyone a hard time. Don't go AWOL again.''

"Okay," she says. "But I don't want to be there indefinitely.''

"You won't be," he says. "Just don't blow it now. All you have to do is hang on nine more months. Then all this is behind you and you're on your way to college. It's almost over. Can you hang on nine more months?''

She takes a sip of Coke and says weakly. "I'll try.''

The next day at school, Olivia explains her predicament to Braxton. While he leaves to attend a meeting, he lets her use his office. She closes the door, calls her social worker and county social services and sets in motion the move to yet another foster home—her thirteenth residence in the past five years. Although resigned to her fate, she remains in a surprisingly upbeat mood. Despite constant obstacles, she does not stay despondent for long. She usually brims with energy and ideas, laughs easily and is generally so high-spirited people are surprised when they discover her background.

On a Friday morning, Olivia misses Little's class because her social worker has found a new home for her. Olivia stuffs all her belongings into a few green plastic garbage bags and drives to her new residence: a four-bedroom foster home, where five other girls and the foster mother live. From a distance, the foster home, which is only a few miles from Crenshaw, looks like a standard beige, Southern California ranch-style house. But a closer inspection reveals the fortresslike security measures. Stucco walls and a rusty, six-foot-high metal fence with spiked tips encircle the house. Each window is latticed with thick bars, and at the front of the house there is a heavy, steel-mesh security door. The house faces a major thoroughfare—with no stop signs or traffic lights nearby—and a constant stream of cars race by at breakneck speed.

Olivia's social worker orders her to sell her Volkswagen because she has no driver's license and no insurance. Instead, Olivia parks the car at the top of a hill near the house. Every morning she tells the foster mother she is walking to the bus stop, and, instead, climbs the hill and drives off to school—if the car starts.

The Volkswagen is not much to look at, just a battered, rusting, nineteen-year-old Bug with torn upholstery, a mangled bumper, and only one headlight. But to Olivia, it is a prized possession. She lovingly washes the car each week. She buys magazines that feature custom Volkswagens and studies them in bed at night. She spends afternoons at auto part shops, shopping for gold hub caps and chrome shift knobs that will give her car a little flash. Her friends cannot understand why she is so attached to such a wreck, why she continues to drive it and risk arrest. But for a girl who has never owned anything that could not fit in a plastic garbage bag, who never received a gift that she cared about—from someone whom she cared about—who never bought anything for herself, except clothes, this car signifies more to her than just transportation.

A few days after she moves into the foster home, Olivia's car breaks down again. I drive her and her best friend Julia to the foster home because Olivia has to pick up a book. She rings the bell. No one answers. Suddenly a girl inside the house shouts, "I'm calling the police!" Another girl yells, "I'll kill you, bitch!"

The foster mother lets Olivia in the house. Several girls argue at the top of their lungs. One girl in the hallway screams at another girl for stealing her clothes. In the kitchen, a girl sprawls on the floor, eyes shut, hands over her ears, sobbing. Another girl in the living room, whose father is dying of AIDS, accuses her roommate of betraying a confidence by telling everyone. She grabs Olivia by the shoulders.

"My dad has HIV and TB," she says, tears streaming down her face. "It's true. I'm not ashamed. But why does she have to tell everyone?" she says, pointing to a girl across the room. "Why does she have to put my business on the street?" She shakes Olivia and begins sobbing.

Olivia leads her over to the sofa and tries to calm her. The sofa is gold crushed velvet covered in plastic. The coffee table is made of wood burl, with a matching wood burl clock on the wall. On the opposite wall looms a large, black velvet Jesus, who graces the bedlam below with a beatific look.

Wide-eyed, Julia glances around nervously. "These foster homes," Olivia tells her, "are always like this. There's always a lot of yelling and dissension and fights over stealing. There's always a lot of craziness. Night and day." She opens the door to her bedroom and sees her roommate curled up on a bed, eating caramel corn and watching cartoons. The dim, musty room is a mess: the floor is strewn with shoes, hair brushes, and empty cereal boxes. The orange carpet is ripped and stained. A broken mirror leans against a wall. A small desk is covered with Olivia's makeup, shampoo, detergent, and a few school books. A floor lamp with no bulb teeters in the corner. Olivia's roommate has cut pictures of rap stars from magazines and taped them to the walls. A cascade of socks, T-shirts, and blouses topples from the roommate's chipped dresser. Green plastic garbage bags, filled with Olivia's clothes, surround her bed.

Olivia sees that the clothes in one of her bags, which she had neatly folded, are in a jumble. "Did you go through my things?" she asks her roommate in an even tone.

"I didn't touch yo' motherfucking shit!" screams her roommate, a tall, skinny, gap-toothed girl with wild hair. "You fucking bitch!" She leaps off the bed and charges Olivia, fists clenched, eyes flashing.

Olivia holds up a palm and says calmly, "Slow down. I'm not violent. I don't like to fight. I just want to know."

The roommate stops suddenly, startled by Olivia's sangfroid. "I ain't gone through nobody's stuff. But some motherfucker done gone through mine and stole my toothpaste and my sponge."

"Don't get so defensive," Olivia says. "Calm down. It was a simple question."

The roommate returns to her cartoons. Olivia finds the book and heads out the door.

FOUR

VENOLA

MY RAINBOW IS WAITING FOR ME

Now that Olivia has returned to foster care, she no longer taxi dances full-time to support herself. But she still needs spending money and cash for gas and clothes, so she works at the club a few days a week, usually on weekends. She now can study in the evenings, but she finds it impossible to accomplish anything at the foster home. So she drives over to a nearby Taco Bell, nurses a cup of water, and studies late into the night, while the winos and street people and crackheads wander in and out.

Theft is a problem at the foster home, and Olivia, who has the nicest clothes and most expensive cosmetics, has lost a number of items, including a watch, perfume, blouses, skirts and toiletries. At night, when she drifts off to sleep, she curls up and clutches her purse to her stomach.

Despite warnings from her social worker and foster mother, Olivia has not sold her car. Still unreliable, it has caused her to be late to a number of classes. She does not have the money for repairs, so she decides to enroll in auto mechanics, an unusual course selection for a gifted magnet student. Olivia is the only girl in the class, and has charmed the teacher into working on her car. He often gives the other students assignments and then shifts his attention to the many repairs Olivia's Volkswagen requires.

A few mornings after Olivia moves into the foster home, the Volkswagen's brakes stutter and fail, and she brings the car to class. While the students are trying to solve a mathematical equation to determine the size of an engine, the teacher raises Olivia's car on the hoist. The other students struggle with the equation, but Olivia whips out a calculator, solves the problem in less than a minute, and joins her teacher.

Olivia is dressed in a colorful, floral-print skirt, orange top, and black high heels. As usual, her outfit violates the school dress code on several counts. And, as usual, she has managed to evade the administrators who wander the halls looking for dress-code scofflaws. Her high heels violate the "no open toe and heel" edict. Her short skirt violates the "no more than four inches above the knee" rule. Her orange top violates the "only black, dark gray, navy, blue, and white" color mandate, which was instituted to prevent gang members from showing their colors. The dress code, to further discourage gang activity, also bans "bandannas, all blue or red shoestrings, sagging pants, belt buckles with initials, beepers, and backpacks with gang or tag writing."

Olivia paces beside her car, shielding her eyes from the bright morning sun with a cupped hand, while the auto shop teacher grunts and sweats beneath the Volkswagen, adjusting the brakes, his hands and wrists shiny with grease. He notices that the front bumper is mangled. "We can take care of this later," he says. "You've got nice clothes on so we'll have some of the young men in the class pound it out for you."

Suddenly, there are several loud pings, which sound like bullets hitting the other cars on the lot. Olivia crouches beside the Volkswagen. The teacher waits a few minutes, then warily climbs out from under the car. He determines that some students on the top floor of an adjoining building are throwing rocks down at the cars. He hustles into the classroom and calls security. While he waits, a student in the back, who is about six feet six, will not do his math equation, will not sit down, and will not stop talking. The teacher hands him a piece of paper and says, "Write your name down here." The student writes, "Bugs Bunny" and continues clowning around. When the school policeman arrives, the teacher tells him to deal with the obstreperous student first and then investigate the rock-throwing incident.

"I want him out of here right now," the teacher says, pointing to the student. "Tell the dean I want to see his parents during third period. The meeting, *this* time, will be at *my* convenience, not theirs."

The guard escorts the student from the class and the teacher follows them outside. When he leaves the classroom, a few students toss chalk at each other. One student overturns a trash can and kicks it around the room. Other students pound their desks, sing rap songs, and hurl books at one another. The teacher returns to the class and attempts to quiet the students. They ignore him. Finally, in frustration, he throws a block of wood across the room. It hits the wall with a loud thwack. The din subsides, for a moment. Then a surprised student calls out, "What you doin', man?"

"If you don't like it, tell your parents!" the teacher shouts.

Olivia, who is accustomed to gifted classes, is so irritated by the clamor that she stalks out of the classroom. I give her a ride to a donut shop near campus where she orders breakfast—chocolate milk and a chocolate donut. Before eating, she closes her eyes briefly, nods her head, and says grace to herself. For years, she was ordered to say grace at group homes, and it is now second nature to her. She devours her donut, lights a cigarette, and sips her milk. She then returns to pick up her car.

The next morning in AP English, the students continue reading *The Crucible,* out loud, with great dramatic flair. Little is pleased the class is engrossed in the play. Last night, two male students who were doing their homework together were so engaged by the assignment that they looked up Little's phone number and called her so they could discuss their interpretations of the play with her.

After the students read another act, Little lectures on Sen. Joseph McCarthy's rise to power and the anticommunist hysteria in America during the time. She draws parallels between seventeenth-century Salem and America in the late 1940s and early 1950s, between the witch hunts conducted by the Puritans, and the hunt for Communists conducted by McCarthy.

"Russians were the threat in the 1950s," Little says. "What is the threat today?"

"Gangbangers!" one girl calls out.

"No," Little says, irritably. "To our national security."

A dozen hands shoot up at once.

"Saddam Hussein," one student calls out.

"How do we really know what's a threat today?" another student asks. "In the sixties, they said Martin Luther King was a threat to national security because he was a Communist. Now we know it was just disinformation put out by the FBI."

"They're saying the same thing about Louis Farrakhan today," a girl responds.

While the discussion rages, Venola, a small, slender girl dressed boyishly in jeans, sneakers, and a white T-shirt, continually waves her hand, but Little does not notice her because Venola sits in the back corner of the class. When the class resumes reading *The Crucible*, Venola, who looks hurt, walks up to Little and slips her a note. "I don't understand how you could pass me up today in class when I had so many important things to tell my fellow students," Venola wrote. "I must have been mistaken when I thought you perceived me as a valuable student in your class."

After Little reads Venola's note, she halts the class. Little, who was Venola's tenth grade English teacher, announces: "I love Venola Mason with all my heart, and we go way back. But now she's going to kick me to the curb because I made one error of judgment. So I'm going to sit in Venola's seat now and she's going to take my place and take as much time as she needs to give her opinion."

Venola stands up and without a hint of self-consciousness addresses the class. "I believe in God," she says. "But there are deceivers out there, like some preachers who are always talkin': 'Jesus, Jesus, Jesus,' but who just want money and power. They take advantage of people's beliefs. They take something good and twist it. Some people follow them blindly. But I believe that God gave us dominion over ourselves. He gave us the ability to choose the path of righteousness or the path of sin, to make decisions for ourselves. When people forget that they have that choice, and instead blindly follow some preacher or some philosophy, we get things like McCarthyism and Salem witch hunts.''

Satisfied, Venola turns to Little and nods. She returns to her seat.

Venola was nine years old when her mother, Paula, decided to leave Louisville to get away from Venola's father, whom she had never married. They had split up several years before, but he would not provide child support. While Paula was working at a film processing plant, he would stop by the house, laze around all day, drink beer, and eat all the food in the refrigerator. When she would lock him out at night, he would park his car by the door, honk the horn and shout, upsetting the children.

Paula decided the only way to resolve the situation was to move across the country. So she and her children hopped on a Greyhound bus and arrived in Los Angeles three days later. Paula had $200 in her pocket. She found a night job as a combination waitress-dishwasher-busboy-janitor in a small restaurant. The family shared a tiny room in a South-Central boardinghouse and slept in a single bed. After they moved in, the gas, electricity, and water in the boardinghouse were shut off because the owner had not paid the bills. Paula, who was supporting three children on the $125 a week she was making at the restaurant, could not afford to move.

In the morning, she slipped into a neighbor's yard, turned on a hose, and filled a basin with water, so her children could wash before school. She walked them to school, caught a few hours' sleep, and in the afternoon walked them home from school. At dusk, she grabbed a shopping cart that she hid behind the boarding house, and canvassed the neighborhood, gathering scraps of lumber and branches. She sawed and chopped the wood into little pieces, dropped them in a hibachi and fired it up on the front porch. With a small pot and pan, she fried fish and cooked pinto beans, rice, and neck bones. After dinner, she heated pans of water on the hibachi, washed her children, and tucked them into bed.

Before Paula left for work, she cut more wood and built a fire in the room's tiny fireplace. The other women in the neighborhood watched in amazement as she scurried about, from dawn until dusk, cooking, cleaning, chopping wood, washing her children, escorting them to and from school.

Paula recalls the women shaking their heads and muttering, "Them country women are something *else!*"

Venola was in the fourth grade during this time, and although Paula did not pay much attention to her daughter's education, Venola excelled in school. She was placed in gifted classes and always strived for As. When she would get a B on a test, she would come home crying, even though Paula would tell her she was delighted with the grade.

Paula eventually saved enough money so the family could move into a two-bedroom apartment. "I'll never forget our first night there—it seemed like a big mansion to me," Venola recalls. "It was like heaven."

By the time Venola enrolled at Crenshaw High School, Paula needed two jobs to support her children. During the day, she worked as a private-duty nursing assistant and, at night, at a convalescent hospital. She returned home, exhausted, at midnight. At the end of each week, Paula handed over her paychecks to Venola, who paid the bills and balanced the checkbook. When the balance would drop precariously, Venola would admonish the rest of the family, "No more spending until the next paycheck!"

Because of her busy routine, Paula never went to an open house at school, never talked to Venola's teachers. Still, Venola continued to excel. Even as a young girl, it was clear to her that school was the only way to ensure she never would have to work double shifts every day like her mother. She would not let anything sidetrack her from her ultimate goal— a college scholarship.

"I was too tired from working to contribute anything to Venola's schooling," Paula says with a shrug. "It all came from her. I haven't seen one of her report cards since the tenth grade. She tell me, 'Oh, Mama, I'm doin' fine.' I just take her word for it. She been making her own decisions for a long while."

While Paula says she cannot take credit for Venola's academic success, she still is extremely proud of her. When Venola writes poems or essays for class, Paula brings fifty copies to the convalescent hospital and hands them out to coworkers and patients.

In an autobiographical essay, Venola wrote:

My neighborhood houses gangsters who don't seem to care about their future. They make living here uncomfortable for me. I have to watch what I wear because some colors are offensive to them. They will attack males I invite to my house . . . because they want to make sure they are not from rival gangs. When I go to my friends' houses I see prostitutes and drug dealers on the corners conducting business. Feelings of sadness overcome me . . . What makes South-Central L.A. so complicated is the fact that good-hearted, honest people share the same streets with drug users and thieves . . . which causes daily anxiety for those of us who want to get ahead . . .

I have chosen to grasp opportunities that come my way and to make the most of them, no matter what the cost . . . I know that my rainbow is waiting for me on the other side, and I won't stop until I see its colors.

Paula has strived to support her family without public assistance. A few years ago, she moved her family out of the two-bedroom apartment and into a three-bedroom apartment, in a less rundown neighborhood. But their new residence was dank and dark, in the back of the building, like their previous apartments. It faced a cluster of telephone poles, and Paula could see the rats, big as cats, running along the phone lines.

The summer before Venola's junior year, Paula finally achieved her dream: The family rented a small house, with the help of a Section 8 federal housing subsidy. Railroad tracks snake beside the house, which is bordered by a weed-choked patch of dirt. But the small bungalow has a large picture window in the living room and is airy and light filled. The walls are covered with pictures of Jesus on the cross and the Last Supper.

"Now we right out in front," Paula says proudly. She points out the window and says, "I can see the cars driving on by. Oh, man. It's an improvement. We like the Jeffersons," she says, smiling, her gold front tooth glistening in the afternoon light. "We keep movin' on up."

Now that Venola is a senior, Paula sees all her daughter's hard work paying off. Every week Venola receives another college recruiting letter. College admission officers are on the lookout for bright black students, and they flag the ones with solid PSAT (Preliminary SAT) scores. After Venola scored a 1200 last year, she began receiving letters. One of her dresser drawers is filled with pamphlets, course catalogues, and videos sent to her from colleges such as Wellesley, Georgetown, and Stanford. Venola dreams of attending a small, private college in the East, but she is practical enough to know that she may not have the luxury of choice. When people ask her where she is going to college next year, she replies, "Whoever gives me the most money."

During this arduous year, Venola will have to juggle work and school and still maintain her grades. Every day at 3:00 P.M., after school, she boards the bus to her job as a nurse's aide at the convalescent hospital where her mother also works. When her shift ends, Venola waits at the bus stop and does not arrive home until about 9:00 P.M. Her mother is still at work, so Venola grabs a hamburger or taco at a fast-food restaurant and tries to squeeze in a few hours' homework before nodding off. The next morning she is up early, so she will have time to catch the 7 o'clock bus.

Venola tries to read as much as she can during her little free time. She is one of the few students in her AP English class who reads for pleasure, which is one reason she scored better than most of her classmates on her PSAT test. Venola reads because whenever the family moved, Paula always walked her to the neighborhood library, ensured she obtained a library card and checked out stacks of books. During the summer before her senior year, Venola's goal was to read twenty books by the end of the year. By mid-September, she has read fourteen—most of them popular novels by black authors such as Terry McMillan and Walter Mosley. After she finishes a book, she neatly writes the title and the author in a notebook she keeps beside her bed.

While some ambitious students at Crenshaw can be ruthless and devious in their pursuit of As, Venola is a favorite among her teachers because her interest in learning is genuine and because she has such a sweet, unaffected, ingenuous manner. Whenever Olivia, for example, misses a class or comes in late, Venola always tries to help her. She knows Olivia's life is not an easy one, so she lends her the assignments and lecture notes she missed.

At the convalescent hospital where she works, Venola is loved by the patients. She enjoys talking to the elderly patients and listening to their

stories. She learned so much about the Great Depression from her conversations with a Jewish patient named Bertha and a black patient named
Melba that she wrote a paper on their experiences for her U.S. History
class.

At school, during lunch and during nutrition period, Venola does not
hang out on the quad with the other students. She tries to finish homework
assignments in the library or type papers in the computer science classroom. When Venola's neighborhood friends ask her why she is always
studying or working or reading, why she does not like to hang out, she
tells them, "You have to navigate your *own* future. If not, you'll end up
with nothing."

Scott Braxton considers students like Venola a gift. They do their work.
They plan for their futures. Their home lives are relatively stable. They rarely
waver from the path that begins at Crenshaw and ends at college. Braxton
regrets he must spend so much time helping high-maintenance students
like Olivia and Toya because he has little time left for self-reliant students
like Venola.

During the past week, Braxton has called numerous child-care centers
in search of an affordable one for Toya. But the child-care centers that
are affordable are far from Crenshaw, and the ones that are close to
Crenshaw are expensive. Braxton suspects that locating a child-care center
for Toya violates some school district edict, or puts him in a position of
legal liability. But he does it anyway. He eventually finds one for $265 a
month, only two blocks from the high school, and reserves a spot for
Toya's baby.

Braxton officially enrolled Toya in her classes last week. Now he has
to coax her to school. He calls her and tells her about the child-care
center. Toya, however, says she does not know if she can afford $265 a
month. Time is running out, Braxton tells her. There is only a week and
a half left in September. If she is going to return to the gifted program,
Braxton tells her, she had better do it now because if she delays any
longer she will be too far behind to catch up.

Toya tells him she will let him know soon.

*   *   *

Toya is living in a dilapidated apartment in a blighted, industrial section of Watts, across the street from a furniture manufacturing plant and surrounded by cabinet factories, auto repair shops, and other rundown apartment buildings. In front of Toya's two-story building is an enormous, sliding, black metal security gate and, above it, a plastic sign: MOVE IN SPECIAL—$295. The tan stucco is crumbing off the building, the paint is peeling off the front doors, trash is scattered along the entrance, and the address is sloppily spray-painted on the front of the building.

To reach her apartment, Toya walks through the security gate; past a long strip of stained asphalt that reeks of Lysol; past a rusting, abandoned stove; past the apartments blaring—alternately—salsa or rap; past the parking lot where discarded auto parts are strewn about; past a corrugated-metal fence covered by huge swirls of savage graffiti. Her front door faces a box factory that churns and thrums all day. The apartment building lies directly beneath Los Angeles International Airport's flight pattern. Toya and her neighbors are taunted all day by the sleek, silvery jets that constantly pass overhead, on their way to distant and exotic destinations.

Toya and her cousin share the apartment's single tiny bedroom. They both sleep on narrow cots that flank the baby's crib. By the front door, there is a small kitchen with a chipped linoleum floor. The living room walls are almost bare, with only a few small pictures of Toya's son, who is now about six months old, and her late mother.

During the O.J. Simpson trial, Toya became enamored of the name, Kato Kaelin. She changed the spelling slightly and named her son Kaelen. As Toya bounces Kaelen on her knee, she talks—above the din of the trucks rumbling by and the airplanes roaring above—about her life during the past few weeks, since school started. When she is stuck at home and Kaelen is napping, she often reads the dictionary. She scans the pages, searching for words she does not know, desperate for some intellectual stimulation. On other days, she and Kaelen spend the afternoon at the public library in Watts, and, after reading to him, she leafs through books about science, anatomy, or grammar, books that serve as simulacrum for the rigor of the classroom. In the mornings she often boards the bus to a racetrack in nearby Inglewood because Kaelen likes to watch the horses limbering up.

Despite the upheaval in her life, despite her difficult circumstances,

Toya has maintained her equanimity. And her dignity. Her apartment is immaculate. She takes good care of Kaelen, who is a bright, happy baby. And while she currently is in academic limbo, she has not abandoned her dream of college.

Toya hopes to return to Crenshaw, hopes to put Kaelen in the child-care center Braxton found for her. But the center charges $265 a month, and the most she can afford right now is $215. She is trying to figure out a way to obtain another $50 a month. She knows she does not have much time.

FIVE

MIESHA

MY TALENT IS PERSEVERANCE

During the last week of September, after several sultry weeks of school, the students can feel summer slipping away. The mornings are no longer bright and cloudless, with luminous blue skies. A miasma of fog shrouds the city at dawn now and does not burn off until midmorning. During lunch, the quad no longer bakes beneath a bleaching, unforgiving sun. The light is softer now, buttery and muted. In the early afternoon a soft breeze blows in from the ocean. The subtle Southern California fall is approaching.

This week, there is a flurry of gang activity. After school, near the campus's front steps, three 11th Avenue Hustlers stab and beat a member of a gang—loosely affiliated with the Rollin 60s—called Penn State. Members wear athletic gear with PENN STATE UNIVERSITY emblazoned on it, but not because they identify with the school's highly ranked football team. The gang's name is an acronym for Pussy Eatin' Nasty Niggas Sucking Titties and Tasting Everything.

Two hours after the Penn State member is attacked, a Rollin 60—a former student—is shot by a member of a rival Blood set, the Van Ness

Gangsters, while hanging out with a group of other 60s a few blocks from Crenshaw. Now school officials are concerned that gang battles will metastasize and spill onto campus. Principal Yvonne Noble sends out a memo to the teachers, detailing the two attacks and a third incident. A teacher confiscated a student's pager—which is prohibited on campus—and the student attacked her. He was arrested and expelled. The principal stated in her memo: "The purpose of this information is . . . not to alarm anyone. I just think you need to be aware of incidents that might negatively impact some of our students, and be prepared to offer the school environment as a refuge . . ."

The next morning before AP English, a group of students are talking about the mounting gang tension. Little decides to integrate the incidents into *The Crucible* discussion.

"Who knows exactly what happened?" Little asks.

A dozen students raise their hands. Several talk at once.

"A guy got shanked in front of the school," one student says.

"I heard he just got shot," another says.

"No," a third student says. "He got hit with a pole and *then* he got shot."

Sadi, who is wearing a baggy DKNY sweatshirt and oversized cords, mumbles to a student sitting next to him, "I knew all them dudes."

A girl calls out, "*He* didn't get shot. The guy in front of the store and a couple of 60s got shot."

"Okay," Little says. "There's an important parallel between these gang attacks and *The Crucible*. When the play opens, there is a report that the girls in the forest were dancing naked, flailing about, drinking blood, chanting to the devil, engaging in all kinds of witchcraft. Because of that report, a lot of people are executed. But let's examine what the *actual* facts were . . ."

After separating rumor from reality in *The Crucible,* the class discusses all the speculation and supposition surrounding the two gang attacks. Little then gives a brief lecture on the concept of group hysteria, the part it played in *The Crucible,* during the Communist witch hunts, and on campus in the wake of the gang violence.

"My brother wants to leave Crenshaw now," a soft-spoken girl in the back row says, staring at her desk. "He's in the ninth grade and has only been here a few weeks. But he's heard so much talk, he thinks it's a lot worse here than it really is."

Little directs the conversation from rumors to outright lies and the role that lying plays in *The Crucible*. "What kind of lies do all of you tell?" she asks the class.

Two girls—the best friends Little vilified in a previous class for chatting and disrupting her lecture—raise their hands.

One says, "I got ahold of three different bank cards and got cash from all of them."

Her friend says, "I signed a phony check for $1,000 and I got caught. I'm payin' it off now."

"How do you justify that?" Little asks.

"God died on the cross for my sins," the girl says. "God knows all."

Olivia interjects, "Just because God knows what we're going to do before we do it doesn't mean there isn't free will."

The other girl responds, "The point is, no matter how big our sins, Jesus forgives us."

Although she has been calm all morning, Little suddenly grows agitated. Her eyes darken and narrow. She purses her lips. She slams her fist on the desk. The girl's comment reminds Little of one of the great vexations of her life—how the black community embraced O.J. Simpson after he murdered his wife. Even though Nicole Brown Simpson was murdered several years ago, the issue still inflames Little, and she still rants about it during class.

"He takes the life of a woman and then everyone says, 'We forgive you.' Well, murder's not forgivable!" she shouts, stamping a foot.

"Miss Little, all that's between God and O.J.," a student says.

"Then I hope that God gives O.J. a wrath he'll never forget. Because that man slaughtered his wife!"

She whirls around and jabs a forefinger at the two best friends, who are chatting and giggling. "Jesus Christ," she shouts. "Will you two *ever* shut up!" She turns back toward the class and says, " 'Thou shall not kill' is a commandment from God. You don't get to slip and slide on that and tell the church, 'I'm a black man and white America has made me a victim, so whatever I do is forgivable.' "

Sadi responds, "If 'thou shalt not kill' is a commandment from God, and America is supposedly a God-fearing nation, why do we have the highest homicide rate in the world?"

"The system is corrupt!" a student shouts.

"Mark Fuhrman planted evidence!" a girl screams.

The class erupts in a burst of yells and whoops and laughs and charges and countercharges. Instead of trying to quiet the students, Little shouts, "WE'RE TALKING ABOUT THE TRUTH! THE TRUTH! THE TRUTH!"

Finally, the din subsides. Little sits on her desk, smooths her hair into place, and takes a deep breath. "Let me tell you why I'm so impassioned about ethical issues that we discuss in this class," she says softly. "My goal is to use the literature we study here as an instrument to make you see the importance of valuing all human life, as an instrument to transform your lives and build your value systems.

"I want to use the literature to show all of you that in each of us is a little of all of us. I want you to embrace that idea in the characters we study, and even in Nicole Brown Simpson. The idea that—in each of us there is a little of all of us—is the key to what I'm trying to teach. It transcends racial differences. It's what this class is all about."

The students listen, nodding their heads, surprised by the somber timbre of her voice, intrigued by her message. Now that she has their attention again, she points to the homework assignment that she wrote on the blackboard before class: "*The Crucible* presents various views of the nature of authority. What are some of these views, and which characters represent or promote them? As opposed to some of the flawed concepts of authority, what does Miller imply through the action is the source of true authority?"

Little asks the students who has the authority in their lives.

Sadi says, "My mom and my minister."

One girl calls out, "God is the ultimate authority in my life. I've been saved."

Olivia says, "Me. I'm the ultimate—and the only—authority in my life."

A tall boy with a buzz cut says, "My conscience is the ultimate authority over my life. If I have something and someone with a gun wants it, they may think they have authority. But if I don't choose to give it to them, I still have the authority."

The class erupts into laughter.

"You be dead, fool," a few students shout in unison.

Miesha raises her hand. She wears faded denim overalls and a sleeveless white T-shirt. Little ribbons are tied to the end of her long corn rows. "My brother is my role model," she announces to the class. "*He*'s the authority in my life."

Miesha was four years old when her brother, Raymond, began taking care of her. Her father lived in Texas. Her mother obtained a job as a Los Angeles bus driver, constantly worked overtime, and often returned home late at night. Raymond, a fifteen-year-old high school student at the time, took charge of his little sister.

When Miesha enrolled in elementary school, Raymond prepared breakfast for her every morning. He helped dress her. He brushed her hair. He walked her to school. In the afternoon, he walked her home. At night, Raymond cooked a full dinner—pork chops and corn, or chicken and rice, or spaghetti, or other dishes she liked. When Miesha complained that she missed her mother, Raymond would explain that their mother worked so hard—up to sixty hours a week—because she cared about them and wanted them to have a decent place to live, food on the table, and nice clothing. Raymond vowed that he would fulfill the role of the conscientious and caring parent.

So it was Raymond who always emphasized to Miesha the importance of school. It was Raymond who helped Miesha with her homework each night. It was Raymond who attended parent-teacher conferences, dance recitals, and school plays. It was Raymond who baked chocolate chip cookies, pound cake with chocolate icing, and pineapple upside-down cake so Miesha would have something to bring to school bake sales. It was

Raymond who rewarded her with dinner at a restaurant and a movie after an outstanding report card.

And when Miesha misbehaved at school, it was Raymond who met with the teachers. Although Miesha was a precocious student, some of her teachers complained that she was "mouthy." Without scolding his sister, Raymond convinced Miesha to show more respect for her teachers, to tone down her comments in class. And Miesha always listened to him. Raymond did so much for her, cared so much about her schooling, that she did not want to disappoint him. And the one way she knew how to repay him was to earn As in school.

But during Miesha's last year of elementary school, she grew increasingly angry and rebellious and her grades slipped. When she broke the house rules, she felt the sting of her mother's thick black bus driver's belt. Raymond was no longer around to serve as a buffer. He had graduated from high school, rented his own apartment, and was employed as a security guard. Miesha decided to move to Texas and live with her father. But she still felt close to Raymond, and they talked on the phone several times a week. Miesha still counted on Raymond to help her when she had difficulty with her math homework, and they solved the problems together on the phone.

In the ninth grade, Miesha, who did not feel welcome living with her father and stepmother, returned to Los Angeles and enrolled at Crenshaw. Her mother was still working extremely long hours and Raymond, again, assumed the role of surrogate parent. Now that Miesha was a teenager, Raymond did not want the social scene to distract her from school. He warned her that there would be a lot of peer pressure for her to fail, that other girls in the neighborhood would try to convince her it was uncool to be a top student. He repeatedly emphasized that she should never be ashamed of her intelligence or her ambition.

Raymond had always tested well and was a gifted math student, but he rarely studied and drifted through high school. By the time Miesha was in high school, Raymond was working for Pepsi, building displays in liquor stores. He did not want Miesha to repeat his mistakes.

In the tenth grade, Toni Little was Miesha's English teacher. Little was put off by Miesha because she seemed like such an angry girl and was so recalcitrant and argumentative in class. Miesha, who is five feet two, may have looked like a petite, pretty cheerleader, but she walked around Crenshaw with an attitude. At Crenshaw, there are more fights on campus involving girls than boys, and Miesha never backed down. Little will never forget the sight of Miesha squaring off against a much bigger girl in the quad. The girl insulted her, and Miesha removed her earrings—the traditional pre-fight ritual—and was on the verge of charging the girl, when Little broke it up.

Although Miesha often was disruptive in class—chatting with her friends, arguing with Little when she tried to discipline her—she always did her reading, always completed her homework assignments, always received high grades on the tests. Still, Little was exasperated by her behavior and threw her out of class a number of times. Finally, Little called a conference with Miesha and her mother. Little told Miesha's mother, who had come from work and was wearing her bus driver's uniform, that it might be best if Miesha transferred to another class.

Miesha began crying. She told Little she did not want to leave the class and promised to change her behavior. And she kept her promise. Little never had another problem with her. By the end of the year, she was one of Little's favorite students. Little thought of her as "my little intellectual." She respected Miesha because, although her writing sometimes lacked polish, her essays were thoughtful and incisive. She respected Miesha's tenacity and her determination to get the grades necessary for a college scholarship.

By her junior year, however, her mother's financial problems made it difficult for Miesha to sustain her record of academic excellence. Miesha's mother owns a home in a well-kept, working class neighborhood, where the lawns are neatly mowed and the shrubbery pruned. She had slipped into debt, however, and struggled to pay the monthly house mortgage, car loan, and all the other bills. Miesha needed money to support herself and to help her mother. During her junior year she had two jobs and worked forty to fifty hours a week. After school, she worked as a salesclerk at a clothing store, and at night as a waitress at a restaurant. She returned home every night after eleven, completed her homework, and awoke the next morning at six.

Miesha wrote about her junior year in an autobiographical essay:

My mother was having financial problems and I felt obligated to help in any way possible. At the time, I was already holding a job as a waitress, just . . . for my personal needs. Suddenly that money wasn't enough.

I soon found myself needing to make a critical choice: Should I get another job? There were many difficulties to be faced if I wanted to take on the responsibilities of the extra work. I needed to determine whether or not the demands of a second job would interfere with my academic performance, whether or not there were enough hours in the day to even get enough sleep . . . I decided to take on the extra responsibility.

After filing my priorities, with school coming first, everything started working out for me. I always managed to find time for each of my academic courses . . . No one would have ever assumed that I was struggling day to day . . . Never did I bring any of my domestic problems into a classroom.

The hardships that I have faced for the past year have taught me that I can overcome any obstacle in my life's path. At the same time, I learned to be thankful for everything that I've been blessed with. God gives everyone a talent, and it is up to each individual to focus on that talent and perfect it.

I believe that my talent is perseverance.

During that difficult year, Miesha still earned all As both semesters. At the end of her junior year, she was ranked fourth—with a 3.9 grade point average—in a class of 356 seniors.

As Miesha begins her senior year, she is a candidate for class valedictorian. Her mother's financial situation has improved, so Miesha dropped the waitress job. Still, her senior year is extremely hectic. She now works thirty hours a week at the clothing store. And she is a cheerleader this year, largely because Raymond encouraged her to try out. He wanted her senior year to be memorable; he wanted her to experience and enjoy every aspect of high school. Now he frequently stops by the house and helps her with her routines.

It is hard to imagine Raymond, who still works for Pepsi, doing a cheerleading routine. He is a singer and drummer in a small band and he has the ultracool mien and manner, the languid grace of a jazz musician. He has a deep throaty voice, a mustache and goatee, and his stage name— Cherry Red—is tattooed on a muscular bicep.

"I remember *all* her routines, and when she forgets one, I'll show her what to do," he says, laughing. "I'll do the routine myself right next to her, right there in the living room."

After Miesha briefly tells the class why Raymond is her role model and the authority in her life, a student turns to Little.

"How about you, Miss Little?" the student asks. "What's the authority in *your* life?"

"I'll tell you at the end of the year," she says. "But for now, I'll tell you that I love my three little dogs. I give them clean sheets. I give them good food. I pay the vet for them. They are a very important part of my life."

The student looks mystified. Little says, "Let's talk about who has authority over the Puritans." She discusses Calvinism and how the Puritans viewed the authority of God, but stops in mid-sentence when she is distracted by the roar of a lawn mower in the quad. She groans loudly, raises her arms, and shakes her palms—fingers outstretched—at the heavens. She marches across the classroom, yanks the cord on the Venetian blinds, and angrily shoves open a window.

"STOP IT!" she screams. "STOP IT. STOP IT! STOP IT!"

The students exchange *there she goes again* glances. The gardeners ignore her. She slumps in a chair, looking helpless and beleaguered. A student who walks in late picks a most inopportune time to ask Little to sign a field trip slip, excusing her from class. Little grabs the slip and waves it in front of the class. "I'm sick of all this extracurricular stuff. We've got the choir and the basketball team and everything else, except what matters. Look at our nice outfits," she says sarcastically. "Look at us on television. All that's very *niiiice*," she says, drawing out the word derisively.

"I don't care about all that. All I care about is that in this class we've only got ten kids who can write an essay that's competitive." She sits on the edge of her desk and surveys the class. "That's where the rubber meets the road."

A girl in the back calls out, "You got an *attitude*, Miss Little."

"You bet I've got an attitude," Little says, furiously wagging a fore-finger at the student, like a metronome at warp speed. "I'm angry. I'm a radical. You all know that. So I'm going to raise hell about this. We spend all this money on security officers, and we still have fights and stabbings all the time.

"There's all this money for basketball uniforms and choir robes, but I can't even get the textbook for this class that I need. I can't get the Xeroxing I need. In these Valley high schools, there's a huge machine and you copy anything what you want. Here, you've got to wait days. Well, I'm sick of spending my own money at Kinkos, so you can have copies for everything. I've got three darling dogs that need food. I won't spend my own money on copies anymore." She crosses her arms with a flourish. "I just won't do it."

She has riled the class up and they begin stamping their feet and chanting, "We want money! We want books! We want copies!" A few students saunter to the front of the room and toss quarters and dimes and dollar bills on a desk.

When Little collects about seven dollars, she calms the class down and returns to the issue of authority in *The Crucible*. The discussion soon drifts to authority and the "crutches" in modern America. The students talk authoritatively about a number of federal programs, including Aid to Families with Dependent Children (AFDC), Section 8 housing and general relief.

"Is welfare and general relief the same thing?" Little asks.

Now the students lecture *her*, and detail the various federal programs, who qualifies and how much money the programs pay.

"In my family, there's no chillin' at mama's," a girl says. "As soon as you can—you jet."

"My cousin just stay at home every day, livin' off AFDC," another girl complains.

"AFDC doesn't pay enough to do anything," Sadi says. "I know *that* firsthand. That's why I *got* to get an education."

SIX

MAMA MOULTRIE

I TOUCH LIVES

Little's battle with the English Department chairwoman, Anita Moultrie, is like trench warfare—long periods of quietude punctuated by brief, violent salvos. This, however, is a one-sided war, with Little usually the aggressor and Moultrie merely counterattacking just to hold her ground.

The flurry of back-and-forth memos—which is the only way they now communicate—has temporarily subsided. But it is inevitable that the tension between the two will, again, roil the academic waters because they are inextricably entwined. Moultrie and Little are the only two English teachers in the gifted magnet program, and all the gifted students in Little's AP English class were taught by Moultrie during their junior years.

The gifted students alternate English teachers at Crenshaw—Moultrie in the ninth and eleventh grades and Little in the tenth and twelfth grades. Ideally, the two teachers would together create a four-year plan for their students. Ideally each year would build on the previous one and, ultimately, culminate for the seniors in the AP exam.

Instead, the two teachers are on separate and distinct tracks, parallel that will never meet. Little and Moultrie are both forty-one, but they are antithetical in every other respect. Little lives alone with her three small dogs. Moultrie and her husband have five children. Little lives on the Westside. Moultrie lives in the neighborhood where she teaches. Little often is aloof, can be prickly after class, and usually avoids involvement in the personal lives of her students. Moultrie is like a surrogate parent.

Little employs the Socratic method, peppering the students with questions so, eventually, they make most of the salient points. Moultrie is the star of her class. She is a commanding, charismatic presence; she does most of the talking and the students fill their notebooks with her interpretations and musings.

Moultrie's and Little's divergent philosophies about who the students should read and what should be emphasized in class represent two poles in academia today. Little teaches a few modern works in her tenth- and twelfth-grade classes, but the reading lists are dominated by dead white males—and females—Dickens, Joyce, Shakespeare, Brontë, Melville, Faulkner. The reading list for her AP class contains no works by black writers. Little feels the students should learn about their culture and their race at home and at church. By focusing on the classics, Little feels the students will be better able to compete at college and on the AP exam. The classics, she feels, will enable them to embrace universal themes; enable them to understand the essence of what she is trying to impart: In each of us is a little of all of us.

Moultrie teaches some classics in her junior English class—such as *The Scarlet Letter*, which all eleventh-grade teachers at Crenshaw are required to teach—but she also feels it is important to expose her students to black authors. And she frequently integrates current events and societal issues into her discussions.

"Some teachers here are not part of the community; they just drive in, teach, and drive on home," she tells me, easing into a chair after class. "I live here. I care about these kids. I consider myself an extension of the family. These are my children, my people. These kids represent my community, my race. I live in the 'hood. I see these kids when I take my children to McDonald's, or go to the market, or I walk into the post office.

"In my class, I want them to learn literature and grammar, but I want them to leave my class with more than that. I consider my teaching to be a calling from God—a ministry. I feel he has entrusted the lives of these children to me. So I take the teaching of my students very seriously. I don't just disseminate information; I touch lives. I want to build their self-esteem. I want to prepare them psychologically and emotionally for life.

"We study some great, white authors, but children of color need to know there are great writers who look like *them*. They need to see our history is not just one of despair and slavery and entrapment and chains. They need to take pride in their culture. They need to gain inspiration in seeing a history of greatness in the African American writers. Some of these writers, like my students, came from impoverished backgrounds. They can be role models.

"Our community here is very isolated and segregated. But when students leave here, they're going to enter a white-dominated society. Not everyone's a racist in that society, but they're still going to be encountering plenty of racism. People will judge them by the color of their skin. I want them to turn that around and use their intelligence and integrity to give people the correct impression of who they are. But to do that they need to be prepared. And my role, I feel, is to help prepare them."

On a September morning, after the eleventh graders have filed into Moultrie's classroom, she says cheerily, "Good morning, class." A few students mumble a reply. She shakes her head in disgust.

She tells the class that she and her husband run a South-Central party company where they rent equipment and provide entertainers for childrens' birthday parties, festivals, and carnivals. It is the largest black-owned party company in Southern California, she says, and they would never hire anyone who addressed them like that.

"You're sixteen years old now," she says. "You'll be applying for jobs. You need to know how to conduct yourselves. You're the gifted students. You'll be the doctors and lawyers and accountants in this community. I want you to get used to looking grown-ups in the eye and addressing them properly.''

She places a hand on a hip and cocks her head. ''This is Mama Moultrie speaking now. So I want y'all to listen to me. I'm going to tell you something that's going to have a big impact on your future. Affirmative action will probably be eliminated here in California.''

She tells the class that in early November, Californians will vote on a ballot measure, Proposition 209, that, if passed, will end affirmative action in the state. ''This proposition probably will pass,'' she says. ''The few crumbs they've tossed our way, they'll soon be taking away. This shows how hypocritical some people are. They say they care about equality, but they want to take away every program that helps foster equality.

''So when affirmative action's over, who do you have? You have *you*. There's nothing else for you to count on. Fortunately, all of you have the wherewithal to go out and kick butt. Even so, what this means is that getting into college is going to get a lot tougher. By the time all of you apply for college, you won't be getting any help whatsoever. So you best be able to make a good impression because many of you will be interviewing for college scholarships next year.

''How do you think these college officials will react if they see you stumble into the interview, eyes downcast, mumbling, 'Hey, wha's up?' But let's say you march in, look them in the eye, say, 'Hello, I'm so and so. How are you?' Do you think it'll make a difference?''

A few students nod.

''Hel-*lo!*'' she shouts, accentuating the second syllable. ''Will it make a difference?''

''Yes, Mrs. Moultrie,'' the class says in unison.

She instructs them to stand up, look at the student next to them in the eye and say, ''Hello, how are you?'' The other student, she tells them, should look them back in the eye and respond, ''Fine thank you. How are you?''

For the next fifteen minutes, as they practice, Moultrie wanders through the classroom, dispensing advice. She tells a girl, ''We tryin' to get you a job, girlfriend. Speak up!'' She then tells a boy, ''No slouchin'. And pull those pants *up!*''

''Before that interview, men, take those earrings off,'' Moultrie says.

"And ladies, never wear pants. No loud colors. No neon yellows and greens. And not too much jewelry.

"And, everyone. Always answer questions in complete sentences. And none of this, 'I be wantin' this job.' There's nothing wrong with talking like that, just don't do it in an interview. We, as people of color, have our own way of speaking. And that's fine.

"When I see my mother, I don't say, 'Hello, Mother. May I embrace you?' she says primly. "Naw. I say, 'Hey, Mama, wha's happenin'? Gimme some sugar.'

"It's called situational language. With your friends, you can talk how you want. But in job interviews and in scholarship interviews, you have to speak standard English."

Moultrie is wearing a long, flowing skirt, an African pattern stippled with bright, primary colors. Her beaded earrings and copper and mahogany necklace are also of African design. As she strides up and down the rows, her onyx and brass bracelets jangle softly. She is a prism of varying personas. Moultrie frequently preaches at her church, so when she is passionate about a subject, she often assumes the sing-song delivery, the swaying, animated gestures of the minister in the grip of divine inspiration. Other times, she uses the precise language and diction of the traditional high school English teacher. But when she wants to jolt her students and insure they pay attention to a particular point about literature or life, she uses the vernacular of the street.

When Moultrie's class finishes practicing their introductions, she introduces some of the works they will be reading this year. "When you learn about slavery in the history books, who are you learning it from? Who wrote those books?" She offers a little palms-up gesture. "Eurocentric white males. In *this* class you'll be reading *Jubilee,* and you'll be learning about slavery from an African American writer, a woman who tells the story from the perspective of a slave.

"You'll be reading *Native Son* and will learn about blacks moving out of the South to Chicago, into the slums and projects. You'll read about a young African American male, a gangbanger. That's right. They had gangs then, too.

"You'll be reading *Othello,* a great play where the protagonist is a man of color. Last year our class went to the theater and saw the play. Othello was played by a brutha, and the brutha was *bad*." She smiles slyly. "He looked like Luther Vandross. And he had a voice like, like, like," she says, struggling for just the right adjective, "like *some*body."

She ends the class by telling the students, "You're all brilliant. You're wonderful. And I'm a fine teacher. I'm a fabulous teacher." She extends both her arms and wiggles her fingers. "Can I get an amen?"

"Amen!" the class shouts in unison.

"You're my amen corner," she tells them. "I'll be countin' on you."

During the next class, Moultrie wants to put *The Scarlet Letter*—the first novel her students will read this year—in a historical context. So she gives the students a brief multicultural history of how North America was settled.

"This is a straight-from-the-hip historical analysis," she tells the class. "This may not be what you learned from your third-grade history teachers. I'm going to tell you how it *really* be. Now you all know about Christopher Columbus. We celebrate him. We have a holiday for him. We all learned he sailed the ocean blue in 1492 and discovered America."

She walks across the room and grabs a student's jacket and another student's pen and another student's notebook. "Did I just *discover* your jacket, your pen, and your notebook?" she asks, glancing from one student to another. She crosses her arms, arches an eyebrow, and flashes them a skeptical look. "What I did isn't *discovering*. It's STEALING! How do you discover something that already exists? How do you discover a place that already has people living there?"

She points to a student. "Let's say I went to Steven's house. And his family's real nice. They give me dinner, let me watch television, give me a place to sleep. I like hangin' out there so much, I decide to *take* their house. I take Steven and his mama and the rest of his family and throw them out of their own house. Is that right? Hel-*lo*!

"Well, Columbus *did* prove the world wasn't flat. He deserves credit for that. He was a navigator, he had his three ships and he had his homeboys with him. He came upon Native Americans. He called them

Indians because he thought he was in India. So we're celebrating someone who got *lost!*

"But Columbus is a young buck and he goes back to his homies and tells them he discovered this new world . . . Well, more than a hundred years after Columbus returned to Europe, some Europeans returned to settle America. Now stay with me because this ties in to *The Scarlet Letter.*"

Moultrie segues into the class a brief lecture on the Puritans and the religious persecution they faced in England. She then tells the class how the Native Americans helped the Puritans after they arrived in America.

"Yet look at how the media has demonized the Native Americans. They've been traditionally portrayed as savage, coldhearted, barbaric, lacking morals. And look at all those cowboy movies. What color did the good guys wear and what color did the bad guys wear? You got it. The media projects anything that's bright and white as good and anything black or of color as bad.

"Look at these beauty magazines like *Glamour.* You rarely see an African American woman or a Latina in there. They're trying to tell us we're not beautiful? But I know we all look *fiiiine.* Am I right, sisters? Absolutely."

She points to a girl in the front row. "Are you wit' me? Am I right, baby girl?" The student nods emphatically.

Moultrie draws parallels between how Americans treated the Indians, stealing their land and consigning them to reservations, and how the Dutch settled South Africa and eventually created apartheid. She discusses the history of slavery in America, as well, but is interrupted by two teenage boys in the hall, shouting and laughing.

A constant irritant at Crenshaw are the "hall walkers"—groups of boys who cut class and meander through the halls, dodging the school police, scrawling graffiti, disrupting classes, and picking fights. No matter how many security officers patrol the campus they never catch all the hall walkers. Most teachers, like Toni Little, simply close their classroom doors to reduce the distraction. But Moultrie, who feels a responsibility to maintain quiet hallways, always keeps her doors open.

"Come on, my bruthas!" she shouts to the hall walkers, whose jeans sag so low, their boxers are visible. "Come off that stairwell. Do you think it's appropriate for you to be standing there, disrupting my class?"

They shrug and shuffle off. She mutters, "Look at these young African American men. They're wasting their lives. Let me show you how ridiculous the mentality is today." She walks to one side of the room. "I'll give everyone here red rags." She walks to the other side of the room. "I'll give everyone here blue rags. Now you two sides can go kill each other." She shakes her head sadly. "Now that's pathetic. Bruthas killin' bruthas.

"Let me tell you about a former student of mine, James Avery. James loved Mama Moultrie. He took a cooking class here and he would bring me cookies and treats all the time. We became very close. He ended up working for our company. When he was eighteen, he became a father. My husband and I kept telling him, 'You got responsibilities now. You got to watch who your friends are.' He'd tell us that some of his homies from the 'hood were in a gang, but *he* wasn't. He was just *friends* with them.

"Well, James was standing in front of a house with some of his so-called *friends* and someone came by and shot him. And he lay there and bled to death in front of his mama."

She walks to a corner of the room and for a moment stares out a window. She turns around, her eyes flinty, and says, "I watched this young man get buried. I watched them throw dirt over his grave. My last memory is his mother stretched over his casket, cryin', 'Please don't put my son in the ground. Please let me have one more look.' "

She taps a piece of chalk on the blackboard. "Mama Moultrie says, 'Choose your friends wisely.' You may not be doing anything wrong, but you still may be in danger. Hel-*lo*! Hel-*lo*!

"Men," she shouts, raising an arm. "If you get to twenty-five and you're still alive, you've beaten the odds. A quarter of our men are in the criminal justice system today. Only 20 percent are in college.

"Sisters," she shouts, lifting the other arm. "We have to *love* our brothers. We have to *nurture* our brothers. Because they'll be the fathers of your children. There's no reason you have to be single mothers and raise your children alone. We have to bridge that gulf.

"Can I get an amen?"

"Amen!" the girls shout.

"Y'all listen to me now. 'Cause this is Mama Moultrie talkin'."

* * *

Moultrie explains to the class how Nathaniel Hawthorne lays the foundation for *The Scarlet Letter* in the introduction. He writes that while he worked in a customhouse, he discovered a faded scarlet *A* and a story written on sheets of "ancient yellow" parchment, which serves as the basis for the novel.

Moultrie reads a section of Hawthorne's introduction: "This old town of Salem—my native place, though I have dwelt much away from it, both in boyhood and maturer years possesses, or did possess, a hold on my affection . . ."

She puts the book down and asks the class, "Now don't you get tired of hearin' your mama fussin' at you all the time? I know I did. You can't wait to go away to college and leave L.A. behind. But you'll see that years later, L.A. will still have a hold on you. You know what I'm sayin'?

"I moved away from my home town, Oakland, a long time ago. And I been livin' in L.A. twenty years. But when I drive into Oakland," she pauses, takes a deep breath, and sighs slowly. "Well, there's somethin' about comin' home. Home is where the heart is. It's also where the fried chicken, black-eyed peas, and cornbread is."

Moultrie reads another sentence: "On some such morning, when three or four vessels happen to have arrived at once,—usually from Africa . . ." She nods and says, "You know what these are, don't you? Slave ships. Remember, we talked about that."

She reads another sentence: ". . . the Collector, our gallant old General, who, after his brilliant military service . . . ruled over a wild Western territory . . ." She pauses and points to a husky boy wearing a white polo shirt. "You know who they took this Western territory from?"

"The Indians," he replies.

"Right. Now Hawthorne tells us in his introduction that his ancestors were Puritans, but he's still gonna be diggin' up some dirt on these Puritans. You're going to be reading *all* about that. And when you read, pay close attention to the language. Hawthorne is famous for his language and his imagery." She reads from the introduction: ". . . There never was in his heart so much cruelty as would have brushed the down off a butterfly's wing."

She shakes her head in admiration. "Listen to the beauty of that language. It's wonderful.'' She reads another section: ''. . . They seemed to have flung away all of the golden grain of practical wisdom . . . and stored their memories with the husks.'' She smiles and says, ''That's wonderful imagery.''

She reads the section of the introduction that details how Hawthorne discovered the pile of parchment: ''Unbending the rigid folds of the parchment cover, I found it to be a commission, under the hand and seal of Governor Shirley, in favor of one Jonathan Pue . . . Surveyor . . .''

''Who else is a surveyor?'' Moultrie asks.

''The dude who's talkin','' a student named Marcel responds. ''He's writin' about what's happenin' in the 'hood.''

''You mean Hawthorne, the narrator,'' Moultrie says.

''Yeah,'' Marcel says.

''Remember, writers don't do anything by accident,'' Moultrie says. ''So you know the color of the letter *A* is significant. You all with me? The Puritans didn't wear red. Because even in biblical times, red was associated with sin.'' She draws from her years as a Sunday school teacher and quotes a passage from Isaiah: ''Though your sins be like scarlet, they may become white as snow.''

She looks out at the class. ''Does everyone know what adultery is?''

''Cheatin' on yo' man,'' a girl says.

''Or yo' woman,'' Moultrie adds. She picks up the book and reads, ''My eyes fastened themselves upon the old scarlet letter, and would not be turned aside. . . . I happened to place it on my breast . . .'' Her tone is theatrical, almost melodramatic. ''I experienced a sensation not altogether physical, yet almost so, as of burning heat; and as if the letter were not of red cloth, but red-hot iron.'' She places the book on her throat and swoons, knees buckling. She reads, with breathless intensity, ''I shuddered and involuntarily let it fall upon the floor.''

She puts the book down on her desk and says, ''He's telling the reader that something drew him to that letter. It was strange and intriguing and he had to look into it. He had to follow through with this.

''Y'all beginning to see the light? Okay then. Stay with me on this introduction. When we get into the first chapter you're going to see how these Puritans sock it to Hester Prynne. They really give her the blues.''

* * *

Before moving on to the first chapter, Moultrie discusses one of her *bêtes noires*—the movie *Dangerous Minds*. "You have brilliant minds. Not dangerous minds. When I see movies like that I get infuriated. I want to slap someone," she says, punctuating her irritation by clapping her hands once. "All those students hip-hopping in class, jiving, gang-banging, tapping their feet, running up and down the aisles, cursing, and punching walls.

"The media *does* project a negative image of children of color. You can't get a camera down here to save your life if something good's happening. But if there's a shooting, they're all over the place. The media has tremendous influence, so that's what white America sees. That's their only image of African American students. They'll say, 'Look at those raggedy old kids of color.' Because of images like those, parents send their kids on the bus two hours away so they can go to school in the San Fernando Valley and get out of the inner city. Well, I'm right here in the inner city. And I'm an excellent teacher. And you're right here. And you're excellent students.

"Because of images like that people cross the street and hug their purses and wallets when they see our young men." She grips her shoulders, feigning fear. "They follow us down the aisles at the department stores to make sure we're not stealing. Michelle Pfeiffer should come on down here," she says, jabbing a forefinger at the floor. "She'll get the surprise of her life. Because she won't find anything dangerous in *this* classroom. Except my *attitude*."

Moultrie and her husband own a business and she teaches full-time, heads the English Department, and has five children—including an eight-month old baby—two dogs, a rabbit, two cats, a turtle, and a mother-in-law at home. On Sundays, she leads a Bible-study group at her church. In order to juggle her manifold duties, she has to be exceedingly well organized. She demands that her students be organized, too. Each student in her class must buy a notebook and divide it into six sections: table of contents, class work, homework, notes, test, and writing assignments. She periodically grades the notebooks.

Before every class, she writes on the blackboard the names of the students who are celebrating birthdays that day and effusively wishes them a happy birthday. Then she neatly lists on the blackboard the points she will cover during the period. Each class begins with a writing assignment, which is graded. The assignments often are based on news that impacts the black community or on African proverbs. In September, students write essays on topics, including: the murder of Tupac Shakur; growing up without a father, and gun control.

In addition to the three writing assignments a week, there are frequent exams, homework assignments, and projects due. Some of the projects are unorthodox and include creating a children's book for black students in South Africa and interviewing family members or neighbors and chronicling the racism they have endured. If students do not turn in assignments, or cut class, or perform poorly on their exams, Moultrie often calls their homes at night and talks with their parents.

Moultrie's class meets from 10:30 to 12:30, Monday and Wednesday mornings, and for about fifty minutes on Friday morning. Most teachers head to the faculty cafeteria during the fifteen-minute morning nutrition break and the afternoon lunch break. Some lock their classroom doors and eat in privacy. Moultrie, however, wants her classroom to be a sanctuary for the students, so she keeps her doors open and eats at her desk. Some students, seeking a respite from the quad, join her. Others stop by to confide in her or ask for advice.

Moultrie's eleventh-grade English class immediately follows Little's AP class and, in structure and style, is a diametric opposite. In Little's class, there are just a few exams and a few papers due. Her class is designed along the lines of a college course.

Little disparages Moultrie's daily writing assignment because it is not based on the literature. She also criticizes the assignment because Moultrie does not emphasize the formal essay structure Little taught the students in the tenth grade, a structure replete with thesis statements, topic sentences, supporting paragraphs, and concluding assertions. Little feels Moultrie's approach does not properly prepare them for the AP exam or for college.

Every aspect of Moultrie's class infuriates Little. She denigrates the daily discussions about race and racism and social inequities. She dismisses the children's books that the students create and the other unorthodox projects because she feels they do not belong in a literature classroom.

She is exasperated when she hears that Moultrie refers to herself in class as Mama Moultrie.

"I'm not their damn mama," Little often says with disgust. "I'm their English teacher."

As September comes to a close, and Moultrie's class begins reading the first chapter of *The Scarlet Letter,* and Little's class finishes *The Crucible,* Braxton worries about the uneasy relationship between the two teachers. He fears the dispute will intensify, disrupting and undermining the program—and the students. If that happens, he knows he will have to intercede. And for a man who assiduously avoids confrontation, he knows that he probably will have to confront Little in the hopes of negotiating an uneasy detente.

Before Moultrie taught in the gifted magnet program, Little had complete control and autonomy. She taught all the gifted tenth, eleventh, and twelfth graders and implemented a progressive, three-year plan. In the tenth grade she taught the students the rudiments of literary criticism. For three years she expected them to write traditional essays, using the formal structure she taught them, employing the literary terms she made them study, explicating the works in the way she instructed them. Little often was innovative in her lectures and her assignments, but the foundation of the class was traditional.

Then Moultrie arrived two years ago and began teaching all the eleventh graders. Moultrie included many black authors in the reading list. She assigned students some projects that were more political than literary. And the daily essay assignments she gave the students were relatively free form and did not build on what Little taught them in the tenth grade.

A more diplomatic teacher than Little might have transcended her differences with Moultrie. A less obdurate personality might have forged a compromise. But for Little, the dispute was not merely professional, it was personal. Little immediately viewed Moultrie as an interloper, someone who was sabotaging her teaching plan. After Moultrie was elected department chairwoman, Little was apoplectic.

Before Little arrived at the school, no Crenshaw student had ever passed the AP English exam. During Little's first year, about half the students in her class passed, an unusually high percentage for an inner-city high school. During the past few years, however, her students' pass rate has been slipping steadily. Little contends this is because students are not getting the preparation they need in the eleventh grade. Several Crenshaw teachers, however, contend that her teaching has deteriorated. She still can be an inspiring lecturer and engender a passion for literature in her students. But she is more easily distracted in class now, other teachers say, spends more time digressing on unrelated subjects, and does not have the same focus and drive as when she arrived.

When Moultrie began teaching in the gifted program, Braxton had hoped Little would take her under her wing. Little was accustomed to teaching gifted children and Advanced Placement classes, had attended many seminars, and had a wealth of teaching aids and background material. Braxton had hoped Little would share her resources with Moultrie and gently direct her. This venture, however, soon ended in disaster. Little viewed Moultrie as resistant to her overtures, as stubborn and hypersensitive. Moultrie viewed Little as supercilious and considered her approach condescending and insulting. Moultrie usually is affable, friendly, and quick to laugh and joke with other teachers, which is one of the reasons her colleagues voted her department chairwoman. But there is a steely reserve behind her bonhomie. Braxton soon gave up trying to get the teachers to work together.

At the end of September, a student walks into Braxton's office and tells him that during class Little criticized Moultrie's teaching ability. He removes his glasses and massages his temples. He feels a headache coming on. Braxton has a young child and an infant—a full night's sleep is now impossible—and a ninety-minute commute to and from work every day. He can never recall a September as stressful as this one. First there was Olivia, who finally returned to school. Then there was Toya, who did not. Then there were the fights on campus, the stabbings, the shooting, the security sweeps during lunch. And now he has to contend with the Little-Moultrie conflict.

He peers outside his office and sees a half-dozen students and several parents waiting to see him. He massages his temples again. All these difficulties, all of this turmoil, he thinks. And there are still eight months of school to go.

PART TWO

FALL

SEVEN

TONI LITTLE

LEARN TO COMPETE

A broiling, bone-dry Santa Ana wind rips through the desert, howls down the mountain passes, through the inland valleys, into the city, and onto the ocean, dissipating the fog and rippling the waves, before fading out, miles offshore. The calendar may say October, but in Southern California, these Santa Anas provide a reprise of summer.

It is 8:00 A.M. and already warm in Little's classroom. She opens a few windows. Not a hint of fog, not a shred of cloud, not a trace of smog can be seen. The winds have swept the skies, blown the smog to the ocean, and left a broad swath of turquoise in the central city.

On this Monday morning, Little decides to prepare the students for the AP exam by assigning them an in-class essay that was used in a previous AP exam. Little figures this will help her gauge the level of the class.

She writes on the blackboard: ''The passage below is from an autobiography. After reading the passage carefully, write an essay analyzing how the author uses juxtaposition of ideas, choice of detail, and other aspects of style to reveal the kind of person she is.'' Little then scribbles a passage from the autobiography of Beryl Markham, an English aviator who chronicled her years in Africa.

Little taps the chalk on the board and asks the class, "Who knows what juxtaposition is?"

The class is silent. She prods them, and a few students speculate on a definition, but it is clear no one knows what the word means. Little underlines the word with an angry backhand slash. "Kids from throughout the country, kids you'll be competing against, know this word." She taps the chalk on her desk. "Didn't you write essays in the eleventh grade?" she asks accusingly. "You're supposed to bring your knowledge from the eleventh grade to this class. And this is something you should have learned.

"Last year, did you analyze style? Did you analyze structure? Or did you just write about the story?"

The two best friends who have tormented Little in past classes are whispering and giggling again.

"I don't find anything humorous about this!" Little thunders. She had a rough weekend and is peevish this morning. Her three dogs all had a virus and threw up several times on the carpet. She was up with them until early Monday morning.

Little points to one of the girls, who is violating the school's dress code by wearing a top with a bare midriff. "Get rid of that gum." She points to the other, who is violating the school's dress code by wearing a short skirt. The girl sips a soda. "You're like a baby with your bottle. I'm not going to play your little-girl games anymore. Grow up!"

The girl drops her head and sulks, so Little says, "It's not that deep! Just pay attention."

Little flinches when she hears a door open and scowls as she watches Venola try to unobtrusively slip into her seat. Little walks over to Venola and chastises her for coming to class late, but stops midsentence when Venola hands her a note that reads:

> Ms. Little,
>   I am very sorry for being late and disturbing your class. I was late because the bus I usually ride was too crowded this morning and it passed

me up. I then had to wait on the next one. I will do my best to prevent
these things from happening in the future. Thank you.
    Most sincerely,
    Venola.

Little reads the note, nods to Venola and says, "That's okay *this* time.
But I'm sick of students drifting into class late, day after day. Let's try to
show a seriousness of purpose in here."

Ten minutes later, when Olivia wanders into class, Little rolls her
eyes and mutters, "What's the use?" During the past few weeks, Olivia
has been a half-hour late most mornings. Sadi always asks her why she
does not simply get up a half-hour earlier. But no matter how early she
sets her alarm, something at the foster home always seems to delay her.

There is only one bathroom for six girls. Sometimes she has to wait
up to an hour before the shower is empty. Sometimes, if she does manage
an early shower, she has to wait again to get back in the bathroom so she
can brush her teeth or fix her hair. Sometimes a girl at the foster home
picks a fight with her. One night she had to sleep in the cramped backseat
of her Volkswagen because she arrived home late, and the foster mother
had locked the house and would not answer the door.

Because it is so warm this morning, most of the students, including
Olivia, are wearing shorts and T-shirts. Olivia usually is fashionably attired
and carefully coiffed. Today, however, she is wearing white shorts, a polo
shirt, white canvas tennis shoes, and her hair is pulled back in a ponytail.
Without her high heels, her hair swirled atop her head, her makeup, her
elaborate, color-coordinated outfits, there is a vulnerable, innocent quality
about her. On this rare occasion Olivia looks like a seventeen-year-old girl.

As Olivia searches through her backpack for a notebook, Little walks
over to a file cabinet and removes a stack of work sheets that explain
literary terms such as, "exposition," "denouement," "rising action,"
"climax," and "resolution." She passes the sheets out to the students and
tells them, "The kids in middle America know these literary terms. They
can crank it out. You better study this work sheet so you can learn
to compete."

Little tells them they have forty minutes to write their sample AP

essay. She returns to her desk and begins reading the students' papers on
The Crucible, their first major essay of the year. The first few essays she
reads depress her.

This year, school counselors encouraged more students from outside
the gifted program to enroll in AP classes. The counselors believe that
these students, who have excelled at Crenshaw, need a more rigorous
English class to prepare them for college. But they have an academic
background different from their classmates, and most did not have Little
in the tenth grade nor Moultrie in the eleventh. Some of them simply do
not write well enough for an AP class.

The essay assignment was: "In many novels and plays, a recurring
theme in literature is the classic war between a passion and a responsibility:
For instance a personal cause, a love, a desire for revenge, a determination
to redress a wrong or some other emotion or drive that may conflict with
moral duty. Choose a character in *The Crucible* who confronts the demands
of a private passion that conflicts with his or her responsibility. In a well-
written . . . essay, show clearly the nature of the conflict, its effects upon
the character, and its significance to the work as a whole."

One student, with two mistakes just on her title page, wrote: "The
Curcible, written by Author Miller." Little scrawled on the page, in red
ink, "Yikes!" Another student wrote on the title page: "The Crucibles."

Not all of the students outside the gifted program wrote substandard
essays. Many, however, lack, rudimentary writing skills, and Little has to
devote an inordinate amount of time to these essays, making notations,
suggestions, and emendations.

Little knows that no matter what she teaches, some of these students
will never pass the AP exam. She just hopes that by the end of the year
she can, at least, teach them to write at the level of a high school senior.

On Wednesday morning, the Santa Anas have died down, but it remains hot and an inky layer of smog rises with the morning light. There are
no horizons today, just a sienna haze encircling the city, a chemical curtain.

Little's despair has lifted. She still has not graded the essays, but she
has scanned those of Miesha, Venola, and a few other favorite students.
They bore little resemblance to the first few essays she read. These students

remembered the structured essay format she emphasized in the tenth grade, and they remembered the literary terms she taught them.

She asks Miesha and several other students to read their essays to the class. A few of the students lower their eyes and shake their heads shyly. But Miesha, who enjoys the spotlight, steps right up to the front of the class. *"The Crucible,"* she reads, "presents various characters who are involved in a personal war with themselves . . . John Proctor . . . confronts the demands of a private passion that conflict with his responsibilities as a husband and as a citizen of his community. His determination to redress the wrongs he committed . . . helped mold the outcome of this play . . ."

Little convinces a few other students to read their papers. When they finish, she beams proudly. During the entire class nothing breaks her exuberant mood. Even when Olivia wanders in late, Little remains upbeat and enthusiastic.

After class, Little spots an assistant principal in the hallway. Little stops her and says, excitedly, "I had a great class today. I was so down at the beginning of the year. I was thinking, 'This is a *gifted* class?' I was wondering where they dug up some of these kids. Did they grab them off the street? But some students read their essays in class today. They were excellent. It really renews my faith. Some of them can compete with kids anywhere."

During the next class, Little decides to initiate a discussion of religious and ethical issues. She had emphasized religious themes when discussing *The Crucible,* partly because she noticed that whenever the discussion drifted toward religion, it galvanized the class. During her years of teaching, Little has discovered that certain ideas, issues, or themes resonate with different classes. This class, Little senses, is particularly attuned to religion and spirituality. So Little decides that religion and spirituality will be the thread that connects the works they will study this semester.

In one of her favorite works, James Joyce's *A Portrait of the Artist as a Young Man,* Little will explore the protagonist's alienation from his family, his country, and his religion. During winter break, the students will read *Wuthering Heights,* and Little will delve into how spirituality is portrayed through the ghost of one of the characters.

Little selects a relatively modern play for the next work the class will study—*Inherit the Wind,* a fictional rendition of the Scopes "Monkey" trial. Many of the students belong to black churches that have a strong tradition of religious fundamentalism. Little figures they will identify easily with the issue of religion clashing with the scientific world.

Little walks over to the corner of the room, pats a stack of novels and asks, "Can literature influence you as much as the Bible? Can we learn lessons from literature that might be different from the lessons in the Bible, but just as valuable?"

A girl in the corner who had been scribbling a note to a friend stops and says, "For me, the only book that has any value is the Bible."

A girl who is dressed in black and wearing skeleton earrings says, "You shouldn't base your whole life on one book. There are so many different works that can bring authority to your life," echoing a theme— authority—that Little had emphasized in a previous class.

Little asks the class, "Is knowing the difference between right or wrong innate, or does it have to be taught?"

A girl with dyed blond cornrows replies, "I come from a single-parent home. My mama didn't tell me much. But I knew when something was right or wrong. I used to fight all the time. Nobody told me it was wrong. I knew it was wrong, but I did it anyway."

The girl in the corner says, "Homeboy knows it's wrong to shoot. Nobody's got to tell him that."

Little's question sparks genuine interest and enthusiasm. The discussion builds slowly, with Little guiding it, and picks up momentum. Now, about half the students are furiously waving their hands. Others shout out their answers. A few stand up, shake their heads in dissent, and argue.

After twenty minutes Little, holding both hands above her head like a referee, quiets the class and says, "Who did the Puritans look to, to pattern their lives? Should we just follow what was passed down to us, without questioning? Where do *you* look to pattern your lives? If you read twenty classic novels since the tenth grade, do you have a greater advantage to determine what is right or wrong? I think you do. I think this literature *does* build character. I regard it as holy."

She introduces *Inherit the Wind* to the class by reading a passage from

the play that addresses the issue of lying: ". . . Whenever you see something bright, shining, perfect-seeming—all gold with purple spots—look
behind the paint! And if it's a lie—show it up for what it really is!"

Little sets the play down on her desk and says, "I had a student last
year and his brother is in prison for murder because of a lie." Sadi, who
knew the brother, nods in assent. They both joined the All Out Kickin'
It Gangsters in the eighth grade and became close friends.

Little crouches beside a girl in the front of the class and says, "I know
you were friends with Timothy. Tell everyone about it."

"I was friends with him and his brother," the girl says. "They lived
a block away from me. What happened was, Germaine was out one night
when somebody got killed. This other guy shot someone. Police found
out. They took Germaine and the shooter in for questioning. The shooter
blamed Germaine. Everyone in the 'hood knew the other guy did the
shooting. But he got off scot-free. Then he disappeared."

Little points both index fingers at the class. "Stand up and tell the
truth. I hate liars. Some people have no morality." She waves a copy of
Inherit the Wind. "*Here* is one place you can learn morality. In literature."

She jerks her thumb toward the hallway. "I just went to an English
Department meeting and I can't believe how some of these teachers regard
literature. One teacher says she sets up her class like the *Ricki Lake Show*.
They're reading *The Great Gatsby*, and she has her students play Gatsby
and Daisy and Tom, and they all sit up there, answering outrageous questions from the class, like a talk show. Another teacher says she gets her
class involved by dealing with the novels like they're sitcoms."

She grimaces and purses her lips, as if she has just tasted something
foul. "That's insulting. We don't have to turn this class into a talk show
to get you interested. We don't have to dumb this down. Do we?"

The students shake their heads.

"Let's get serious and read, read, read. Let's hold this literature in
high regard. Let's give it the respect it deserves."

The students resume reading *Inherit the Wind* during the next class.
Little wants to encourage more students to participate, so she asks a quiet
boy in the corner to play the part of Reverend Jeremiah Brown leading a

prayer meeting. Most students in the class play their parts with great enthusiasm, but the boy's reading is awkward and dispirited, so the class revolts. This is a *preacher,* the students grumble to Little, and this student's portrayal bears little resemblance to the fire and brimstone preachers they see in church.

"Let *me* play the part," Miesha asks. "My mama's been takin' me to church for the longest. I *know* how to preach."

Little nods her head, and the boy looks relieved. Miesha then transforms the part of Reverend Brown—a white minister preaching to Tennessee crackers—into a black preacher banging a bible in a South-Central church. Miesha is the best actress in the class, and she plays the part to the hilt. She reads the lines, but she also improvises and adds her own interpretation to the role. She draws out the vowels, her voice quavering. She breaks the words down, sometimes pausing at each syllable for dramatic effect. She lowers her voice to a gravelly rasp. She shouts. She waves her hands above her head, praising the glory of God.

"Brothers and Sisters . . ." Miesha says, "The Lo-ord's word is *how*ling in the wind . . ." She lowers her voice and, in a mock baritone, intones, "*Yay* uh."

"I hear it!" a student calls out.

"I see it, Reverend!" another student shouts.

"And we be*lieve* the word . . ." Miesha says. "*Yay* uh. Yes, we do."

"We believe it, sister . . ." a student shouts.

"In the beginning," Miesha whispers theatrically, "the earth was without form and void." She looks around, wide-eyed. "And the Lo-ord said—" She pauses, pounds her desk with both fists, and bellows, " 'Let there be light!' "

"Let there be light," a student calls out.

Miesha whispers, "And there *was* light. . . ."

"Amen! Amen!" the class calls out.

"And the Lord said—" Miesha waves a hand and shouts, " 'Let there be Firmament . . .' "

"Preach it," a student shouts.

Miesha jumps out of her chair, holds out her hands and asks the class, "Do we be*lieve* in the Word?"

"Yes!" the class roars in unison. "We believe."

"Do we be*lieve* in the *Truth* of the Word? I'm talking the *Truth*, here. Yeah-uh."

"Yes! We believe in the truth."

"Do we *curse* the man who denies the Word? *Yeah*-uh. Do we *curse* that man?"

"Yes! Curse that man."

"Do we *cast* out this sinner in our midst?"

"Yes! Cast that sinner out!"

"Do we *call* down hellfire on the man who has sinned against the Word?"

"Yes! Hellfire on that man."

By now the class is swaying and humming and stamping their feet, responding to each of Miesha's questions, reading from the play and also making up a few lines on the spot. When Miesha finishes, the class cheers, and students call out, "You spoke the *truth*, girl"; "You laid it *down*"; "You *told* it, sister."

Little applauds and says with pride, "Now *that* is acting."

EIGHT

SABREEN

ONE LESS CHILD TO SUPPORT

Braxton slumps in his office chair, looking dazed and disappointed. Toya just called him. She thanked him for all his efforts. She thanked him for not giving up on her. But she told him she cannot afford to pay $265 a month for child care. She has decided to enroll in a Watts high school program for teenage mothers, which provides free child care.

"A couple of years ago, one of our gifted girls who got pregnant went to that program," Braxton tells another teacher. He shakes his head and frowns. "Toya's too bright for that. The intellectual level there is nil." He taps a pen nervously on his desk.

"There was so much that girl could have—" Braxton says, breaking off in midsentence. He stares mournfully out his office door and thinks about the scholarship to Cornell that Toya had to give up over the summer; the scholarships she surely would have been offered this year, but now will be ineligible for; the opportunities that would have transported her far from Watts; the tremendous promise she showed during her first three years of high school; the uncertain future that now awaits her.

Braxton, however, does not have time to brood over the loss of Toya. He has to immediately shift his attention to Sabreen, another gifted senior with an imperiled future.

One Saturday afternoon Sabreen, who was thirteen years old, spent several hours at the laundromat washing and drying the family's clothes. Her mother stopped by to pick her up and became enraged when she discovered that a shirt was stolen from the dryer. When they arrived home, she cracked a broom handle across Sabreen's back and screamed at her.

Sabreen was accustomed to beatings with belts, shoes, and broomsticks by her mother or stepfather. But that Saturday afternoon was the final fillip for Sabreen; she vowed that she would never allow anyone to strike her again. She convinced a cousin to drive her across town to her father's house, and he reluctantly let her move in. He later told Sabreen that when her mother was pregnant, she had wanted an abortion, but he stopped her. Since then, he explained, Sabreen's mother has resented her.

Later, long after she moved out, Sabreen briefly encountered her mother, who said matter-of-factly, "Now there's one less child to support."

Sabreen stayed with her father for a few months but after a heated argument, she ran away and embarked on a dismal journey that landed her in thirteen different residences during the next three years. She lived in foster homes and she lived in group homes. She lived with the family of a friend from school. She lived with a friend's godmother. She lived with a boyfriend's sister's boyfriend's friend. A few nights, she slept in a park.

During a critical court hearing to determine whether Sabreen's mother or father would regain custody of her, neither showed up. The court made her a ward of the county. Although the foster homes were distasteful to her, she felt safe. She did not think a foster mother would beat her.

Despite an unstable, peripatetic existence, Sabreen managed to excel in the classroom. She was classified as gifted, and her teachers wanted her to skip a grade, but her mother refused. They did, however, persuade

Sabreen's mother to send her to a gifted magnet elementary school on the Westside.

Some of the South-Central students detested the hour bus ride to and from school, but Sabreen appreciated the time away from home, away from the beatings, the shouting, the fighting. She enjoyed reading novels without the cacophony of seven children, a mother, and a stepfather jammed into a small apartment. When the bus dropped her off at home, Sabreen would flee to the public library and study until dark.

Because Sabreen lived in so many different foster homes, she attended four high schools in two years. In the beginning of her junior year, she was living in a group home and attending a nearby continuation school. At the time, a dean at Crenshaw asked the vice principal of the continuation school if he could send him one of his troublesome students. The vice principal agreed, under one condition: If Crenshaw, which was overcrowded and not accepting any new students, would let Sabreen enroll.

The vice principal had been impressed by Sabreen's high test scores and eagerness to learn. She was too bright for continuation school. He wanted Sabreen in a high school that offered accelerated classes. He enrolled her at Crenshaw, she excelled there and eventually transferred to the gifted program.

At the beginning of Sabreen's senior year, she was ranked ninth—with a grade point average of 3.74—out of a class of 356 seniors. She was taking all honors and Advanced Placement classes even though she was working forty hours a week as a saleswoman at a Westside store called Bed, Bath and Beyond. But during the first month of school, her life was thrown into turmoil. She was living with a friend's godmother, who was in the process of obtaining foster-care certification. The situation, however, became untenable for Sabreen because the godmother did not like her coming home so late at night from work. Sabreen had no intention of quitting, because she had bills to pay, including her car insurance and registration fees. So in September she went AWOL. She moved in with a twenty-five-year-old friend, who had an apartment in Long Beach, about twenty-five miles from Crenshaw.

It had been difficult enough for Sabreen to attend all her gifted classes and work full-time. But during the first few weeks of school, she was stuck, every morning, on the San Diego Freeway, fighting traffic for up to an hour, driving from Long Beach to Los Angeles. At night after work, she had to make the long drive home. She had been rising every morning at 6:00 A.M, returning home at about midnight, and trying to finish her homework during her breaks at work.

In early October she missed several morning classes. She was not able to complete all her homework assignments, including her essay on *The Crucible* for Little's class. Sabreen spent many hours in Braxton's office, frustrated, exhausted, and confused. "I feel like I went from a child to an adult, with nothing in between," she told him one afternoon.

Sabreen, who is tall and slender, dresses neatly in slacks and prim blouses—her work clothes. Her father is black, her mother half black and half Hispanic. Sabreen has high cheek bones, almond eyes, and wavy hair, and new classmates always try to guess her provenance.

Despite the pressure of work and school, she remained enthusiastic about learning. In class, she was interested and energetic, animated by her love of ideas. She always participated in class discussions and excitedly waved her hand and shouted out opinions. School, as it had been for many years, provided an escape for Sabreen, a place for her to feel a sense of accomplishment.

Still, the combination of a full-time job, demanding Advanced Placement classes, hours commuting on the freeway, and a tenuous living situation often overwhelmed her. Last spring, she had such severe stress-related stomach aches that her doctor thought she had an ulcer and she was briefly hospitalized. Sabreen knew she could not afford to be hospitalized during her senior year. She had too much to do.

The only person she felt comfortable talking to about her life, the only person who she felt was truly interested in her problems, was Braxton. Many times during the past month she sat in his office and cried. All Braxton could do was listen to her, encourage her, and try to keep her in school another week.

Sabreen knew that her life was unmanageable, but she refused to return to county supervision because she could not bear the thought of another foster home. So she procrastinated, knowing that eventually—inevitably—her social worker would track her down and force her to make a decision about her future.

On this October morning, Sabreen's social worker marches through the front door at Crenshaw, down the hall, up the stairs, and into the gifted magnet office. Braxton calls Little and tells her to send Sabreen to his office. Sabreen suspects why she is being pulled out of class. She prays as she walks to Braxton's office, asking God to watch over her. She is terrified that there will be police officers in Braxton's office who will transport her to a county shelter, far from Crenshaw, and she will have to drop out of school.

When Sabreen walks into Braxton's office and sees the social worker, a tall, blond, stern-looking woman with glasses, she is relieved that there are no police and relieved that she has been caught. She feels like the fugitive from justice who, upon apprehension, knows that a life of unrelenting vigilance—and constant anxiety—has finally reached an end.

The social worker tells Braxton that her supervisor wants to pull Sabreen out of school and have her locked up at a county facility. Braxton tries to dissuade the social worker, telling her that Sabreen is very committed to school and is on track to graduate in June, even though she has been AWOL. It would be a shame, Braxton says, to interrupt her studies. "Sabreen's having a tough time right now," he says. "But she's a bright girl and college is in her future. What does she have to do to make sure she can continue here at Crenshaw?"

The social worker states the conditions: Sabreen has to return to county foster care. Immediately.

Sabreen exhales wearily. She knows she has no choice but to acquiesce. She agrees to go wherever the county sends her. Sabreen tells the social worker that she knows the county sometimes discharges seventeen-year-olds from the county foster care system.

"I wish I could live with a parent, but I can't—that's reality," Sabreen says. "So I might as well get an apartment and be on my own. Officially."

The social worker tells her that in order to be "emancipated" from the system, there has to be a court hearing and the judge has to make the decision. She is welcome to pursue that avenue, the social worker tells her, but until then, as a ward of the county, she has to follow the rules.

A few days later, Sabreen moves into her new foster home, a modest pink stucco house with a tar-paper roof and a patch of ivy instead of a front lawn. The house is located just south of Imperial Highway, a depressed thoroughfare that belies its regal name and bisects some of the city's poorest neighborhoods. Sabreen's foster mother, in addition to looking after three foster children, runs a day-care center from her house, and a half-dozen children scamper about the living room. The furniture is chipped and the windows are covered by iron bars. The floor is strewn with toys, books, plastic trucks, and small blackboards. Cartoons blare from the television set. The smell of fried bacon permeates the house.

Sabreen's bedroom has a narrow cot with a mattress so worn the springs ripple the surface. A threadbare sheet covers the window. The dresser is battered, and in the corner of the room another bed lists at a forty-five-degree angle. The wall socket has no safety cover. A dank smell emanates from the moldy, stained carpeting.

Sabreen cries when she sees the bathroom: the tub has a dark ring of dirt around it, and the shower door is opaque from grime. She decides she would rather go AWOL again than bathe or shower here. Unfortunately, it is too late to find another place to sleep tonight.

The next morning, before school, she calls her social worker.

"This isn't going to work," she says, describing the bathroom to her.

"Why don't you clean it?"

"I don't have time."

Sabreen's social worker tells her she has no other option. After her first morning class, Sabreen rushes to Braxton's office and bursts into tears. He hands her a box of Kleenex.

She dries her eyes and says, "That's it. I can't take these places anymore. I'm splitting. I've got a job. I'll rent my own apartment. I don't care if they arrest me and throw me in juvenile hall."

"Damn it," Braxton says angrily. "You've got too much ability to throw it away now. You got this far. You can't chuck it all now."

He finally calms Sabreen down, and she trudges off to class. After school, she returns to the foster home and scrubs the bathtub and cleans the shower door. Lost in thought, she devises a plan to finagle a court hearing and convince a judge to free her from county supervision. To emancipate her.

The following Saturday, many of the Crenshaw seniors will be taking the Scholastic Aptitude Test, but Sabreen is so overwhelmed with work and moving and her many personal crises that the exam is the last thing on her mind. Like Olivia, Sadi, Miesha, Venola, and virtually every student in Little's class, she will walk into the exam room without any preparation.

The parents of many middle-class students pay for SAT preparation courses. These students spend months—and sometimes years—gearing up for the exam. They study an extensive array of SAT books, interactive CD-Roms, and on-line preparation material. One Southern California SAT preparation firm, based in suburban Orange County, offers night classes for students that start as early as the seventh grade. The parents of these students know that small numerical swings can be crucial in determining their children's futures. By contrast, many Crenshaw parents never attended college, are not familiar with the SAT, and do not push their children to prepare. And the idea of paying Princeton Review $1,400 for a ten-week—four days a week—summer preparation course, or even $745 for a six-week course, is simply not within the ken—or the budget—of most students in South-Central.

Those students whose parents can afford private tutors have an even greater advantage over the Crenshaw seniors. One of the most exclusive and expensive one-on-one tutoring services in the country is Advantage Testing, which operates centers in eight cities, primarily on the East Coast. The average cost of an Advantage tutor in Manhattan is $175 for a fifty-minute session. Most of these students pay between $5,000 and $8,000 a year. If the acclaimed head of the firm, Arun Alagappan, tutors the student, the cost is $415 a session. Alagappan recommends that his students sign up for two sessions a week for an entire school year. This can cost more than $25,000 a year—more than the annual family income of many of Little's students.

The mean gain for the students Alagappan tutored in 1997 and 1998, he claims, was 266 points. Expressing concern about the inequities in America's high schools, Alagappan says he offers his services pro bono to about 15 percent of his students. The mean gain for these students—most of whom are from the inner city—is slightly more than 300 points, he says. They benefit most from the tutoring because they are starting at a lower point. "Instead of just *reviewing* fundamentals," Alagappan says, "you're often *teaching* fundamentals."

Advantage Testing can charge premium prices because the tutors are so well qualified. Alagappan is a graduate of Harvard Law School, and many of his tutors—some of whom earn more than $100,000 a year—also have graduate degrees from prestigious universities.

Alagappan teaches the students much more than just test-beating gimmicks. For the math section of the SAT, he teaches the underlying principles of algebra, geometry, and arithmetic that comprise the foundation of the exam. He has meticulously analyzed published SAT exams and assembled about 200 frequently asked questions, as well as a glossary of about 80 terms. He also teaches students a number of mnemonic devices, such as TACOS: The total area minus the cutout equals the shaded region.

For the verbal section, he teaches principles of logic that help students with the analogy and sentence-completion sections of the exam. He also drills students on how to summarize the thrust of a paragraph in a sentence, which aids them on the reading-comprehension section. He has composed a list of about 3,000 vocabulary words that have appeared on more than one SAT exam. And he provides a special word list to students from Manhattan, who tend to have problems with farm words—such as bovine, arable, gander, and hutch—and church words—such as hymn, heathen, chapel, and pagan.

While students across the country intensively prepare for the exam, most inner-city students—students who need the most SAT preparation—receive the least amount of help. Most of the seniors in Little's class have jobs, and some, like Sabreen, work forty hours a week. They return home from work late at night. The next morning, they awake exhausted and drag themselves to the bus stop by 7:00 A.M. so they can arrive at school on time. The students have little time or energy left for SAT preparation.

Today, with affirmative action under assault, a student's SAT score is even more critical. Given the discrepancy of SAT tutoring available to students, college admissions are becoming even less meritocratic.

While the SAT is designed to predict freshman grades, the exam's ability to forecast later success is questionable. What it more accurately reflects is a student's socioeconomic background. For all ethnic groups, the higher a parent's educational background and income the better the student's SAT score. For a host of complex reasons, blacks score lower on the SATs than whites, Asians, and Latinos. Although the gap has narrowed during the past few decades, this year black average scores trail those of whites—434 to 526 on the verbal test and 422 to 523 on the math.

Since World War I, when the average test score for white U.S. Army recruits was higher than blacks, social scientists have struggled to understand the divergence between black and white results on standardized tests. The gap on virtually all scholastic aptitude tests appears before kindergarten and persists through high school. Some social scientists blame the decline of the black family and a culture of poverty. Others argue that standardized tests are racially biased. Some point to societal inequity, including segregated and inadequate schools, unequal job opportunities, and a long history of racism.

Even when black and white students have the same family income, blacks still trail whites. College-educated black parents often were the first in their families to attend college and grew up in homes with few books and little academic tradition, which has an impact on their children's test scores, some researchers contend.

Other minorities have endured prejudice and hardship, but the black experience in America is sui generis. Orlando Patterson, author of *The Ordeal of Integration*, offers this succinct description of black history in America: ". . . Two and a half centuries of slavery, followed by a century of rural semiserfdom and violently imposed segregation, wanton economic discrimination, and outright exclusion of Afro-Americans from the middle and upper echelons of the nation's economy . . ."

Andrew Hacker, author of *Two Nations,* contends that blacks do not test as well as other ethnic groups because of their social isolation, which affects black Americans of all classes. "Surveys of neighborhoods and schools show that black Americans spend more of their lives apart from other groups than even recent immigrants," Hacker writes. "One outcome of this isolation is that they grow up with less sustained exposure to the rules of 'linear reasoning' that are expected on SAT and IQ tests. To be sure, blacks with middle-class jobs generally adapt to this regimen. Even so, their children tend to move among members of their own race, where they develop alternative intellectual styles. The result is that black modes of perception and expression become impediments to performing well on the official menu of standardized tests."

The college environment often is a greater predictor of whether minority students will graduate than their SAT scores, according to an exhaustive affirmative action study that tracked 45,000 students. The study, published in 1998, revealed that black students whose SAT scores were in the lowest category listed—under 1,000—graduated at higher rates, the *more* selective the school they attended. Highly selective schools, the report explains, have greater resources and provide more financial aid, personal attention, and support services, including mentoring and other programs. Some Crenshaw gifted students score well above 1,000, but their scores still are considerably lower than those of the middle-class students whom they will be competing against. Without affirmative action, many of the Crenshaw seniors would see their college applications to elite universities rejected.

Some of the seniors have taken the SAT before. Olivia scored 1,160, which is impressive considering she was hustling for tips until 2:00 A.M. at a taxi-dancing club, was virtually homeless, and had never studied—or even seen—an SAT prep book.

Venola, who works at a convalescent hospital every day after school, hopes to attend a small private college in the East. She knows she needs to raise her SAT scores, however, in order to have a chance for a scholarship. The first time she took the SATs, she walked into the exam room cold and scored about 1,000. A neighbor of Venola's, who had attended college, decided to help her. She paid for three ninety-minute SAT tutoring sessions for Venola. (A standard $700 Stanley Kaplan review course is about thirty-six hours.)

Six weeks later, Venola took the test again. She scored one hundred points higher.

NINE

AFFIRMATIVE ACTION

TO TREAT SOME PERSONS EQUALLY, WE MUST TREAT THEM DIFFERENTLY

In late October, fall finally arrives in Southern California. The air is cool now, the sky overcast, with shreds of fog clinging to the tops of the jacaranda trees. Seagulls crisscross the Crenshaw campus, their white breasts iridescent against the gunmetal gray sky. They catch gusts of wind, float on updrafts, and glide high above the quad.

On a misty Monday morning, Little stomps into the room, ignores the greetings of some students, and glowers into her coffee. A few students exchange nervous glances and one mutters, "Miss Little got her *attitude* on today." When students begin to argue over who will read the parts in *Inherit the Wind*, Little snaps, "I'm not in the mood for this." She flashes the class a forbidding look.

The students divvy up the roles and play their parts for a few minutes until they are interrupted by a girl who walks into the classroom and hands Little a note. Little had previously complained that the drill team, which was using a room down the hall to change, was too noisy. The coach of the drill team, who is seeking to resolve the dispute, sent the note.

When the girl leaves, Little shouts, "That evil serpent can't get away with this!" She raises an index finger. "Don't you see what's behind this note? Can't you see what she's trying to do to me? This is harassment!"

The class grows impatient. This is a dispute they do not understand and do not care about. So as Little grumbles about the note, the students ignore her and resume reading the play.

A few minutes later, Little notices that Curt, a tall boy wearing a Lakers sweatshirt, is whispering to a girl sitting next to him. She walks over to his desk and shouts, "I'm trying to run a class here!"

Curt says, "I just wanted to find out one thing related to this class and I asked—"

She pounds a palm on his desk. "I'm sick of your antics! I'm sick of your gabbing! You always want it to be about me, me, me. When you make a point in class, everyone has to listen to you. Then it's important. But when someone *else* is talking, you could care less. Well, I'm tired of it. You better get it together. Because no one's catering to you anymore. The world doesn't revolve around you. Maybe I'll just stop calling on you in class. Let's see how you like *that* . . ."

She continues to denounce Curt for several minutes, so vehemently that he and his classmates are stunned. After all, Curt is one of the most conscientious students in the class and one of the top students at Crenshaw. And his offense was minor. They know, however, that this is the wrong day to cross Little. One girl in the back of the class, exasperated by Little's screed, says, "Calm down, Miss Little. It's over."

Little will not relent, so the class, again, simply resumes reading the play, raising their voices above Little's until she returns to her desk. For the rest of the class she sits and scowls while the students play their parts.

Later in the week, her mood still has not improved. When a student wanders in late, Little loses her temper.

"This is *not*," she says, slicing the air with a karate chop, "a serious class. I'm trying to teach literature here, and I'm offended by how casually some of you take this class. I'm not interested in floaters and errand runners and playgirls. What's wrong with some of you? This is AP lit. Why aren't you serious?"

Little borrows a television and VCR from a teacher down the hall and pops in the movie version of *Inherit the Wind*, starring Spencer Tracy. While the students watch the play, the phone rings. It is Miesha, calling from the administration office. She asks to speak to another student.

"I need to get something from her to give to my mother," Miesha tells Little.

"I'm not interested in your errands!" Little bellows into the phone. "You should be in class right now."

"You're just watching a movie—"

"*Just* watching a movie? *Just* watching a movie?" she repeats, louder this time and with more indignation, She slams the phone down.

Miesha arrives thirty seconds later, out of breath. After class, Little leans over, grabs Miesha's desk with both hands.

"Have I *ever* wasted your time in class? Did you ever consider that this will enhance your understanding of the play? How can Spencer Tracy *ever* waste you time? Every time I see him in this part, I have a greater understanding of the play."

Little shakes the desk. "What's *with* you."

"I'm sorry," Miesha says.

Little continues to lambast her. Miesha stands up and says sullenly, "I *said* I'm sorry. I can't give you blood."

As Little paces and mutters, Miesha walks out.

All the students have left the classroom except Danielle, who is the top-ranked senior and the front runner for class valedictorian. She walks up to Little and says, "Miss Little, I'm worried about you." She studies her face and asks, "Are you okay?"

Little dismisses her with a wave. "Oh, I'm all right. Don't worry about me."

Danielle wanders off to her next class, still bewildered by Little's rage. She remembers how Little used to fume and lose her temper in sophomore English. But Danielle believes that this year Little is more mercurial and short-tempered; she seems to treat every minor transgression as if it were a catastrophe. Danielle fears that Little is on the verge of a nervous breakdown.

After Danielle leaves, Little dashes down to a patio behind the teachers' cafeteria. Jittery and frazzled, she lights a cigarette and takes several quick, nervous drags.

"I've got to get off this low road," she tells me, exhaling sharply. "I know I've got to stop taking everything so personally. But my passion carries me." She finishes her cigarette and immediately lights another. "For better or for worse."

Little stays after school every day to tutor students, and it is here, in her nearly empty classroom, where she finally relaxes. Without the pressure of a room overflowing with students, Little has an entirely different personality. The AP students who are not confident about their writing stop by after school and Little patiently goes over their essays with them. One girl, who has missed almost two weeks of class, lingers by the door, timorous and intimidated. But instead of the tongue-lashing she expected, Little listens to her problems, cracks a few jokes, and encourages her. Little tells her about the upcoming exam on *Inherit the Wind* and urges her not to miss class.

A few minutes later, Danielle stops by. She is a soft-spoken, serious girl, that rare selfless teenager. "I've been thinking," she says, looking uneasy. "And I'm still worried about you."

"It's okay, Danielle," Little says.

"It's just not worth it," Danielle says. "Why get so upset about these little things?"

Little shrugs.

A friend of Little's, a young female teacher, walks by the classroom and calls out, "Want to go to dinner tonight?"

Danielle pats Little's shoulder. "You do that. Go to dinner. Have a good time. Forget about all this."

The next week, on Tuesday, November 5, Californians vote on an anti-affirmative-action ballot measure, Proposition 209. Moultrie's comments to her class at the beginning of the year prove prophetic because the measure is approved. The proposition, in essence, ends affirmative action in California and will have a cataclysmic impact on collegebound inner-city students. Proposition 209 says: "The state shall not discriminate against, or grant preferential treatment to, any individual or group on the basis of race, sex, color, ethnicity, or national origin in the operation of public employment, public education, or public contracting.'' For Crenshaw students this means that California's public universities and state colleges will no longer take race into account in order to increase minority admissions. The proposition, however, does not go into effect for undergraduate admissions until next year. So the students in Little's class will be among the last group of California seniors to benefit from race-based preferences. But many of the freshmen, sophomores, and juniors in the gifted program—and their parents—are worried, and Little's seniors know that in four years, when they apply to graduate programs, the end of affirmative action could have critical consequences for them.

California is not alone in ending affirmative action. Last spring, a federal appeals court ruled that a white candidate to the University of Texas law school was a victim of racial discrimination because many black and Latino applicants were admitted despite having lower grades and test scores. Texas now bans affirmative action in admissions, outreach programs, and scholarships. The U.S. Supreme Court refused to review the decision. But given all the attention focused on the Texas case, and California's track record as a bellwether for political trends, black and Latino leaders across the country are concerned about the impact on other states. They fear that two critical dominoes have just fallen in what they anticipate will be a protracted war against affirmative action.

Most colleges and universities across the country still base their affirmative-action programs on a 1978 U.S. Supreme Court decision involving Allan Bakke, a white engineer in his early thirties who was rejected by the University of California at Davis medical school. Bakke's age probably was a major impediment. But he also knew that the medical school's admissions policy worked against him because sixteen of the one hundred places in the first-year class were set aside for minority applicants. To make room for them, higher-ranked white applicants such as Bakke were rejected. The policy was implemented in 1968 because the first class at the medical school, which was chosen on the basis of only grades and test scores, contained not a single black or Latino student. Nevertheless, after

Bakke was rejected, he sued the medical school for discriminating against him because of his race.

A state court and the California Supreme Court both ruled that UC Davis's admission program was unconstitutional and violated Bakke's right to the equal protection of the law. The university, however, appealed and the case went to the U.S. Supreme Court. Bakke won the battle, but staunch opponents of affirmative action felt he had lost the war. By a 5-4 majority, the Supreme Court ordered him admitted to the medical school and struck down the school's racial-quota admission system. But the Court approved the idea of considering race as a "plus factor" in admissions in order to foster a diverse student body.

Justice Harry A. Blackmun concurred with the decision in an oft-quoted opinion: "In order to get beyond racism, we must first take account of race. There is no other way. And in order to treat some persons equally, we must treat them differently."

The Bakke decision meant that public colleges in California and across the country were prohibited from setting aside a specific number of slots for minorities—quotas—but they could still give minorities an edge in the admissions process in order to promote "diversity" in the student body. The decision endorsed affirmative action, but narrowed its scope.

In the years following the Bakke decision, the UC Davis medical school admitted fewer blacks. Yet many of those affirmative-action students who *were* admitted to the medical school turned out to be just as competent doctors as the other students, according to a comprehensive study conducted by two UC Davis medical professors. The study, published in the *Journal of the American Medical Association*, concluded: "An admission process that allows for ethnicity and other special characteristics to be used heavily in admission decisions yields powerful effects on the diversity of the student population and shows no evidence of diluting the quality of the graduates."

The study, which spanned from 1968 to 1987, reported that about 45 percent of the students who were accepted as a result of affirmative action, despite lower grades and tests scores, were white. These students were given preference because of "characteristics . . . other than race that were deemed important," including leadership qualities, poverty, or overcoming physical disabilities. But more than half of the students given preference were "underrepresented minority students." The results of this study are significant because of the shortages of doctors and dearth of health care services in many minority communities.

During the first two years of medical school, the students who entered through special admissions lagged behind in the basic science courses, but by their third year they began to catch up in medical and surgical clinical courses. On the National Board of Medical Examiners test—taken while in medical school in order to obtain a license—these students had a higher failure rate and more often repeated the exam before passing. After graduation, however, both the regularly and the specially admitted students had "quite similar" experiences in residency training programs and were "equally likely to receive honors evaluations."

An editorial in the *AMA Journal* praised the authors of the study for demonstrating that "the number of fully qualified individuals in the applicant pool is much larger than formerly was thought. They show that UC Davis applicants who qualified for the special admission program . . . had excellent outcomes that were comparable to those admitted the usual way . . . Some specially admitted students have not been successful, but the count is small compared with their overall numbers and their potential to increase medical care to patients most in need."

Almost two decades after Bakke, the decision remained influential. During the 1990s, however, foes of affirmative action began complaining that University of California campuses were giving minorities a greater advantage than merely the "plus factor" delineated by the Bakke decision.

Many Californians mistakenly believed that universities in the state routinely accepted unqualified black and Latino students and, as a result, were forced to reject hordes of qualified whites and Asians. The reality is that every high school senior whose grades and test scores place them in the top eighth of the state's high school graduates is admitted to a UC campus, although it might not be their first choice.

The greatest controversy has surrounded the competition for the limited number of spots at UC Berkeley and UCLA, the most selective campuses. Although the average minority student was accepted to these two campuses with test scores and grades substantially below the average for white students, it is not as if they were grossly unqualified. (The year after Proposition 209 went into effect, and affirmative action was eliminated, eight hundred of the black and Latino students who were rejected from Berkeley had 4.0 grade point averages.)

Many prominent foes of affirmative action, such as Stephan and Abigail Thernstrom, authors of *America in Black and White,* contend that minority students, with lower grades and test scores than white students, should not be admitted to elite institutions because they will not be able to compete and, ultimately, will be demoralized and stigmatized. This argument, however, has been refuted by the most extensive affirmative-action survey ever conducted in which the authors studied the academic records and the postgraduate lives of 45,000 students at twenty-eight of the nation's most selective universities over twenty years. The study, which focused primarily on white-black comparisons, was published as a book, *The Shape of the River: Long-Term Consequences of Considering Race in College and University Admissions.*

The study reported, for example, that the graduation rate among black students who entered elite colleges in 1989 was 75 percent, with another 4 percent transferring and graduating from other colleges. While this percentage was lower than that of the white students at these same schools, it was significantly higher than the 59 percent graduation rate for white students at Division I schools across the country. The study also found that black students earned advanced degrees at the same rate as other students at elite universities and professional degrees in law, business, and medicine at an even slightly higher rate. These black students also were more likely than their white classmates to be involved in civic affairs after their graduations.

The book was written by economist William G. Bowen, a former president of Princeton University, and Derek Bok, a political scientist and former president of Harvard University. They contend that graduates of these selective institutions comprised "the backbone of the emergent black middle class." The authors concluded that they are in favor of affirmative action at elite universities, not to redress past wrongs, but because it will benefit the black community, it will enhance the experiences of whites who are exposed to racial diversity during their college years, and, in the long run, it will enrich American society.

"A mandate to ignore race in choosing applicants would require that more than half the black students attending these selective institutions be rejected," the authors wrote. "Would society be better off as a result? Considering the educational benefits of diversity and the need to include more highly qualified minorities at the top ranks of business, government, and the professions, our findings convince us that the answer is no."

The assault on affirmative action could have significant long-term consequences for students rejected from prestigious universities because of the practice of "grade weighting" by some postgraduate programs. This policy, which is common in the top tier of law schools nationwide, gives greater weight to the grades of applicants from elite colleges and universities. UC Berkeley's prestigious Boalt Hall School of Law, for example, gives applicants from schools such as Yale, Stanford, and Harvard extra points in the admissions process, while students from schools such as Howard University, a historic black college, and California state universities, which are less expensive and less selective than the UCs, have their GPAs lowered. (In the fall of 1997, the faculty at Boalt Hall eliminated grade weighting in the wake of a complaint filed with the U.S. Department of Education's Office of Civil Rights by the Mexican American Legal Defense Fund, the NAACP Legal Defense Fund, and other groups.)

General Colin L. Powell, whose own career in the army benefited from affirmative action, has expressed his admiration for the quality of Bowen and Bok's study and how absurd he regards the argument that blacks at top universities will be stigmatized by affirmative action. "I would tell black youngsters to graduate from the schools magna cum laude," he has said, "and get one of those well-paying jobs to pay for all the therapy they'll need to remove that stigma."

In the mid-1990s, two obscure California academics laid the groundwork for Proposition 209 by drafting an initiative that prohibited all racial and gender preferences in California employment, contracting, and education. The authors, however, did not have the political savvy, the clout, nor the money to get their initiative on the ballot. Their timing, however, was impeccable because Gov. Pete Wilson joined their cause just as he was preparing to announce his bid for the 1996 Republican nomination for president.

Wilson's sudden, vehement opposition to affirmative action, and his efforts to parlay this divisive issue into the White House, appeared to be a cynical act of political opportunism. When he was mayor of San Diego, one of his 1979 campaign flyers stated: "Pete has been a strong supporter of the affirmative action efforts supported by the minority community. He believes that America's minorities have been handicapped for years by inadequate housing, education, and job opportunities, and he has dedicated his efforts to alleviating these problems." Later, as governor, Wilson signed into law a number of bills with affirmative action clauses.

This was not the first time Wilson flip-flopped on an issue for political advantage. When he was running for governor, Wilson promised not to raise taxes. He eventually signed the largest tax increase in state history. While he campaigned for reelection as governor, he promised California voters he would not run for president. The next year he launched his presidential campaign. He centered his campaign around Proposition 187—an initiative that would deny public services and education to illegal immigrants—and on the hustings, Wilson constantly railed against illegal immigration. Yet when Wilson was a United States senator, he had resisted efforts to penalize employers who hired undocumented workers, in an apparent effort to curry favor with wealthy farmers and agricultural concerns.

So when Wilson suddenly changed positions on affirmative action— and even went so far as to file suit against California to end affirmative-action programs that he once embraced—few were surprised. He was joined in his anti-affirmative-action campaign by Ward Connerly, a conservative black businessman who was a major financial supporter of Wilson's and had been appointed by him to the University of California Board of Regents. The campaign manager for Proposition 209 acknowledged that trotting out Connerly as a visible spokesman for the cause—and later employing him as the proposition's campaign chairman and pitchman— was a cynical ploy to use affirmative action to defeat affirmative action.

In 1995, Wilson and Connerly persuaded the Board of Regents—most of whom were appointed by Wilson or his Republican predecessor—to prohibit the use of race and gender as a criteria in admissions decisions. The University of California, which had taken its battle in support of racial preferences all the way to the U.S. Supreme Court in 1978, now was an explicit symbol of the anti-affirmative-action movement.

After that stormy UC regents' meeting, Wilson held a press conference and announced that "the people . . . who play by the rules deserve a guarantee that their children will get an equal opportunity to compete for admission . . . regardless of their race . . ."

Wilson and the University of California regents were embarrassed when, a few months after the regents voted to end affirmative action, it was revealed they had been running their own surreptitious affirmative-action program for years. But this affirmative-action program did not benefit disadvantaged and impoverished students. This affirmative-action program benefited the children of rich and influential white people, the people who Wilson contended "play by the rules."

It turned out that Wilson, Connerly, and several of the regents who had voted to eliminate affirmative action had been using their position and clout to obtain admission to UC campuses for the children of family, friends, neighbors, and business associates, some of whom were then admitted ahead of better qualified applicants. One angry regent, Ralph Carmona, denounced these backdoor methods as affirmative action "for the rich and famous," and "preferences based on power and privileges."

An extensive *Los Angeles Times* investigation revealed that during the previous fifteen years, more than eighty current and former public officials made hundreds of requests to UCLA, seeking admission for well-connected students. More than two hundred of these students were admitted to the university after initially being rejected. Another seventy-five were admitted ahead of hundreds of others with better SAT scores and better grades who were rejected. Many of these requests were channeled through UCLA staff members responsible for fund raising. A nephew of a wealthy Saudi Arabian sheik, whose abysmal SAT score of 700 was well below UCLA's standards, was rejected by admissions officials. His father, however, was considered a prime target for the school's upcoming fund-raising campaign, so the UCLA chancellor, Charles E. Young, overruled his admissions staff and the student was accepted. (He ended up attending a college on the East Coast instead.)

The investigation also revealed that a lobbyist employed by the University of California and his aides gave special consideration to well-connected students applying to UC campuses throughout the state. During the past decade, more than a hundred politicians and other public officials made more than a thousand requests for admission, housing, and other assistance to UC campuses.

The chancellor of UC Berkeley said Connerly passed two requests— for the children of friends—directly to him. Both students were admitted, including a community college student with a 2.60 grade point average. Wilson recommended several dozen students to graduate school campus admission officers over the years on behalf of the children of friends or members of his gubernatorial staff, his press spokesman acknowledged.

Regent Leo Kollogian, who voted to eliminate affirmative action, conveyed this high-minded sentiment to a reporter: "To me, when you give preferential treatment, you're not exercising equal rights . . . That's not the way I understand the Constitution to be." Yet the *Los Angeles Times* investigation later revealed that Kollogian had, during the past decade, made thirty-two backdoor requests to UCLA. Three of his lobbying efforts were on behalf of his business partners' children. One, who had a 3.45 grade point average and a 790 SAT score, was admitted ahead of 6,000 other students with better grades and test scores.

Right after the regents voted to end all racial preferences, Wilson intoned somberly at a press conference that from this "historic" point forward, the integration of the University of California would occur "on the natural." On the natural, however, apparently does not apply if you are the child of a wealthy white developer, or politician, or potential contributor to the university. Only the descendants of slaves, farm workers, Native Americans, and the impoverished, whose parents have no wealthy friends, must compete on a playing field that is purported to be level.

Despite Wilson's sudden conversion on the affirmative-action issue, his presidential campaign proved to be a debacle. But his legacy lingered. Proposition 209 passed by a 54 to 46 percent majority.

The substantial support for the proposition, however, was a bit misleading. While most Californians strongly opposed numerical quotas and preferences, polls indicated that voters supported affirmative action by a slim margin. The wording of Proposition 209 capitalized on this ambivalence, because while the initiative specified ending all "preferential treatment," it made no mention about abolishing affirmative action. Exit polls revealed that many voters had been confused about the exact intent of the initiative. Even the name of Proposition 209 was misleading: the California Civil Rights Initiative. The initiative also had the advantage of a better-funded, more sophisticated campaign operation than its opposition, and it benefited from an antiminority movement that had been gaining momentum.

In *The Shape of the River*, Bowen and Bok debunk the myth that a significant number of qualified white applicants to colleges are rejected because of special admissions policies that favor blacks. The authors studied the admissions policies of five universities and determined that because the numbers of black students admitted through affirmative action was relatively small, "even if white students filled all the places created by reducing black enrollment, the overall white probability of admission would rise by only one and one-half percentage points . . . Thus nearly as many white applicants . . . would still have been disappointed."

It is also a myth that before affirmative action, the admission process at America's colleges and universities was untainted by preferences, that it was a pure meritocracy. In fact, college admissions at universities never were based entirely on merit. Children of privilege have always benefited from their own brand of affirmative action. The difference is that while there has been little attention paid to preferences given to the privileged, affirmative-action programs for the disadvantaged are widely denounced, exhaustively examined, morally scrutinized, and frequently challenged in the courts by those who claim to be defenders of equality and protectors of the Constitution.

At Ivy League schools and many other elite universities, the children of alumni—known as legacies—have a decided advantage. A 1991 report by Berkeley's Institute for the Study of Social Change asserted: "In American higher education, far more whites have entered the gates of the ten most elite institutions through 'alumni preferences' than the combined number of all the Blacks and Chicanos entering through affirmative action."

Alumni preferences began in the early 1900s to curtail the enrollment of the sons of Jewish and Catholic immigrants who began applying to elite universities. This practice has endured, particularly at Ivy League and other prestigious schools, primarily because it is a highly effective fund-raising tool. In 1988, 280 of 1,602 Harvard freshman had fathers who had attended the college—more than one in six. If legacies had been admitted to the 1988 freshman class at Harvard at the same rate as other applicants, the number of alumni children would have dropped by almost 200—a figure that exceeded the total number of blacks, Latinos, Puerto Ricans, and Native Americans entering through affirmative action. The U.S. Department of Education's Office of Civil Rights conducted a two-year investigation into Harvard's admissions policies in response to complaints that Asian American applicants were admitted at a lower rate than whites, despite better grades and higher test scores. The office concluded that the admissions policies were "legally permissible," and explained that whites were admitted to Harvard at a higher rate than Asians because of the number of students at the college who were legacies and recruited athletes—who had SAT scores about 130 points below the nonlegacy group. Both groups had small numbers of Asians.

Alumni preferences endure at other elite institutions as well. At the University of Virginia, 57 percent of alumni children applicants are admitted, compared to 36 percent of all other students. At Stanford, alumni children are admitted at twice the rate of other applicants. While many of these alumni children have qualifications—as well as opportunities— that exceed other applicants, there is still no question they have a distinct advantage.

In addition to children of alumni and athletes, applicants from underrepresented regions of the country and the children of the very wealthy are routinely given special preference. Institutions do reap some benefits from this practice. Admitting alumni children and children of the rich helps fund-raising. Admitting athletes can raise revenue and enhance a school's reputation. Admitting students from underrepresented states, such as Nebraska and North Dakota, helps develop a national presence.

"How do the reasons for affirmative action stack up against reasons for other admissions?" wrote Barbara R. Bergmann in her book *In Defense of Affirmative Action*. "The reasons for affirmative action are far more compelling: helping to cure the country's racial cleavage, improving the parity of blacks in the job market, encouraging blacks and whites to know each other on campus, and giving a hand to many young black people who grew up in bad environments.

"If we are going to eliminate special admissions to selective schools, we should start with those special admissions that have the weakest justification . . . After [affirmative-action opponents] have succeeded in eliminating special admissions for alumni children, athletes, Nebraskans, the wealthy, the well-connected, and friends of the dean, they will have acquired the moral standing to raise their voice against affirmative action."

TEN

SABREEN

A DOLL AND A TEDDY BEAR

The teachers and administrators at Crenshaw are all talking about Proposition 209 and speculating on how it will affect the students. Although Little voted against the proposition, she does not address the issue in her class. When the school's college counselor, Cassandra Roy, stops by to remind Little's students about college application deadlines, she discusses the implications of the proposition. Roy claps her hands several times until she has everyone's attention.

"Listen to me. All you young African Americans are entering a new world. Affirmative action is over in California. The free ride has screeched to a halt. This is going to have a big impact on all your lives. This year it won't affect you, but it will affect you very soon after that.

"Don't think that because you're a beautiful black or brown person, someone's going to cut you some slack. Forget it. In the very near future, color will no longer mean anything."

Roy, who grew up in South-Central, talks to the students like a skeptical aunt who, while fond of her nieces and nephews, lets them know she is hip to their tricks. She raises an eyebrow and says to the class, "Listen, my babies, my angels, I see you out there on the quad, scrunched up with your girlfriends or boyfriends. Instead of all that foolishness, you all should be working on your college applications and college autobiographies.

"The deadlines are coming up. The Cal State deadline is November 30, and the University of California deadline is the Wednesday before Thanksgiving. Like Curtis Mayfield sings, 'People get ready. The train's a comin'.' If you don't meet your deadlines, people, the train's gonna leave you at the station.

"We down to the hard money now. You don't take care of business now, those colleges will close the door on you. I'm not saying this to scare you. It's the truth."

Several teachers are discussing Proposition 209 with Braxton in his office. Braxton holds conservative views on a number of social issues, and he is an acolyte of a conservative black talk show host in Los Angeles named Larry Elder, who opposes affirmative action. Elder graduated from Crenshaw and bills himself as the Sage From South-Central. He frequently argues on his show that discrimination is not nearly as bad as many blacks contend and that minorities too readily see themselves as victims and avoid taking responsibility for their problems.

"I agree with Elder on many positions," Braxton tells the other teachers, "I even agree with him on affirmative action—in theory. But I disagree with him in practice. The reality is so much more complicated than the anti-affirmative-action crowd acknowledges. I wish we were farther along than we are. But look at SAT scores. A lot of our kids just don't have the scores they need. But the playing field isn't level when they take the test. And look at the incredible obstacles many of them have to overcome just to get through high school. I've seen so many of our kids get into college as a result of affirmative action and thrive. I know there are problems with affirmative action. It's not perfect. But the bottom line is, we still need it."

As the teachers head off to class, Braxton stops one of them and asks her if she can help Toya. Although Toya has dropped out, Braxton still worries about her. He tells the teacher that when Toya left Crenshaw he was concerned because the high school program for unwed mothers she planned to attend would not properly prepare her for college. Now, he tells the teacher, he fears she will not return to high school.

Braxton talked to Toya this week. She told him she could not enroll in the unwed-mother program because her legal guardian, her aunt, lives in one school district and the program is in another. Braxton tells the teacher, "You used to teach there. Can't you make a phone call and try to get Toya into that program?"

The teacher shakes her head. "That girl's got to learn the consequences of getting pregnant. You can't do everything for her," she tells Braxton in a scolding tone.

"I know, I know," he says, looking sheepish. "But she's *gotta* finish high school."

"What she *gotta* do," the teacher says, "is take care of business for herself now."

The teacher heads off to class. Braxton stands up and stares out his window, lost in thought, still troubled about Toya. His reverie is interrupted by a call from Sabreen, who has missed the past few days of school. She tells him that she detests her foster home, wants to schedule a court hearing as soon as possible, and convince a judge to emancipate her. Then she wants to marry her boyfriend, who lives in Riverside, which is about an hour east of Los Angeles. She will either attend school there or drop out and take the General Educational Development (GED) test and earn a high school equivalency degree.

She cries and chatters nonstop, jumping from topic to topic. She seems emotionally fragile to Braxton, as if the pressure is finally breaking her down. He tells her before she does anything rash—such as drop out of school or go AWOL again—she should meet her guidance counselor. She agrees to stop by school in the afternoon.

At 3:15, Sabreen arrives at the gifted magnet office, wearing bib overalls and a red flannel shirt. Braxton pulls out a folder with her transcripts and test scores. "You *know* a student is well-traveled and has been to a lot of high schools when you see this," Braxton tells Sabreen, waving the worn, dog-eared folder.

"Yeah," Sabreen says, smiling, "but my grades are the bomb. Read 'em and weep."

Braxton and Sabreen walk down the stairs and gather around a conference table with her counselor, Charles Oshiro. He studies her file for a few minutes.

"Do you know," Oshiro tells Sabreen, "that it's illegal to work forty hours a week and go to high school?"

"Gotta pay the bills," she says.

Oshiro turns to Braxton and says, "I can't believe she's taking these classes and working full-time. Some of these kids here amaze me. I've got a fourteen-year-old, a ninth grader, who has her own apartment. She's another one who wants to be emancipated. No mother or father. Gets $500 a month in Social Security."

Oshiro cradles his head in his palms. "What are we going to do with her?" he asks Braxton.

"I just don't want to lose her," Braxton says.

"Why do you want to drop out of school?" Oshiro asks Sabreen.

"My social worker says if I get my GED it will help me get emancipated. It'll show them I'm ready to get out on my own. I want out of the foster home. I want to be with my fiancé. We're going to get married pretty soon."

"How old is he?" Oshiro asks.

"Twenty-one."

"What's he do for a living?"

"He works in a warehouse."

Oshiro shakes his head. "No money in that."

Sabreen drops her chin to the table and stares off into the distance, looking despondent.

"You want to go to college?" Oshiro asks.

"Definitely."

He glances at her test scores and whistles in admiration. "You can be anything you want to be, as bright as you are."

"What do you want to do?"

"I want to be a doctor."

"That's twelve years of school. Can your fiancé handle that?"

"Yeah."

"It's hard to be married and go to med school. My son went to med school and he was working seven days a week for years and years. He didn't get any sleep. He got one day off a month. But it was worth it. Now he's got a five-bedroom house."

"That'll be me," Sabreen says. "I'm going to get a Lexus, too."

"Keep your goals high. That's great. You're a very bright young lady. I don't want you to drop out. But I hear you've been missing a lot of school lately. You have too many distractions. You've got a full-time job, a boyfriend, honors classes."

"I'm wearing down this year," she says.

"Your priorities are wrong," Oshiro says. "You need to put your energy into school."

"But I love my job. And I have to work. So I can't quit." She waves a hand impatiently. "Look. I need to find out from you what my options are."

Braxton asks him, "Did you ever have a seventeen-year-old who got emancipated?"

"One student. But I'm not sure about all the details with the county." He faces Sabreen. "Look, you're a bright young girl and we all want to help you. We think it would be best for you to stay in school. Can't we persuade you to do that?"

"I don't know," she says. "But I need to talk to someone who can fill me in on all this emancipation stuff."

Oshiro recommends another counselor at Crenshaw who is more knowledgeable about county regulations. He will set up an appointment for her.

By Friday, Sabreen is no longer interested in another counseling session. She has made up her mind: she will drop out of Crenshaw today. Her social worker helped her arrange an emancipation hearing, which is scheduled for next week. Sabreen will try to convince a judge to release her from county supervision. She still is unsure if or where she will attend high school.

Braxton is extremely unhappy that she is dropping out, but he knows there is nothing he can do or say to change her mind. So he gives her a hug and tells her he will miss her. He wishes her luck and asks her to call or write.

"You've really helped me a lot," Sabreen tells him. "Thanks for being there for me."

Although this has been a hectic and emotionally draining week, Sabreen still managed to turn in—albeit late—her essay on *The Crucible*. It was neatly typed and entitled "The Plight of Abigail." Now she must visit Little's class a final time—to obtain a checkout slip from her.

"Isn't there any other way to solve your problems?" Little asks.

"My life's just too hard," Sabreen says. "I can't do it anymore."

Tears stream down Little's face. She denounces county social services for not providing a better environment for Sabreen; she denounces a society that does not care about girls like Sabreen; she denounces over-worked social workers who did not spend more time resolving Sabreen's problems. Finally, she decides to write a note to Sabreen's next high school English teacher. If there is a next high school English teacher.

"Sabreen is an exceptional thinker with a state-identified gifted intellect," Little writes. "I am very saddened by what happens to gifted children who are underserved by the system. It turns out there's very little that I can do to change the things that thwart the . . . academically able students . . . While Sabreen missed several days of class, she wrote passionate and well-structured essays . . ."

After signing the letter, Little hands it to Sabreen, who is sniffling. Little hugs her and begins to cry. Sabreen, after composing herself, hands Little a tissue and tries to comfort her.

"I'll be okay, Miss Little. Don't worry about me. I'll be back in school. Somewhere. You can count on that."

Sabreen arrives at the children's court on a Tuesday morning, shortly before eight o'clock, carrying a cup of McDonald's coffee in one hand and a white purse in the other. She is wearing black slacks and a white rayon blouse. In an effort to convince the judge of her maturity, her hair is parted low and swept to the side—the most sophisticated hair style she could devise.

The hallway on the fourth floor, where Sabreen's case will be heard, swarms with parents and children and social workers and attorneys and translators. The din of a dozen different languages fills the hallway. Cartoons blare from six mounted television sets.

Grimacing, Sabreen shifts uneasily in a plastic chair. "My stomach hurts," she tells me. "I'm nervous." She launches into a long monologue, without pause, eyes fixed far off into the distance. "I wish I could just go to high school and go to parties and dances," she says. "I wish I had the perfect parents, the perfect family. I wish I could come home from school, do my homework and watch TV and relax. I wish I could live the life of a typical seventeen-year-old. But it's not like that. So I have to deal with it.

"I didn't want to leave Crenshaw. School has been my life. I used to do anything to delay going home. I'd stay after school. I'd go to the library and read books. My life would be falling apart, but I'd tell myself that I was smart. School would help me survive. I'm surprised I'm not a drug addict today. I guess school saved me from that. When I checked out of Crenshaw I was really sad. When I walked out that front gate for the last time, I was teary-eyed. But what could I do? I just walked down the steps to the parking lot and went to work.

"I didn't want to drop out. This was my last year. But I was at the end of my rope. I'd had enough. I guess I have a seventeen-year-old body and an adult life." She closes her eyes and says, "I just can't do it anymore. I'm so tired."

Her court-appointed attorney walks over and interrupts her. "Get ready. Just tell the judge what you told me. Make it simple."

"What're my chances?" Sabreen asks.

"They don't like to let children go before their time," he says. "But it's up to the judge."

Sabreen's father does not show up for the hearing. But her mother waits across the room with a friend. The friend walks over to Sabreen and says, "I work with your mother and every time she talks about you she cries. I want to give you a book."

She hands Sabreen a book entitled, *The Gift of Forgiveness*. "This book," she says, "changed my life."

"I won't read it," Sabreen says, avoiding the woman's gaze. "So don't bother."

"Can I have a hug?" the woman asks.

Sabreen shrugs. The woman bends over and hugs her. Sabreen sits stiffly.

After the woman walks off, Sabreen says, "My parents completely destroyed my life. They lost custody because they never bothered coming to court when it mattered." She frowns. "They came to the first two hearings. But they missed the third one. That was the key hearing. The most important one. How hard is it to come to court?"

She shakes her head. "I don't care what my parents say. I'll never come home. Ever. And I'll never hit my kids. Ever."

Her lawyer strolls over and says to Sabreen, "Your mother's lawyer wants to know something: Will you agree to talk to your mother?"

"No!" Sabreen replies sharply.

At about 10:00 A.M., Sabreen's lawyer escorts her into the courtroom for the hearing, which is closed to the public because she is a juvenile. She returns fifteen minutes later clutching a yellow teddy bear in one hand and a doll in the other. Her eyes, hooded and teary, tell the story.

She collapses into a chair. She puffs up her cheeks, and exhales in a sudden burst. "The judge said that she could see that I was capable," Sabreen says, in a weary monotone. "But she said that if something happens to me, if I'm injured in some way, the court is liable. She said she'd emancipate me in March, on my eighteenth birthday."

She holds up the teddy bear and the doll. "There were big piles of toys next to the judge's table. She said I could pick two."

She stares at a blaring television for a few minutes, nodding occasionally. "Okay," she says resolutely, as if she has made up her mind about something. "Now we go to plan B.

"On Sunday I packed up all my stuff at the foster home and moved in with my cousin in Riverside. Man, was I glad to get out of there. With that day-care center she was running, it was always noisy, kids screaming, her daughter yelling. If I'd work late, the next morning I'd get woken up by music or the TV. I don't care if I have to sleep on the floor. I want my own place."

Sabreen recently arranged for her cousin to be named her legal guardian. Her new plan is to tell her social worker she is moving in with her cousin. Instead, Sabreen and her boyfriend will rent an apartment in Riverside this week and get married within a few months. The chain store where Sabreen works has a shop in Riverside, and she has obtained a transfer there. Next week, she will look into attending high school near her apartment.

"Everyone says to me, 'Why you getting married?' 'Why you leaving high school?' But they don't understand. I don't have any parents. I don't have anyone to take care of me. So this is something I have to do. This is the best way I know to look out for myself."

She stands up and walks down the hallway, clutching the teddy bear and the doll, tightly holding on to the last vestiges of an evanescent childhood.

ELEVEN

LATISHA

STOLEN CHILDHOOD

On this cool, crystalline morning, a brisk breeze blows in from the ocean, stripping the lavender jacaranda petals off the trees that line the school's front walkway. The breeze sweeps the petals across the lawn and they bounce and bob like purple buoys on a green sea.

To the north of the school, towering stands of palm trees undulate in the wind, their waxy fronds glistening in the sunshine. In the distance, daubs of puffy clouds mass over the Hollywood Hills. Gusty winds have dissolved the haze, so the large white letters of the HOLLYWOOD sign are sharply etched against the olive drab hills. The sign may represent glitz and glamour to America, but across town in South-Central it seems a world away and remains a stark reminder to residents how truly cut off they are from the rest of the city, how little they share in the prosperity that Hollywood generates.

In Little's class, the breeze rustles the blinds, scattering motes off the slats, which are velvety with dust. Little closes the blinds and then tells the class that she has just finished grading their *Crucible* essays. While a few of the essays were excellent, she says, many students are still making rudimentary writing errors.

She taps the stack of essays and says to the class, "Why are so many of you still writing in the past tense? Why don't you know that big works—like plays and novels—are underlined and small works are in quotations? Why don't you know that a comma always follows a transitional phrase? I thought I taught you all that in the tenth grade? Some of this can be remedied. Come to tutoring after school. We'll work on it. You need to know these rules. When you get to college, you have to know how to write."

Little gives each paper two grades: one for content, the other for writing style. When she hands the papers back to the students, they groan, or grin, or look embarrassed and stuff them in their backpacks, or show them around and exchange high fives.

There are a handful of As. Curt, who Little vilified last week for talking in class, received an A+/A-; Danielle, the student who was concerned about Little's emotional health, received an A/B+; Miesha received a B+/A-.

As Little passes out the essays, Olivia is worried about her grade because she wrote the paper in a rush and missed several classes during *The Crucible* discussions. For days her braces had irritated her gums, which were now infected, and her teeth ached. Olivia signed up for a program that provides free orthodontics, but all the work is done by UCLA dental students. Her car was out of commission that week, and she rode several buses in order to reach her morning appointments at UCLA. She had to return several times before someone could properly adjust her braces.

On Friday, the following week, her *Crucible* paper was due. She began writing it on Thursday at her foster home, but several girls were fighting and screaming and she could not concentrate. She drove to the library nearby, but it was closed. She tried writing at Taco Bell, but the piped-in music was so loud she could not concentrate. She finished the paper in the office of a student-run business at Crenshaw.

Olivia, who is wearing black and white checkered slacks and matching checkered cap, taps her black high heels nervously as she waits for her essay. When Olivia sees her grade, she throws her head back and laughs. Sometimes, when she laughs, her eyes still contain a wary reserve, as if she is unable to fully experience a moment of true happiness. Now, however, her eyes glitter with merriment. She looks like a teenager again.

Olivia received the highest grade in the class—an A+/A.

"A reoccurring theme in literature," Olivia wrote in her opening paragraph, "is the 'classic war between a passion and a responsibility' . . . John Proctor . . . confronts the conflict of his . . . private passions and his commitment to society. In this conflict his individualism and inner struggle become manifest and are also significant to the work as a whole . . ."

Little wrote beside the grade: "This is a superbly written essay. You have presented your ideas with aptitude and force. Bravo!"

The students who received As on this essay can share their achievement with a parent, grandparent, or older brother or sister. Olivia has no one. Her foster mother does not care about the essay; the other girls at the foster home do not care. So Olivia, knowing it might be her only chance for some adult acclamation, runs up to me after class, grinning and waving her paper, and exclaims, "Look! Look at my grade!"

As the class files out, Little approaches Sadi, who, two years ago, was one of her best students. He received a solid B on the paper, but Little was disappointed. A gifted poet like Sadi, she feels, should have written a stronger essay.

"Your essay flowed well," she tells him. "But where's your passion? Don't be afraid of presenting more abstract thought. In the tenth grade you had tons of abstract thought. You had real passion then, too. Now you're backsliding. Your writing is clear, but you're losing your voice, your strong opinions. Don't be a floater. Put something of yourself into these essays."

Sadi nods, a guilty look on his face. He knows she is right.

After class, Sadi walks down to Braxton's office to ask for his help. He had a dispute with the auto mechanics teacher, who threw him out of class and will not let him back in. It is too late to drop the class, and although it is a nonacademic, elective course, an F on his transcripts could hurt his chances for a college scholarship.

Sadi tells Braxton that when he finished his assignment in auto shop, he slipped on his head phones and listened to his CD player. The teacher was irritated that Sadi was listening to music in his class, so he grabbed the CD player. Sadi grabbed it back. The teacher sent him to the principal's office.

After Braxton listens to Sadi's explanation, they walk across campus to see the auto mechanics teacher. "I remember when this guy was a knuckleheaded ninth grader," Braxton tells me, putting a hand on Sadi's shoulder. "Every time there was some kind of fight on campus between gangs, and there was a big crowd, Sadi was always in the middle of it."

Two tattooed gangbangers in corn rows pass by.

"Hey, Sadi," one says. "Wha's up?"

"Not much," Sadi says.

"Sadi's one of those pivotal kids," Braxton says. "He knows all the thugs."

Sadi grins. "That's 'cause I used to *be* a thug. But all my friends who are still alive are in jail now. My mom had to put a block on the phone 'cause I was getting so many collect calls from jail."

"When I ran for student-body president at Dorsey," Braxton says, "all my thug friends worked for me and got me elected. Thugs vote too."

"I didn't know you went to Dorsey," Sadi says. "My mom went there."

They stroll across a sidewalk, beside a wall covered from top to bottom with blue, spray-painted gang graffiti. When they enter the auto mechanics class, Braxton sees Olivia in the lot behind the class, beside some students who are fixing her Volkswagen.

"Olivia only comes to class when she needs her car fixed," Sadi says.

Braxton covers his mouth to suppress a smile. The auto shop teacher, Daniel Vidaure, spots them and Braxton attempts to resolve their dispute. "Sadi's a very bright individual," Vidaure says. "He gets his work done quickly. But he can't listen to music here. When he started to walk out of class, I told him not to leave. He walked out anyway. He's out of control."

"*He* was trippin'," Sadi says, motioning his head toward Vidaure.

Braxton points to the door and tells Sadi to wait outside. Braxton listens to Vidaure for a few minutes and nods sympathetically. "We can't have that kind of behavior," Braxton says. "But what can I do to get him back in your class."

Braxton schmoozes with Vidaure for a few minutes, and he finally convinces him to let Sadi return to class next week. As Braxton and Sadi walk back across the campus, Braxton asks him about his recent college tour. Sadi and a group of other Crenshaw students have just returned from a one-week tour of black colleges in the South. A student business raised the money for the trip.

Sadi tells Braxton that before the tour he had no idea where he wanted to attend college. Now he has decided to attend Clark College in Atlanta. Sadi, who has won numerous speech tournaments reciting his poetry, was impressed with Clark's speech program.

"And being there made me realize," Sadi says, "that there's something I like about going to college with my own kind."

"You better get serious this year if you want a scholarship," Braxton says. "I hear you're not pushing it in some of your classes. This semester, you know, is critical."

"I know," Sadi says wearily. "I know."

"On the football field at the University of Arizona, in the end zone, are the words: 'Bear Down,' " Braxton says. "That's what you should be doing now. Bearing down."

On a Friday afternoon in mid-November, on the Crenshaw football field, the team is playing its archrival, Dorsey High School. The schools are more than football rivals. Crenshaw is a Crip school, and Dorsey is Blood territory. Now, games between the two schools, only a few miles apart, are no longer played at night, because of gang violence.

Five years ago during the closing minutes of a Crenshaw-Dorsey night game spectators were caught in the crossfire of a gang shootout and two were wounded. The gunfire at the Dorsey stadium lasted several minutes and players, who had dropped to the ground, could hear the bullets hitting the goal posts and could see bullets kicking up divots in the grass. The spectators fled the stands.

Two years earlier gunfire again cut short a Crenshaw-Dorsey game. No one was injured, but more than twenty shots were fired outside the Dorsey stadium.

Before this year's game, about twenty policemen patrol Crenshaw, swiveling their heads, scanning the stands and the street, searching for signs of trouble. Every few minutes, a squad car cruises by.

The game between the two schools is called the Roscoe's House of Chicken & Waffles Bowl because the restaurant sponsors a breakfast, with the losing team waiting on the winners. Crenshaw wins this year's game, which is not marred by violence. But attendance is down because many students, afraid of getting caught in a gang shootout, stayed away.

There are no AP English students on the Crenshaw football team, but there are several cheerleaders, including Miesha. Miesha's brother Raymond, who helped her learn the cheerleading routines, has not yet seen her perform at a game. He wanted to watch her today, but she discouraged him. This is her first year as a cheerleader and she is not yet at ease in front of a crowd.

She plans to wait until all her routines are perfect—even if she has to wait until basketball season—before she invites Raymond.

The next work the AP literature students will read is *A Portrait of the Artist as a Young Man* by James Joyce. Little introduces the book by asking the class, "What's significant about novels? Why do we read them? It's because the novel reflects the human condition. A Western story might be entertaining, but it doesn't make it to the level of literature.

"Why do Faulkner's and Fitzgerald's novels have literary merit and teenage romance novels don't? It's because Faulkner and Fitzgerald endure. They tell us something about the human condition. And the human condition is universal . . ."

Little then explains Joyce's stream-of-consciousness style to the class. "Some of your *Crucible* essays were stream of consciousness," she says, sarcastically. "But that's not what I'm talking about."

Little begins telling them about the life of James Joyce. "He was the oldest of ten children . . ."

Two students whisper and giggle, and Little says, "Be careful, I'm Irish."

With her red hair, fair, freckled skin and bright blue eyes, Little certainly looks Irish. And she attributes her quick temper, her sardonic sense of humor, her impetuous manner, to her Irish heritage. Unlike most Americans of Irish descent, however, she is Protestant, not Catholic. She lacks that cultural tradition of guilt, that tendency to look inward when things go wrong.

Little asks a girl in the corner to read the first paragraph of the novel aloud: "Once upon a time and a very good time it was there was a moocow coming down along the road and this moocow that was coming down along the road met a nicens little boy named baby tuckoo . . ."

Of all the works Little assigns to seniors, *Portrait of the Artist* is her favorite. She feels it is important for students in South-Central to identify with Stephen Dedalus—the protagonist—to see that an Irish teenager feels the same alienation that they feel, has the same desires they have, endures poverty, just as they do, has aspirations and dreams, just as they have. She wants them to see that great literature transcends culture and country and, most importantly, race.

"People's identities are shaped by their family, their religion, and their culture," she says. "That's what shaped Stephen's identity, that's what shaped my identity, and that's what shaped your identity. Take any kid from South-Central, add those three elements, and you have a story.

"Now just don't read this book for the grade. There're a lot of life lessons here. You can't read this book properly without inhabiting it. So inhabit it."

At eight A.M., before the next class, Little pulls out her key and is about to open her classroom door when she notices that the door is covered with gang graffiti. The number 55 is spray-painted above NHC. In the middle of the H there is a small X. Sadi translates for her: "That's the 55th Street Neighborhood Crips. The X in the H means that they are scrapping with the Hoovers. That's the Hoover Street Crips."

Little ignores the graffiti, and when the students are seated she explores the theme of alienation in *Portrait of the Artist*. She asks the class, "What if you were born the same person as you are, but somewhere else?"

A girl in the corner misunderstands Little's question and says, "You mean if I found out I was mixed? Then, like, damn, who am I? That happened to me. When I found out my grandma on my Mama's side was white, I was like, whoa. Why didn't you tell me earlier?" She flashes Little a worried look. "I didn't mean it in a racist way, like there's something wrong with white people."

Another girl says, "Yeah, something like that happened to me. I didn't pay it no mind, but I wondered, too. Why didn't I know before."

"If you find out you have a white grandma, so what," Miesha says. "You're seventeen years old. You should have a strong identity by now."

The girl with the white grandmother mutters indignantly, "Hey, if I found out my mama was white and I was dark as mud, I'd trip out. That's some serious shit."

A boy with a mustache and goatee says, "In my family I got whites and American Indians. Don't bother me."

"Can't we get back on the topic," a studious girl wearing a cardigan sweater calls out.

"This *is* the topic," Little says. "This is the search Stephen is on. He is searching for who he really is." She discusses how Joyce uses "epiphany," "sensory impression," and "metaphor."

"Okay," she says wearily. "I hope everyone remembers what a metaphor is."

Sadi raises his hand. "It's like the expression, 'I'm dope as crack.' "

Little appears mystified.

"Dope means cool," Sadi says. "So the expression, 'I'm dope as crack,' means you can't get any cooler."

Miesha shakes her head. "That's not a metaphor, that's a simile." She then defines metaphor for the class.

"Joyce uses a lot of sensory impression," Little says. "Let me give you an example of when I had a strong sensory impression. It was that stabbing in front of school a few weeks ago. I saw the blood gushing out of the kid's face. I saw the kid put his hand to his face. I saw the blood dripping through his fingers. Dripping, dripping, dripping.''

Little tells the students that their next assignment is to write an autobiography, which will help them understand *Portrait of the Artist*. ''I want all of you to use epiphany in your autobiography. Use sensory impression. *Portrait* is a series of episodes, so your autobiographies should be episodic. Joyce has an incredible memory of his childhood. How many of you remember things from your childhoods in such great detail?''

''I remember the day my dad left us,'' Sadi says. He pats his heart and says, ''I remember how I felt.''

Sadi shakes his head and stares out the window, recalling the sense of emptiness that seemed to fill the house, the aching loneliness he felt. He was living with his mother and father in a small cottage behind a house on 16th and Vermont. His great-grandmother lived in the front house. He was five years old when his father left and he did not know why.

Years later, after he was suspended from junior high school yet again, and his mother felt she could no longer control him, she tracked down his father and asked him to stop by and chat with Sadi. This, for her, was a last resort.

He talked to Sadi about the importance of following the tenets of the Muslim religion, avoiding the neighborhood gangbangers, respecting his mother. Sadi listened, but because he was still angry at his father for walking out on the family and because his father's life was not a sterling example of Muslim rectitude, he did not give the comments much credence. By now Sadi was not just a mischievous teenager in need of fatherly counsel. He was running with a hard-core street gang and packing a gun.

''If I'd been around, this kind of thing wouldn't be happening,'' his father said to him.

''Yeah,'' Sadi replied. ''But you weren't around.''

Little pulls out a stack of homework assignments she recently graded and hands them back to the class. But several are ripped, and one is so frayed, and punctured that Little has a hard time determining whose it is.

She laughs and tells the class, ''I've heard students say, 'The dog ate my homework.' But I've never heard a teacher say it. Well, I'm saying it. One of my dogs ate the homework.''

"*Damn,*" a boy says. "Is that a pit bull?"

"That's just my little four-pound dog," she says proudly. "He's feisty."

After she returns the homework, Little tells the class, "The only reason to read Joyce is to figure yourself out. What are the kinds of things that shaped all of you?"

"When I was growing up, my mama was working all the time," Miesha says.

"Go deeper," Little says. "What went on in your childhood to make you the lovely person that you are."

Miesha nods. "My brother is a person I hold in high regard. It's like he raised me. Other people would tell me things, but I didn't care what they'd say. But when my brother would say something, it had an impact. He wouldn't just tell me. He'd show me the consequences of things. He'd show me a girl with a baby or a guy on drugs. He'd say, 'Look at her. Look at him. Look at the way things turned out. That's not for you.' A lot of what I did was for my brother. I had a fear of disappointing him."

"The rest of you," Little says. "What shaped you?"

"Reading," Sadi says. "Reading played a key part in forming my ideas."

Little nods. "I remember a turning point in your life. It was in the tenth grade and you had just finished reading *The Great Gatsby*. You saw something of yourself in Jay Gatsby. That character, that dreamer who had hope at the end of the green light. You couldn't write for shit then. You'd get so frustrated. After I'd mark up an essay, you'd get it back and you'd be so frustrated you'd just throw it down on your desk. Then you got uplifted and, suddenly, you could write. It was like Fitzgerald inhabited your soul. The words began flowing like butter. And you were saved."

She pauses, eyes shining, smiling at the memory. "These authors can save souls. As much as Baptists can save souls. You could have been a gangster. But literature saved you."

Later in the week, after school, Latisha stops by Little's classroom. She has shown minimal interest in the class during the first few months of the semester, and Little viewed Latisha, who has dyed-blond corn rows, as just another cute cheerleader coasting through school. Little is stunned when Latisha tells her that reading *Portrait of the Artist* has been a searing, heartrending experience.

"A lot of the messed-up things that happened in his family reminded me of the messed-up things in my own family," Latisha tells Little. "The things that molded Stephen's personality reminded me of the things that molded my personality. He said he felt like he didn't belong in his family. It's like, dang, I feel like that, too.

"I relate to that stream-of-consciousness thang he has goin' on. I can put myself right in there. It's like, yeah, that boy think like I do. Like I'm not crazy, not a couch case.

"There were so many things I can relate to. Like his family being so raggedy and poor and all. Like him wanting to be a hero to his people by takin' all the money he won from that writing contest and spending it on them. I put myself in his place.

"It's like he couldn't move forward until he went back and dealt with things that happened in the past. That made me think back to things that happened to me when I lived in the projects. Things I don't really want to remember."

Joyce's impressionistic memories of childhood, Latisha tells Little, had a profound effect on her. So many scenes from the book reminded Latisha of her childhood. So many of Joyce's images perfectly captured her own life, such as: "his childhood was dead or lost"; "even before they set out on life's journey they seemed weary already of the way"; "he had tried to build a breakwater of order and elegance against the sordid tide of life."

Joyce's stream-of-consciousness style—his fragmented flashes of memory—has unearthed for Latisha images of her own childhood, painful memories that have long been buried. She has tried writing her autobiography several times in the past few days, but each time she gave up.

"There's somethin' that happened to me, somethin' that molded my personality," Latisha tells Little, her voice tremulous. "But I keep tryin' to write around it. I don't want to put it in my autobiography."

As she sobs softly, Little hugs her and hands her a Kleenex. Latisha wipes her eyes and says she does not want to be misunderstood. She does not want sympathy. She simply does not know if she has the strength to write about a part of her past that, for so long, she has been trying to forget.

Latisha grew up in a Huntsville, Alabama, housing project with her mother, brother, and her mother's boyfriend. The elementary school she attended was composed of mostly middle-class white children and had just been integrated with students from the projects. There was a gifted program at the elementary school and when Latisha was in the first grade she longed to be a part of it. She envied the students because they took field trips to NASA's Marshall Space Flight Center in Huntsville, made model spacecraft for class projects, and put on plays for the school. Although there were no black students in the program, Latisha was not intimidated. Her relatives in the projects had always told her she was a smart little girl.

Latisha asked if she could join the program, but her teachers told her it was only open to students who passed a special IQ test. After Latisha repeatedly requested to take the test her teacher finally relented. The next week her teacher found her in the cafeteria and shouted, in amazement, "You made it!"

But not long after her acceptance—the high point of Latisha's childhood—her world was shattered. Reading *Portrait of the Artist* forced her to confront memories she had spent years trying to forget. Little persuaded Latisha to include this part of her past in her autobiography.

> "*I had become an expert in . . . covering up and keeping one family secret, in particular, hidden,*" Latisha wrote. "*Only recently have I come to understand the impact the continual sexual abuse . . . had. It started when I was less than eight years old and continued until I was in the fourth grade. A man my mother was living with forced me to surrender to sexual activities . . .*
>
> "*I remember on a Christmas in the second grade I woke up early with a lot of excitement because I was hoping for a 10-speed bicycle. I asked if I could open my presents. This man said that I first had to allow him his . . . sexual pleasure. He said that I wasn't to say anything. I did not then understand . . . but somehow I survived . . .*"

The bright, happy girl who had always loved school, who had always been one of the best students in her class, withdrew into a shell of anger and hostility. She instigated fights with other children. Her grades slipped.

By the time Latisha finished elementary school, the abuse had ended, because her mother had split up with her boyfriend. But during junior high school, Latisha had to endure a new horror. Her mother began using crack, and she left Latisha and her brother alone for days at a time.

Latisha often was happier when her mother, who was on welfare, was out of the house, on a crack binge. When she was home she often battered Latisha, who began wearing long-sleeved shirts to school to cover the bruises. When Latisha was in the eighth grade, her mother's relatives decided she would be safer in Los Angeles, where her father lived.

Her father, a security guard, rented a small apartment and there was no room for Latisha. So she lived with her father's sister, who immediately put her to work. Latisha was miserable. She spent all her free time baby-sitting her aunt's children and cleaning the house. She eventually persuaded her father to find a bigger place. He rented a two-bedroom apartment in a three-story complex across the street from a convalescent hospital, and Latisha moved in with him.

When she was in the ninth grade, her father enrolled her at Crenshaw, and when Braxton discovered her test scores, he transferred her to the gifted program. Latisha was lonely during her first two years at Crenshaw. She had few friends and little interest in school. At night she was tormented by the image of her mother's boyfriend, and she downed shots of brandy until she could sleep, until she could eradicate the flashes of memory.

Before school, she often bought a fifth of gin and a bottle of juice at a liquor store. She sat in the back of her morning class, sipping the juice and gin. Sometimes, she just cut school and drank all day. "I'd drink at night so I could sleep," Latisha recalls. "I'd drink during the day to forget. I was just tryin' to numb my soul."

During Latisha's first three years of high school she never once discussed the molestation; she had not told a single person. She was afraid to tell her mother, afraid that she would kill her ex-boyfriend and go to prison. But the effort to keep others from knowing about her childhood, to keep herself from dwelling on the terrible memories, was too much for her. She was an alcoholic at fifteen, and her relatives wanted her to join Alcoholics Anonymous. The next year, she felt as if she were having a nervous breakdown.

Finally, she told an aunt in Alabama about the molestation. During the next few months they talked extensively on the telephone. The conversations helped her enormously, and marked a turning point for her as she attempted to transform her life. Still, she was ashamed. She tried to forget the molestation rather than face it. She quit drinking, she says, "when God jumped into my soul." She regained her enthusiasm for school. She wrote for the student newspaper. She was selected for the cheerleading squad.

Reading *Portrait of the Artist* forced Latisha, once again, to confront her past. And writing her autobiography proved cathartic. It gave her the insight that she could not have prevented what happened, that she did not have to be ashamed, that she could be proud of what she has accomplished in high school.

"I have learned from . . . Stephen Dedalus in *A Portrait of the Artist* to always keep searching for the meaning of life, despite the false appearances . . ." Latisha wrote in her autobiography. "Literature gave me insight into the fact that I am not alone."

Latisha struggled with her autobiography because she found it too painful to chronicle her childhood. Little encouraged her to first jot down all of her thoughts on paper in a Joycean, stream-of-consciousness style. She could then use those impressions as a basis for her autobiography. In a flurry of words, Latisha recounted her past:

When I moved to L.A. . . . had dreams about mom's ex-boyfriend . . . started getting depressed . . . felt violated . . . became an alcoholic . . .

Right now I'm crying thinking about it . . . how could my mom be so stupid, with him beating on her . . . they did drugs together . . . same man raped his own sister . . . mom sold my stuff for drugs . . .

Just talking about it has made me a stronger person and I am determined . . . to be a financially stable person and break the cycle in my family. I'm one of the only ones in my immediate family that hasn't been incarcerated . . .

I slacked for a while, which is reflected in my grades, but I'm back on the beam. I know I need my education . . .

I'm my own parent . . . I support myself financially . . . My childhood has been stolen . . . My point is to overcome this whole thing . . . Physical, mental, sexual abuse has given birth to my strength.

When Latisha enrolled at Crenshaw, her goal was modest: She wanted to graduate without getting pregnant. Her mother had two babies before she was eighteen, and twelve of her cousins in Alabama had babies while in high school. Now, however, Latisha's goals are more ambitious. Her grades are improving. She plans to attend college and study journalism.

This is a hectic year for Latisha. In addition to school and cheerleading, she is managing editor of the school newspaper and works about thirty hours a week, after school and on Saturdays, at a clothing store in a mall. On Sunday, she sells food from a catering truck. She rarely sees her father because he works the graveyard shift, and she arrives home late at night, just as he is leaving. They often communicate by leaving messages on the answering machine. She rises at six every morning, boards one bus, transfers and rides a second bus to a corner near Crenshaw.

Latisha wants to prove to everyone—and herself—that, despite the years of abuse, she can still be a success. That is why she is a cheerleader this year, why she is running the student newspaper, why she is determined to attend college.

And why, when she is named Crenshaw's homecoming queen in November, she is ecstatic. Being named homecoming queen is proof to everyone at Crenshaw—and proof to herself—that she did not allow the molestation to destroy her, that she did not succumb to addiction or crime or teenage pregnancy like so many of her relatives. Latisha feels a passage about Stephen Dedalus in *Portrait of the Artist* encapsulates her own transformation, her own efforts to rise above her childhood and create a better life for herself: ". . . his soul had leaped at the call. To live, to err, to fall, to triumph . . . !"

Writing her autobiography, detailing the molestation, expressing her innermost thoughts, has freed Latisha, unleashed something in her that manifests itself now in class discussions. During the first few months of school, she was aloof in class and rarely participated in the raucous give-and-take of AP English. Now she frequently speaks out, offering her opinion, disagreeing with other students, haranguing Little for not assigning works by black writers.

Although Latisha is a polished writer, she has a slang-filled manner of speaking that the other students refer to as "ghetto," or "eastie." (The east side of South-Central is more impoverished, with a higher percentage of housing projects, slum apartments, and welfare recipients.) Emboldened now, Latisha explicates *Portrait of the Artist* for the class in a kind of literary ebonics.

On a Monday morning, a few days after Latisha's tearful talk with Little, the class discusses one of their homework assignments: "Stephen's father is a source of humiliation to him. Cite the passage that most clearly indicates this fact."

Latisha, who is wearing white jeans, a denim jacket, and denim cap, raises her hand and says, "When Stephen think of his father, he's like, 'Damn! This nigga get on my *last* nerve.' You know what I'm sayin?"

Little appears perplexed. She asks the class, "Can we have a more traditional interpretation?"

After the students discuss Stephen's father for a few minutes, Little asks them, "How many of you feel that you don't belong in your own family?"

"I go back to Alabama and see my people," Latisha says, "and these girls still clowning over guys, still having babies. These guys still a bunch of ballers. I look at them and I'm like, 'Hello! I don't belong to y'all.' "

"What's a baller?" Little asks.

"A baller is someone who's in the game," Latisha says.

"What game?" Little asks.

"You know, makin' money in a way that's not legit. You know, illegal. I ain't callin' anyone out. I just telling you how it is. I come from a family of ballers. But, like Stephen, I'm different from my family. I ain't no baller and I ain't never gonna be no baller.

"And, like Stephen, I got big dreams. I'm like, dang, I want to *be* somebody. You know what I'm sayin'? That's why I'm here right now, in this classroom."

TWELVE

OLIVIA

EASY MONEY

Toni Little trudges into class, tosses her coat on a chair, brews a pot of coffee, and mutters and curses under her breath as she sits at her desk and studies a memo. An emanation of hostility surrounds her, a forbidding aura of steadily rising anger and antipathy. The students keep their distance.

The memo is from the school principal. "Please meet with me and Mr. Braxton on Friday . . . in my office," the principal wrote. "The purpose of this meeting is to try to resolve the personal differences you are having, which is resulting in a rift within the department. I am asking . . . the union rep to also attend."

When the eight o'clock bell rings, Little pushes the memo aside disdainfully and jumps to her feet. "There are *some* teachers here," she tells the class, "teaching African folk tales, when they're supposed to be teaching contemporary American literature. There are *some* teachers here teaching *Othello*, when they're supposed to be teaching contemporary American literature.

"These teachers are never criticized, but everyone is coming down on *me*. Making *me* go to meetings. Disciplining *me*. Taking *me* to task for showing some concern about what is taught at this place . . ."

Little is interrupted when a girl wanders into class late. "I'm tired of this, too. Students wandering in whenever they feel like it. Why can't everyone get here on time? From now on, it'll be ten points off for being late."

She walks to the back of the class, stops in front of a girl chewing gum and holds out a piece of scratch paper. The girl wads the gum in the paper and Little tosses it in the wastepaper basket. "It'll also be ten points off for chewing gum. Got it?

"A few of you, in your papers, described *The Crucible* as a novel. Don't you know what the genres are? Didn't you ever talk about genres last year?"

She approaches one shy girl, who has never taken a class with gifted students before, and asks her, "Do you know what a genre is?"

The girl looks around nervously and says, *"The Scarlet Letter?"*

"No! No! No!" Little stamps a foot in frustration. "Somebody better give me the right answer before I *really* go off."

She whirls around and points to Danielle, one of the school's top students. "Help me," Little pleads.

Danielle nods and says, "Plays, poetry, novels, short stories."

Little emits a sigh of relief. "Is a novel ever nonfiction?" Little asks a boy in the corner.

"Yeah," he says.

"No!" she shouts, as he jerks his head back.

Little stands frozen for about a minute, blinking hard, her hands shaking, her lips trembling.

"Calm down, Miss Little," Latisha says.

"Don't you get it?" Little asks, still distraught.

"Now we do," Latisha says, trying to soothe her.

Midway through the class, Braxton stops by to talk to a student about his college application. But he spots another student, Kevin, who is wearing a black nylon do-rag, a violation of the school's dress code because it can be construed as gang attire. Kevin is a tall, quiet boy, a sprinter on the track team. He recently attended services at a Nation of Islam mosque and is thinking of becoming a Muslim.

Braxton escorts Kevin into the hall. He tells him to remove the do-rag. "No," Kevin says flatly.

Braxton leads him to the principal's office, where Yvonne Noble orders him to remove the do-rag because it violates the dress code. Kevin tells her he does not belong to a gang, he just likes the way it looks.

"I don't care to discuss it with you," the principal says. "Just get it off." Kevin still refuses, so Noble suspends him from school for the day. She tells him if he wants to return to Crenshaw, he has to leave the do-rag at home.

Braxton returns to Little's class after the bell rings, still seething at Kevin's insubordination, one of the rare occasions when he is visibly angry. Now he has to embark on another unpleasant task: he has to discuss with Little the principal's memo and the upcoming meeting.

As he walks into her classroom, Little, without so much as a hello, launches into a fuming monologue. "She's just mad because I said *Othello* shouldn't be taught in eleventh grade. Her class is an American literature class. Well," Little says, staring angrily at him for a moment. "*Othello* is not American literature. Is it? So I tell people the truth. So what? Everyone's going to say that this white girl is down on *Othello,* so get over it. But that's not it. Why do I get ordered to go to a major meeting because I'm telling kids that *Othello* is not American literature?"

"Do you have to say it in front of the whole class?" Braxton asks.

"*I'm* not the problem!" Little says.

"Look," Braxton says, "I just want to create a dialogue between you two."

"Everyone wants to be so niiiice," she says, derisively drawing out the word. "I'm sick of nice. I want those kids to learn. I don't care about nice. I'll quit if this kind of thing doesn't stop. If I have to sue everyone for harassment in order to pay the mortgage, I will. I'm just trying to teach. Why am I being called to the carpet for being the perpetrator? I don't have to put up with this. I simply don't subscribe to her philosophy. We don't agree on what a sound literary background is."

Flushed and breathing hard, Little falls into her chair. "I have a pounding headache," she says. "I'm stressing out."

Braxton sees that Little will not listen to him this morning. He backs up and says, "Uh, I've got to supervise nutrition. I'll talk to you later."

After he leaves, Little tells me, in a confidential tone, "There are two spies in my AP class. They're ratting on me. They're going back to Moultrie and telling her what I'm saying. I know who they are." She throws up her hands in futility. "How can anyone teach in an environment like this?"

Moultrie is mystified why Little is so angry that she teaches *Othello* to her juniors. Moultrie contends *Othello* is in the school district-approved curriculum. Even if it was not in the curriculum, she wonders, why would another English teacher object to students studying Shakespeare? Braxton, who is in his office, trying to devise a way to resolve the dispute, realizes that *Othello* is not the problem, just a manifestation of the problem.

"Miss Little is one of the biggest frustrations I've had since I've been at Crenshaw," Braxton tells me. "With Miss Little, it's always, 'the best of times, the worst of times.' It's always an emotional roller coaster. When she's on, I'd challenge anyone to find an AP English teacher who is more stimulating to the students, who can spark that kind of passion for discussion. She can be such a talented, brilliant teacher.

"But a week later, the class might be totally unproductive. Or she might kick everyone out for something that irritates her. She can be such a difficult, troublesome personality. I've spent more time dealing with her battles, her problems, her irritations than with any one else."

He taps his pen on a folder. "Every attack she makes has some validity. But her approach isn't devised to solve the problem. It's an outlet for her own internal problems." He closes his eyes briefly, drops his chin to his chest, and says, "It's been very, very frustrating."

Braxton often views Little, who was classified as gifted when she was in elementary school, as the typical gifted child. Willful. Impetuous. Brilliant when engaged. Disruptive when bored. Temperamental. Obstinate.

On Friday afternoon, after school, Little reluctantly walks down the three floors from her classroom to the principal's office, sighing and muttering, like a patient on the way to a root canal. Noble, Moultrie, and the school's union representative are waiting for her. The mood in the room is tense. The two teachers are both so angry that they do not greet each other, and, although sitting in chairs side by side, they rarely look at each other. Moultrie, a proud woman, feels that Little treats her disrespectfully and is contemptuous about her teaching ability. Little feels Moultrie is antagonistic toward her simply because she is white.

Noble opens the meeting by telling Little, "We're here because Mrs. Moultrie has received complaints from students and teachers about you."

Moultrie brings to the meeting a list of eleven complaints about Little. The complaints are listed on a single sheet of paper, entitled "Issues of Concern," and Moultrie passes Xerox copies to Noble, Little, and the union representative. Moultrie then reads a number of the complaints, including: "Negative comments made to students about me. Negative comments made to other adults—loud enough for students to hear. Negative and derogatory comments made in the cafeteria. Jeopardizes students' grades, motivation, and self-esteem. Petition behind my back to be ousted as department chair and place herself in that position—"

"I wasn't trying to oust you," Little interrupts. "I simply ran for department chair. So at Crenshaw, if an African American heads a department and a white person wants to run for that position, the white person is trying to *oust* the African American?" Little asks sarcastically.

Braxton slips into the room, about twenty minutes late. Moultrie then tells Noble that she brought to the meeting several letters from teachers and students recounting how Little ridiculed her teaching ability.

"Can I have copies of those letters?" Little asks.

"Teachers and students have come to me because they wanted to speak on my behalf," Moultrie says. "But I haven't mentioned their names and I'm not giving you a copy because you're a vindictive person. I don't want them to suffer repercussions for telling what they saw."

"If I can't see these alleged statements," Little asks angrily, "how do I know they're not trumped up?"

"This whole thing is very unprofessional," Moultrie says. "I don't have to come to work every day and deal with your insecurities."

Noble tells Little, "She's not going to give these statements to you because you *are* vindictive. The kids and teachers know that, and they asked Mrs. Moultrie not to let you see them.''

Little remonstrates, but Noble tells her the matter is not negotiable. She then asks Braxton if it is true that Little told him that Moultrie was ''dumbing down the curriculum.'' Braxton, uncomfortable being thrust into the center of the squabble, hems and haws and finally sputters. ''Yes.''

Little shakes her head and says to Braxton, ''I was having a conversation with you about a book called *Dumbing Down the Curriculum*. Our conversation was much more academic than me simply accusing her of dumbing down the curriculum.'' Little insists she never denounced Moultrie in front of students and other teachers, but admits that she does disagree with many of the works Moultrie assigns and her approach in class.

''Her class has racist overtones,'' Little says. ''Students have come to me and complained that she teaches them that all white people should be suspect after what whites did to them.''

Moultrie denies this. Little ignores her and adds, ''This kind of talk is not conducive to an academic program. This isn't preparing kids for college. If I ran a white agenda here, all hell would break loose.''

When Little stridently rebuts and ridicules Moultrie's list of complaints, Moultrie becomes indignant. She stands up and says to Noble, ''I'll leave it to you to handle this. There's no reason for me to be here. It's not productive because she's not telling the truth.''

Moultrie walks out.

Noble then tells Little that she has to learn to get along with her colleagues, that this kind of internecine warfare has to stop. Noble ends the meeting with a final admonition to Little:

''I don't want to do it,'' Noble says, ''but if I have to discipline you, Miss Little, I will. And if I continue to hear that you're criticizing Mrs. Moultrie, the next meeting between you and me won't be this pleasant.''

A few minutes before the next AP English class, Little stands by the window, glowering at the morning mist. She is still seething about the meeting in the principal's office. ''This is black-on-white harassment,'' she tells me before class. ''That's all it is.''

Kevin wanders into the classroom. Without the do-rag. Little ignores him. Sadi walks over to the window and asks Little if he can be excused from class, because he has to consult the speech teacher about one of his college applications.

"No," Little says, staring out the window.

"But it's about college."

"No."

"But it's important."

Finally, she turns toward him. "Can't you hear what I'm saying?"

"But—"

"No! No! No! No! Students in here have millions of reasons why they have to leave class. I'm sick of it. I will *not* excuse you." She resumes staring out the window. Sadi shakes his head in disgust, returns to his desk, and throws his backpack on the floor.

When the bell rings, Little leads the students to the library for Braxton's annual college pep talk.

"The college application season is here," Braxton tells the students. "Every year our gifted magnet students are accepted to some very fine schools. But it's all contingent upon the senior year. My first year here, one student got a scholarship to a private college back East. But he didn't do well on a required course during his senior year. He got a D. They rescinded his acceptance."

The class groans.

"All of you here are superintelligent," Braxton says. "But some of you don't use your intelligence. All of you can go to college next year. Even those who might have flaked out in the past. But remember, this semester's grades are the last these colleges will see. So work hard!"

Olivia, who is absent this morning, has missed the last few classes. When Little runs into her later in the day in the gifted magnet office, she chastises her. "You're too inconsistent," Little tells her. "You say you've got it together, then you show up late all the time. I'm not the cause of all your problems, and I don't have a solution. All I'm interested in is your performance. But you're not taking my class seriously. Why haven't you been in class?"

"Oh, man," Olivia says. "If you knew where I was."

"Wow me," Little says, looking bored.

"I was in jail."

Little's jaw drops and her eyes widen. "For what?"

"I don't want to say."

Little leads Olivia to the corner of the office, away from the secretaries, and wheedles the story out of her.

A man in his midtwenties, the ringleader of a check-cashing scam, has been approaching Crenshaw students and asking them if they want to make some easy money. A few students, including Olivia, expressed interest. The ringleader buys blank checks from a crackhead, who breaks into post office boxes and steals them. The ringleader gives a check to a student, who deposits it. When the check clears, the student splits the money with the ringleader.

Olivia recruited another Crenshaw student and they went to the bank one afternoon after school with one of the stolen checks. When Olivia's friend tried to deposit the check in her account, a suspicious teller called the police.

Olivia and the other girl were arrested, taken to the police station and charged with forgery. They were told to call their parents. Olivia called a classmate's mother, whom she lived with over the summer and who is still listed as her guardian. The woman picked up Olivia and drove her back to the foster home.

When Olivia's friend was arrested at the bank, she was terrified and ashamed. Terrified at how her mother and father would react. Ashamed at dishonoring her family. Because Olivia has no family, the arrest is merely an annoyance to her.

Olivia's teachers are surprised, and disappointed, by her casual attitude about the arrest. They hoped she would acknowledge that what she did was wrong, would evince some measure of guilt. But Olivia has developed a cocky, somewhat ruthless persona over the years, partly as a defense against what she views as an uncaring world. Since no one ever seemed to care about her, she felt she had to do whatever was necessary to take care of herself.

She tells her friends that this was a victimless crime, and only the bank—which could afford it—stood to lose a relatively small sum of money. And she blithely tells her friends that she is not particularly worried about the upcoming trial, which is scheduled for the first week in December.

Olivia has no prior record and knows she will be tried as a juvenile. She knows her juvenile record will be expunged when she is eighteen. She is convinced that the court will simply let her go with a warning and a brief probation period. She does not expect the arrest to disrupt her life.

Her teachers are not so sure.

THIRTEEN

SOUTH-CENTRAL

A SUNLIT GHETTO

A winter storm from the Pacific Northwest rumbles down to Southern California and lingers along the coast, pelting the city with a torrential rainstorm. The thunder sounds like timpani and the rain that blows against the windows of Little's classroom is a percussive counterpoint, tattooing the glass with the brittle, steady beat of a snare drum.

As the students arrive, they strip off wet coats and dripping backpacks and pat the water off their hair. Little sits at her desk, watching the rain, her mood matching the weather. Scowling, her eyes fixed on the back wall, above the students' heads, she interprets the mythological and religious symbolism in *Portrait of the Artist*. She then discusses original sin and why Jesus was crucified. "What do we do to people who tell the truth?" Little asks. "What do we do to these people, people like Martin Luther King and John and Robert Kennedy? What do we do to people like this? We take them out. We crucify them."

She nods knowingly, reflecting on her recent meeting in the principal's office. She identifies with King and the Kennedys—a tremendous leap, even for Little, who frequently dramatizes and elevates her battles with administrators and her disputes over Xerox-machine access and curriculum choices to epic, life-and-death struggles.

"When Stephen sins, is he concerned because what he does is against the teachings of the Catholic Church? Or is he concerned because it doesn't conform to his own conscience? Get out a piece of paper and write down, 'What is a conscience?' "

Miesha raises her hand and says, "If you're raised in South-Central, you think different about things. You might have a different kind of conscience."

"If you're raised in South-Central," Little says, "and you go against your conscience, what will happen?"

"That could get you fucked up," Miesha says.

"In my neighborhood," Sadi says, "some people will kill you and then go out and eat a sandwich. Your conscience should tell you not to kill people, but these fools be killin' people all the time and they not thinkin' twice about it."

The class then focuses on how conscience plays a part in *Portrait of the Artist*, how Stephen Dedalus is tormented by his conscience, how he is torn between his desires and his religion, how he struggles to create his own identity while questioning his family, his culture, and his church. After a spirited discussion, Little writes a homework assignment on the blackboard: "In an effort to explore the richness of myth—as something more than just a piece of fiction or fairy tale and to realize its relevance to the fabric of humanity—upon completion of this book write what you believe the purpose of life is. Write authentically what it means to you. Avoid explaining or preaching. Don't give me rules and regulations . . ."

When the bell rings, Little walks over to the window and watches the rain pelt the quad. During class she was distracted by the discussion, but now she agonizes about the meeting in the principal's office, and she becomes increasingly agitated.

"When we were talking about religious symbolism in class, I was amazed how few students knew the details of Jesus' crucifixion," she tells me. She rests her forehead against the glass and listens to the rain drumming on the roof. She whirls around and says, between clenched teeth,

"I'm living the crucifixion! I'm being crucified here! It's happening to me! They're taking away my life breath. The life breath of every teacher is authority. They're taking that away from me. They should be saying to me, 'Right on, Miss Little!' Instead, they're persecuting me."

She stares through me for a moment, her lips trembling and her eyes wide. "I'm so tired of a community that cares only about feelings and the love of Jesus. Some of them just want to shake and bake before some preacher, who doesn't give them any information. I'm sick of this feelings free-for-all. I'm not buying into this self-esteem crap. I want to teach correct standards. And what do I get for it? I'm being brought down. They say I'm disruptive and rude. A young teacher would be shaking in her boots. But I won't put up with it. I won't go along with this bullshit." She glances around nervously. "That's why they're going after me."

As the students file into Little's class, the Wednesday before Thanksgiving, they are all in a panic. The University of California applications are due Saturday. The applications require an autobiography, and a few students ask Little for advice. She tells them they already wrote an autobiography when they began studying *A Portrait of the Artist*.

"This is a different type of autobiography," a student says. "This is an application kind of autobiography."

"The same principle still applies," Little says. "Remember what I said when we first started studying *Portrait of the Artist*? Everyone's identity is shaped by their family, their religion, and their culture. So start out by examining what shaped you. What shaped your parents and grandparents? Who are they? Where are they from?"

Most of the students' grandparents are from the rural South. They moved to South-Central during a population boom that began during World War II, when Los Angeles and a number of other cities were the destination in a great migration, a massive transposition of blacks from the South to northern cities.

The Southern California defense production boom began in 1940 and, while white workers flooded into the area to work at aircraft plants and shipyards, black migration was limited because of discriminatory hiring policies. A. Philip Randolph, president of the Brotherhood of Sleeping Car Porters, demanded that defense contractors end discrimination or he would call for a march on Washington and attract 50,000 protesters. Randolph met with President Franklin D. Roosevelt, who was concerned that if blacks protested the nation would appear hypocritical because it was preparing to fight a war in defense of democratic ideals. In June 1941, Roosevelt issued an executive order requiring that defense contractors abolish discriminatory hiring practices.

Before the war, Los Angeles' black population was relatively small—less than 65,000. But as a result of Roosevelt's order, and because of acute labor shortages, blacks poured into the city and landed jobs in war industries. Between 1942 and 1945, about 200,000 blacks migrated to Los Angeles. Many of the new arrivals were confined to a traditionally black South-Central neighborhood, a vibrant thirty-block stretch surrounding Central Avenue. Since the 1920s, "The Avenue" had been the black cultural hub, the center of the West Coast jazz scene, a street bustling with hip nightclubs and thriving storefront businesses.

Historian Lonnie Bunche wrote: "Talk with any Black Angeleno over the age of fifty and he will wax poetic about the richness of black life along Central Avenue, describing the plethora of homes, the wonderful atmosphere and music that flowed from the Club Alabam and the Apex Club, the economic promise of black businesses—whether a bakery, a newspaper, or a beauty parlor, the pride in self that sprang from the bookstores, literary guilds, and community organizations . . ."

After the war, the black population continued to multiply, as black servicemen, who had been stationed at California bases, decided to stay. From 1940 to 1960 the black population in Los Angeles increased 423 percent—the largest increase of any major city in the United States. By 1965, about 400,000 blacks lived in Los Angeles, the fifth largest black population in the country. Despite the enormous population gains, most black migrants were shoehorned into a few traditionally black neighborhoods and were forced to stay within these prewar boundaries because of restrictive housing covenants.

Still, many black immigrants who had been raised amid the segregation and sharecropping serfdom of the rural South, found South-Central—with its stucco apartment buildings, palm-lined streets, pastel bungalows, and postage-stamp front yards—a vast improvement. They soon discovered, however, a new kind of discrimination and a disparate kind of poverty.

Life in South-Central had deteriorated over the years, for many of the same reasons inner-city neighborhoods around the country had deteriorated. The unemployment rate in South-Central was double that of the rest of the city. Much of the housing, which was owned by absentee landlords, was in disrepair. Many of the small businesses also were owned by outsiders. Residents frequently complained about police harassment, beatings, and unprovoked shootings. From 1963 to 1965, sixty black Los Angeles residents—twenty-five of them unarmed—were killed by police.

All the indignation and rage simmering beneath this palm-tree ghetto erupted on a sweltering August night in 1965. A highway patrolman pulled over a twenty-one-year-old man in Watts on suspicion of drunk driving. A routine stop led to an arrest, a confrontation, and then the arrest of the suspect's brother and mother, who had arrived at the scene. A crowd gathered. Angry words provoked scuffles. More police arrived. A riot broke out. When it was over, six days later, thirty-four people were dead, more than 1,000 were injured and the damage was estimated at almost $200 million.

After the riots, commissions were formed, grants awarded, the causes of the riots explored, the efficacy of government programs examined. Although President Lyndon Johnson's antipoverty legislation received much attention, comparatively few jobs were created in Los Angeles. Soon the Vietnam War was diverting funds that could have been used in the War on Poverty. The problems of Watts and South-Central soon receded.

By the mid-1950s, a moldering Central Avenue could no longer attract top jazz acts. A decade later, the Watts riots proved to be the death knell for the Avenue. Most of the neighborhood's businesses never reopened after the smoke cleared, the curfews were lifted, and the National Guard left town.

In the years following the Watts riots, gleaming glass and steel towers were constructed downtown on Bunker Hill, but South-Central neighborhoods continued to deteriorate. During the late 1970s and early 1980s, while heavy industry declined across the country, many large industrial plants in the area shut down, resulting in tens of thousands of lost jobs. Many of the factories that survived moved to suburban sites, far from the inner city, leaving behind a grim pastiche of boarded-up buildings and vacant warehouses. Later, recession and competition from foreign imports led to more plant closings and more jobs lost by black workers.

Years before the Watts riots—and years after the riots—parents in South-Central complained about the condition of the public schools. During the early 1960s, schools in Watts and South-Central were so understaffed and overcrowded that many students were forced to attend half-day sessions. Yet in other areas of the city there were many empty classrooms. Until 1965, Jordan High School in Watts was the only high school in the city without a chemistry laboratory. Supplies were sparse at inner-city schools and buildings were dilapidated. These schools were a dumping ground for substitute, conditional, and probationary teachers. Then, after their teaching skills improved, they often transferred to more affluent areas of the city.

By contrast, California schools, overall, were among the most generously funded in the nation. Six years after the Watts riots, an enrollment survey by the U.S. Department of Health, Education and Welfare found that the Los Angeles Unified School District was "the most segregated in the entire country." A group of black and Latino parents in Southern California filed suit in the state courts alleging that funding for California's schools was unconstitutional because there was such a great gap in funding between the children of the rich and the poor. In 1977, several years after a court decision ordered the state legislature to devise a different system of school funding, a new system was finally enacted.

"As soon as Californians understood the implications of the plan— namely, that funding for most of their public schools would henceforth be approximately equal—a conservative revolt surged through the state," wrote Jonathan Kozol in his book *Savage Inequalities*. "The outcome of this surge, the first of many tax revolts across the nation in the next ten years, was a referendum that applied a cap on taxing and effectively restricted funding for *all* districts."

This referendum, which cut property taxes in California, was known as Proposition 13. It passed in 1978 by an overwhelming margin and ended any hope of significantly improving inner-city schools. One California legislator interpreted Proposition 13 this way: "This is the revenge of wealth against the poor: 'If the schools must actually be equal,' they are saying, 'then we'll undercut them all.'"

While this push for equality in school funding galvanized middle class parents, the referendum's roots ran much deeper. Proposition 13 was the culmination of a widely popular tax revolt that swept California during the 1970s—and spread throughout the nation during the 1980s, paving the way for the Reagan presidency.

Proposition 13 cut funding for California's libraries, universities, children's programs, parks, playgrounds, and, perhaps most importantly, its public schools. Teacher salaries in California have remained competitive, largely because of powerful teacher associations and unions. But there has been a steady diminution in all facets of the public school system since 1978, including counseling services, books, computers, laboratory equipment, arts and music offerings, building maintenance, and numerous academic programs.

Wealthy parents, however, soon found a way around the limitations imposed by Proposition 13. They set up private, tax-exempt foundations to raise money for their schools. In Laguna Beach, a foundation has raised $6 million since the early 1990s. In La Jolla, another affluent community, three foundations provide additional funding for the local high school, one of the finest public schools in the nation. One foundation acquires funds for the school and its classes; another is for college scholarships; a third supports the school's 400-seat theater. The academic foundations contribute about $200,000 a year.

Even in the Los Angeles Unified School District, foundations and parent booster clubs have created a separate but unequal funding source for the city's schools. Parents raise several million dollars every year, most of it concentrated among only a small number of the district's more than 650 schools.

Of the twenty-six schools that raised $100 or more per student, twenty-two were located in the more affluent Westside and San Fernando

Valley. These schools are able to provide students with resources not available to students in poorer areas of the same school district.

A parents booster club at the Westwood Charter Elementary School, for example, raises about $225,000 a year, which pays for teachers' aides and drama, video, music, physical education, and technology programs. Two other elementary schools in the district raise more than $200,000 a year—one on the Westside and the other in the San Fernando Valley.

Today, after about two decades of Proposition 13-imposed limitations, California's educational system has declined precipitously. During the year of the Watts riots, California was ranked seventh in the nation in education spending; thirty years later the state was forty-third nationally. The U.S. Department of Education recently ranked the state's fourth graders tied for last, with Louisiana's, in reading skills and near the bottom in math. Education Week in 1997 gave California's schools a D- in school climate, D- in school resources, both the lowest in the nation and concluded that California's schools, "once [a] world-class system, is now third-rate." Some California politicians attempted to blame the influx of Latino immigrants for the students' abysmal test scores. But all ethnic groups in California—including whites—scored near the bottom in comparison with the same groups nationally.

In addition to Proposition 13, the largest prison-construction program in the history of the United States also has contributed to the state's dire funding shortages for schools. From 1984 to 1995, California built nineteen new prisons, but the state has not built a new University of California campus in almost thirty years. California's "three strikes" law, which went into effect in 1994, created even more of a demand for prison cells. It is the nation's toughest three-strikes sentencing law and calls for a minimum of twenty-five years to life for anyone convicted of a felony after two "serious or violent" prior felonies. The problem is the measure is so broadly worded that a number of nonviolent offenses—including petty theft—qualify as a third strike. The law has been modified since its passage to give judges some discretion, but many of the state prison inmates incarcerated under the measure still received their third strike for nonviolent offenses.

Because Proposition 13 capped government revenue, each decision about spending in the state is a trade-off. More money for the state prison system—with its $4 billion a year budget—ultimately means less money for education.

Long-time white residents of South Los Angeles fled the area following the Watts riots. Then fair-housing legislation afforded many middle class blacks the opportunity to live elsewhere. During the 1980s, the confluence of gangs, drugs, and violence precipitated more black flight, and about 75,000 blacks moved out of South Los Angeles during the decade. Many of those who left were middle and working class black families who volunteered at church and were active politically. They felt that government and business leaders were abandoning their neighborhoods, and they saw more opportunity in outlying areas that had better schools and safer streets. The community was drained of its most active and prosperous residents. The people who remained often were the unemployed, the growing number of single mothers, the elderly, the welfare cases. An influx of Latinos, fleeing a crumbling economy in Mexico and civil wars in Central America, replaced those who left.

Blacks competed with Latinos for increasingly scarce blue-collar jobs. Many employers preferred hiring newly arrived Latinos because they were willing to work for lower pay with no benefits and were unlikely to complain about substandard working conditions. One union local, for example, which organized the predominantly black janitors who cleaned downtown office buildings, was busted by groups of contractors who hired undocumented workers and paid them minimum wage. Almost 2,000 custodial workers lost their jobs and wages plummeted from $13.00 an hour to $3.50. The racial tension in South-Central was exacerbated by the presence of Korean merchants, who bought up small markets and liquor stores.

Adding to this volatile mix was the Los Angeles Police Department. Black and Latino residents protested the department's heavy-handed methods for decades, but LAPD officers, in the model of their chief, Daryl Gates, paid little heed. Officers continued to patrol the inner city like an occupying army, employing a hyperaggressive mode of street policing.

The LAPD assiduously rooted out officers who stole money, took bribes, or used drugs, but traditionally has been lenient on officers who used excessive force. During the 1980s and early 1990s, young black men continued to complain about being stopped for trumped-up reasons, proned out on the sidewalk, sworn at, humiliated. Sometimes guns were put to their heads if they did not move fast enough. And sometimes they were beaten.

On a March night in 1991, two LAPD officers pounded Rodney King fifty-five times with their aluminum batons—while their sergeant and a cadre of more than twenty other officers looked on. People across the nation were shocked when they saw the beating, videotaped by a neighbor, replayed repeatedly on television. But not in South-Central. Everyone knew of a Rodney King in their neighborhood.

These officers fractured Rodney King's cheekbone, cracked his right eye socket, broke eleven bones at the base of his skull, broke his ankle, and struck him with such force they knocked several fillings out of his teeth. In April 1992 they were acquitted by an all-white Simi Valley jury. This was the final affront for South-Central residents, and it set off the worst American urban insurrection of the century. Fifty-one people died and about $1 billion in property was destroyed.

The students in Little's AP English class were in seventh grade during the riots. Now, during their senior year—almost five years later—they see little change in their neighborhoods.

In the frenzied months after the riots, there was an outpouring of concern by residents throughout the city. Hundreds of corporations expressed interest in investing in South-Central. A unique rebuilding effort was created, headed by the private sector, which touted an alternative to the wasteful federal programs of the 1960s. The results of this approach, however, were modest.

Five years after the riots, the rebuilding efforts have, in essence, merely ensured that conditions in South-Central returned to pre-riot levels. Many new jobs simply replaced old ones that disappeared during the conflagration. Many new buildings simply replaced old ones that had been torched. One of three buildings that were destroyed or extensively damaged during the riots have not yet been rebuilt. On these sites, hundreds of vacant lots—surrounded by chain-link fences covered with advertisements for hauling services and handymen—dot the riot area.

While a handful of corporations made good on their commitments to South-Central, many others bailed out after the publicity abated. Government financing was a fraction of what was needed. In more affluent areas of the city that suffered riot damage, the rebuilding efforts has had markedly different results. In Hollywood and the Wilshire district, for example, the thirty buildings that were damaged or destroyed all have been rebuilt.

There has been, however, some improvement in South-Central since the riots. While crime is still a major complaint among residents, homicide rates have dropped, and cocaine use and gang warfare has declined from the peak years of the early 1990s. A handful of corporations have invested in the area, providing jobs and much-needed services. A few investors such as Earvin "Magic" Johnson have launched successful businesses in the predominantly black Crenshaw district. In addition, the continuing influx of Latino immigrants has revitalized some areas of South-Central, fueling the expansion of small businesses and renovation in residential areas. Southern California's economy finally rebounded from the worst business downturn since the Great Depression. And since 1992, there have been two black police chiefs. The LAPD has improved relations with minority neighborhoods and has attempted to institute community policing measures.

But the many promises made in the fervent days after the riots— promises that never were fulfilled—have angered many South-Central community leaders, who now feel betrayed. As South-Central's economy languishes, widening the gap between rich and poor in the city, community leaders warn business owners and local politicians to take heed. No fundamental changes were instituted after the Watts riots and as a result, conditions festered and culminated in the 1992 riots. But while the uprising in Watts was confined to the ghetto, the 1992 riot was a microcosm of Los Angeles itself—sprawling, multi-ethnic, amorphous, both urban and suburban. The riot's epicenter was in South-Central, but there was also rioting in the San Fernando Valley and Pasadena. There were buildings burned on the edge of the Westside. There was massive destruction in the largely Central-American Pico Union area.

If conditions in South-Central are ignored and allowed to deteriorate further, community leaders ask, how destructive and widespread will the next riot be?

While Little's students discuss how they will incorporate South-Central into their autobiographies, Olivia sits in the corner of the classroom, chewing on her pen, staring out the window. This has been a rough week for her. She argued with another girl at the foster home and the girl punched her. Then the girl's older sister grabbed all of Olivia's clothes, threw them outside, and rubbed them on oil stains in the street. Olivia had to take her whole wardrobe to the cleaners. And hearing the other students excitedly talk about Thanksgiving, about spending time with their families, depresses her.

Before class one student asks her what she has planned for Thanksgiving.

Olivia sighs, looks down, and says softly, "I have no idea."

This week, for the first time, Olivia is worrying about her upcoming court hearing. Initially, she was blasé about the arrest. But now, while the other students are collecting letters of recommendation from teachers for their college applications, Olivia is collecting letters of recommendation from teachers for her juvenile court judge. This forces her to think about what might happen at a trial. She now realizes that she might have underestimated the consequences of the crime.

Olivia asks several people at Crenshaw to write letters to the judge, including Little, Braxton, and her AP Computer Science teacher.

Little wrote: ". . . The 'system' . . . didn't serve her highest good . . . Her encounters with group home after group home leave something to be desired. As a result, I am writing to represent a voice for the injustices that may have caused some of the choices that Olivia has made . . . She has risen above so many of the early obstacles that got in her way . . . Consider Olivia's circumstances and the difficulties that she has faced in growing up unsupervised for a good portion of her youth . . . She needs our collaboration."

Olivia's Computer Science teacher wrote: "As a student, Olivia has continually demonstrated outstanding academic, intellectual and personal qualities. . . . She independently creates and develops program designs that illustrate in-depth and broad perception in academic skills. Her problem solutions exhibit originality and are interesting and thought provoking. Olivia has become an indispensable member of the class.''

Braxton wrote: ''First and foremost, I do not condone her behavior in this incident and believe strongly that individuals must accept consequences of their actions . . . Olivia entered our program in the ninth grade and immediately made an impression . . . as a go-getter who made education a top priority. She finished that year with straight A's both semesters . . . Olivia understands struggle, and despite her family circumstances has overcome tremendous obstacles to be in a position to graduate from high school and go to college.''

Olivia's trial is scheduled for early December. She tries to present a blithe and brave facade to her classmates. When she is alone, however, or when she stops by Braxton's office and discusses the case with him, she expresses concern. She still holds out hope that the judge will place her on probation. But she knows there is a chance that the judge will mete out a harsh sentence; she knows there is a chance that next fall she will be in a juvenile jail, instead of a college dorm.

Because of Olivia's uncertainty about her future, because she is focusing on her trial instead of college, she has procrastinated in filling out her college applications. She has already missed the deadline for the University of California. Her teachers hope her legal limbo is resolved soon, before she misses all her other deadlines and sabotages her chance for college.

FOURTEEN

CLAUDIA

SACRIFICE AND PRESSURE

Olivia, who is anticipating a dismal Thanksgiving at the foster home, receives a reprieve. Sadi, who has been friends with her since the ninth grade, extends a last-minute invitation. This salvages her weekend and she joins Sadi and his mother, who was born on the Louisiana-Texas border, for a Southern-style Thanksgiving dinner at their apartment.

The next week, Olivia discovers her trial date has been continued to January 24. She had hoped that her future would be resolved by now, and she is tormented by the uncertainty. Although she missed the University of California application deadline, she still has some college options. The application for the school Olivia hopes to attend—Babson College in Massachusetts—is not due until February.

Olivia's despondency about her case is compounded by the impending holiday season. She is depressed, as she is every year, about spending Christmas at the foster home. This is the most painful part of the year for her, listening to students chatter excitedly about Christmas, seeing all the families shopping at the mall. Christmas always serves as a painful annual reminder to Olivia of what she does not have—a real family.

After English class, Olivia and I walk to her car, and she says, "I get sick of people feeling sorry for me during Christmas." In a mock-sympathetic voice she says, " 'Oh, let's invite poor Olivia. She's got no place to go.' That's what people say every year. I'm sick of it."

Her breakfast consisted of a glass of chocolate milk and a cigarette, so she decides to drive over to McDonald's for something to eat. But her car will not start. After about fifteen minutes, after turning the key a few dozen times, she gives up. She leans her head against the window, closes her eyes and says softly, "Everything's falling apart."

The next week, on a rainy Wednesday morning, Olivia wakes up in such a gloomy mood that she turns her alarm off and drifts back to sleep. This is the third day in a row she has missed school.

Before English class, Sadi asks me, "Have you seen Olivia?" I tell him I haven't.

"I've been paging her for a few days," Sadi says. "But she doesn't answer. I called over to her place one night. I could hardly hear her. The foster mother was yelling at her so much."

Another student who has missed a week of school, Andriana, approaches Little after class. Little is about to rip into her, but when she hears Andriana's excuse, she nods sympathetically.

"I had to go to my grandma's funeral in Louisiana," she tells Little. "We took the Greyhound. So we really didn't spend much time back there. We spent almost the whole week on the bus, getting there and getting back."

Little pats her shoulder and says, "Don't worry about it. You can make up what you missed."

When the bell rings, Little writes on the blackboard: "Stephen Dedalus has certain experiences that produce sudden insights about himself, other people, or ideas. Joyce calls experiences of this kind epiphanies. Write for a half hour, in a stream-of-consciousness style, about the insights or ideas that you came to understand at the conclusion of, in particular, and throughout the book."

Little tells them not to worry about grammar or style or sentence structure. The assignment will not be graded. Just be extemporaneous and uninhibited, she tells them. The students immediately begin scribbling. The exercise frees them—like Joyce—to confront their pasts and explore poignant and painful incidents from their childhoods.

Miesha describes something that happened to her when she was thirteen, an incident she has never spoken about, an incident that gives Toni Little insight into Miesha's prickly exterior, her tendency to distrust people and keep them at a distance. She writes:

My ability to relate to Stephen in his spiritual confusion made me realize that we are the same in many ways. Stephen's first sexual experience made him feel guilty, and therefore he was fearful of the punishment that would be given by God. My first experience, although it was not by choice, was very shameful.

"Don't tell anyone about this, girl," I was told. Doesn't God already know? Doesn't he hate me for letting this happen? Is this my fault? Could I have stopped it? No, I don't think I could have stopped it. So does that mean God wanted it to happen? I thought He was my protector. Where was He then? When this man forced me to lay there and keep quiet while he sexually abused me. Where was He? Where were You? . . . I prayed to my brother, not the Virgin Mary. I prayed to him for the same reason Stephen prayed to her: the sense of forgiveness. He was sympathetic to my situation, and he was neither harsh nor cruel, just like Mary.

I still believe in God, and Stephen does also, but I am a strong believer in my personal savior, my brother, Raymond.

After the students hand in their papers, Little delivers a final, brief lecture on *Portrait of the Artist*. The students will take a two-hour exam on Monday, and Wednesday will be the last class before winter break. When the students return, there will be about two and a half weeks of class, final exams, and then the second semester will begin.

"At the end of the book," Little says to the class, "what does Stephen discover to be the highest truth?" Without waiting for an answer, she says, "The highest truth for him is that he is the creator of his own life.

"Where do you get your sense of self? Are all of you just victims of circumstances and your environment? Circumstances and environment didn't define Stephen. And circumstances and environment don't define you. There is one major lesson all of you can learn from Stephen's struggle. That's the answer to the question of who controls your lives and your destiny."

Little extends her arms toward the class. "The answer is: You do."

As she puts together the exam on *Portrait of the Artist*, Little is plagued by two questions. She wonders if Olivia will show up for class. And she wonders if Claudia will hand in her exam.

Claudia has been an enigma to Little the entire semester. She has never been absent for a class. She has never even been late. She has impressed Little by how articulate she is, how she is always willing to stake out an iconoclastic argument in class, always willing to challenge the orthodoxy of the class, especially on religious themes. While Claudia has completed all the exams, she has refused to turn in a single one. Little has watched Claudia finish the exams, along with the other students. But when Little has collected them at the end of the period, Claudia has just stuffed hers in her backpack and walked out of class.

Braxton is perplexed and distressed by Claudia's behavior. She is one of the brightest students at Crenshaw, classified by the school district as "highly gifted" because her IQ is above 150. And in the ninth and tenth grade, she rarely received a grade lower than an A. But during her junior year, her grades slipped. Braxton had hoped this was an anomaly; he had hoped that Claudia would see how much was at stake during her senior year and become serious about school again.

Braxton was the coordinator for gifted students at Claudia's junior high school and he has known her since the seventh grade. When Crenshaw's gifted program hired him, he recruited her. Braxton has always respected Claudia's passion for learning. She often spent weekends and summers at the downtown library, reading novels or studying subjects that piqued her curiosity. He always enjoyed his conversations with Claudia because of her maturity and her intellectual curiosity. He envisioned Claudia at an Ivy League college.

But now he discovers that Claudia is flunking English. If she does not pass English, Braxton knows, no college will accept her. If she does not raise her grade, she will not graduate from high school. He decides to pull her out of AP chemistry this morning—she has not done much work in this class either—and confront her. Braxton calls the chemistry teacher and asks him to send Claudia to his office for a conference.

Claudia is wearing black jeans, a black jacket, skeleton earrings, and bright green nail polish. She sets her backpack down in Braxton's office and sits in a chair across from his desk.

"Share with me why you're failing English?" Braxton asks.

"I haven't turned anything in."

"I thought you got that out of your system last year. I thought you were going to get it together this year. Why haven't you turned anything in?"

"I just haven't."

"Have you talked to Miss Little?"

"I don't feel I can talk to her."

He sighs. "You and I go a long way back. I know you. I know the learning process brings you pleasure."

"I enjoy being in Miss Little's class," Claudia says. "I enjoy literature. I enjoy the discussions."

"So how did you arrive at this point? Why do you refuse to hand in your work?"

She crosses her arms and shrugs. She does not seem rebellious or angry; her expression is simply impassive, lithic.

"In my eighteen years with the school district, I don't think I've ever run across a case where someone goes in the other direction as fast as you, without a whole lot of emotion. I don't get it. It's freaking me out."

"You don't get what part?"

He leans back in his chair, locks his fingers behind his neck, and says wistfully, "There was this wonderful child I fell in love with in the seventh grade. She always enjoyed the educational journey, the challenge, and the success that came along with the effort. I'm still trying to figure out what happened to that girl after the tenth grade."

"I don't know."

"Your attitude now is, 'I enjoy the discussions, but I'm going to fail.' It's like you've decided that you're predestined to fail. I know you read the literature. I know you pay attention." He shakes his head. "Again, I've never run across something like this. I took some students to Pitzer College a few weeks ago. And you know who I kept thinking of? You. A top-notch private school like that, with small classes and high academic standards, would be perfect for you. A scholarship there is worth $26,000 a year."

He pounds his fist on his desk. "You're frigging denying yourself an opportunity to go there. You're being very self-destructive. Why don't you just do the work in Miss Little's class?"

She looks uncomfortable and jiggles her foot. "I guess I'm lazy. I don't know what else to say."

Braxton stares at her for a moment and then shakes his head in resignation. "So what are we going to do about this English class," he says, sounding irritated. "I don't want to be having this conversation with you in June because you're not graduating. Do I need to pull you out of that class right now?"

"I don't know," she says. "Let me think about it over Christmas vacation."

"You know, Claudia, I wish I had some magic words for you. I wish I could say something that would help you."

"I'm responsible for this," she says. "I know my priorities are screwed up."

"So what are you going to do next year?"

"Maybe I'll go to community college. Maybe I won't go to college. Maybe I'll go to cooking school."

Braxton leans over across his desk and says, "The reason I'm fit to be tied about this situation is that I know what college is like. I'm an adult. I've been to college. I know that you'd thrive in college. With your intellect and love of learning, college would be wonderful for you. That's why it hurts me so much to see you throw it all away."

A flicker of emotion sweeps over Claudia's face for the first time. She swallows hard.

"You okay?" he asks.

"I'm fine," she says, her voice breaking.

"You don't look fine."

They talk for a few more minutes, but it is clear to Braxton that no matter what he says, Claudia is not going to open up to him. He sends her back to chemistry class.

Claudia's mother, Margarita, graduated from college in Guatemala and then taught elementary school. Margarita's father was the manager of a prosperous coffee plantation, and the family had a comfortable, secure life. But one summer, Margarita visited Los Angeles during her vacation and never returned home. She was willing to leave her family, give up teaching, and work in a garment sweatshop, in a country where she did not speak the language. She was willing to sacrifice so much for one reason. She wanted children, and she felt they would have more opportunity in America.

After Margarita moved to Los Angeles, she met a man from El Salvador. They had one child—Claudia. He is a parking lot attendant, and Margarita now works as a maid. They rent a small apartment in a weathered, two-story, chocolate brown building, a few miles south of downtown. The building is just off a major thoroughfare lined with garment factories, knitting mills, zipper shops, warehouses, and tile manufacturers. Claudia lives in a small Latino neighborhood, wedged between factory-lined streets. Her apartment is located across the street from a boarded-up, windowless factory and a few hundred yards from the Harbor Freeway. There is a small homeless encampment in the shadow of the freeway overpass, and the rumble of traffic and grinding gears and screeching brakes creates a constant din and clouds of exhaust.

By the time Claudia was in kindergarten, Margarita had taught her the multiplication tables and how to read and write in Spanish. Margarita had a little magnetic board, with letters and numbers on it, and she would drill Claudia each day. When Claudia was in the first grade, she was so advanced her teacher wanted her to skip three grades. But Margarita refused and Claudia eventually was placed in a gifted program. Unlike some gifted children, Claudia was a motivated student, and in elementary and junior high school always received straight As on her report cards.

In the eleventh grade, however, she lost interest in school and simply refused to do any work. This is when she stopped turning in her exams. She received several Fs, but during the summer before her senior year, she attended summer school and made up the classes she had failed. She was still on track for college. Braxton had thought her phase of teenage rebellion had passed, that it had merely been a temporary lapse after years of academic excellence.

But now, a few months into her senior year, she has lost interest in school again and is in danger of flunking several classes. Still, Claudia is not lazy. She rides two buses after school to reach her catering job near Hollywood, where she works about thirty hours a week. And while she does not do her class assignments, she still scours the library for challenging books and reads widely.

No one at Crenshaw can explain her change in behavior.

One afternoon, when her parents are not at home, Claudia sifts through some of their papers and documents from Central America and she has an epiphany—like Stephen Dedalus in *Portrait of the Artist*, she later realizes. She spots two birth certificates from the 1960s. She searches through the pile of documents and then finds two yellowed newspaper obituaries.

Claudia asks her aunt for an explanation. Claudia discovers, for the first time, that her mother had been married in Guatemala and had two children. One child died at five months and the other at nine months. Later, her husband died.

Now Claudia knows why her mother had been so overprotective. Why she would not let her go on school field trips to the tide pools or the mountains. Why she would always explain, "What if the bus crashes?" or "What if something happens?" Now Claudia knows why her mother wanted her to stay home all the time and study. Why she only wanted her to leave the house to go to school. Now she knows why her mother often seemed so sad, why she scrutinized every detail of her life. Now Claudia knows why she feels so smothered. Now she knows why she needs a respite from the pressures of school and grades and exams and college.

All these insights come to Claudia in a cascade of emotions and self-knowledge. While the newspaper clippings illuminate her past, she is still perplexed about her future. She still has no idea if she will ever regain her enthusiasm for school, if she will attend college in the fall, or if she can even summon up the effort to graduate from high school this June.

On Monday, December 16, a cool, breezy day with weak winter sunlight filtering into the classroom, the students gather for a written exam on *Portrait of the Artist*. The exam consists of a twenty-five question objective exam—true and false and multiple choice—and an essay:

"*A Portrait of the Artist as a Young Man* differs from more conventional novels because it doesn't show Stephen Dedalus's development in a straightforward chronological progression . . . [It's] a series of episodes that at first may seem unconnected but which, in fact, are held together by use of language, images, and symbols. . . . In a well-organized . . . essay explain whether Joyce was successful or unsuccessful in presenting a journey of the inner workings of the main character's mind by using language to tell a story that simultaneously combined mankind's great myths, individual human psychology, and the details of everyday life . . ."

After Little hands out the exams, Claudia, along with the other students, hunches over her notebook paper. Little sees Claudia begin to write. Each student enrolled in the class is taking the exam now—except Olivia. But since Olivia often is a half-hour late, Little still holds out hope that she will wander into class.

By nine o'clock, it is clear that Olivia has blown off the test. Shortly before ten o'clock, Little asks a student to collect all the exams. When the bell rings, and Claudia grabs her backpack, Little steps in front of her.

"Did you turn it in?" Little asks.

"Sure didn't," Claudia says, meeting Little's probing gaze.

"Why not?" Little asks.

"My essay wasn't any good," Claudia says, as she scurries around Little and heads out the door.

On Wednesday, the last day of class before the three-week winter break, Claudia is at her desk, as usual, and Olivia is still absent. Although it appears increasingly likely that Claudia will flunk the class, she has one chance left—the final exam. Little knows that Claudia has done all the reading. Little knows that Claudia writes well enough to earn a high grade on the final, which would enable her to pass the class and stay on track for graduation. But Little has no idea—and at this point, neither does Claudia—if she will actually turn in the final exam.

Little hands out copies of *Wuthering Heights*, which she assigns the class to read during the vacation. After she gives a brief lecture, introducing the novel, a few students ask her if they can complete any extra-credit assignments during the vacation to raise their grades. "I'm willing to negotiate," Little says. "But I'm *not* willing to negotiate with people who say mean things about me." Little raises an eyebrow and nods knowingly, while the students just stare at her, perplexed.

After class she tells me in a conspiratorial tone, "They were just playing dumb. But a few of them knew *exactly* what I was talking about. These are the ones who are snitching on me. They're the culprits. They're being used by the system and being taught that if they inform they'll get Brownie points. It's all hearsay. But I'm *livid* about this. It's a gang bang." She cuts the air with a karate chop. "I'm going to take this thing to the wall. I've had it. I'm sick of this job. I'm sick of this paperwork. I'm sick of this school . . ."

A girl in Little's tenth grade class, who is holding a small camera, approaches us shyly. "Miss Little, can I take a picture of you?"

"No," Little says, shooing her away.

As the girl drops her head and shuffles out of the room, Little tells me, "These kids I inherit are not prepared for a class like this. Only four or five of them even have a chance to pass the AP test. I've got a tough row to hoe. Even though I have a liberated personality and an acid tongue, I deliver services to these kids. That's what I should be judged by. But I'm not." She points to the floor below her. "Braxton's in on it, too. He's playing the game and cooperating with everyone who's against me. I've had it with him."

When Braxton passes Little in the hall, she ignores him, and he realizes that Little now views him, too, as part of the conspiracy against her. A former English teacher, Braxton still has great respect for Little's teaching ability. If he ever decided to return to the classroom, Little is still the first teacher he would ask for resource material and for insight into how to generate enthusiasm for the literature. He recalls a comment a parent once made about Little: "She's crazy. But I'd sure hate to lose her." Now that Little has turned against him, however, and he might have to endure a cold war with her for the rest of the year, he is not so sure.

Exhausted, he removes his glasses and massages the bridge of his nose. His eyes are bloodshot. He realizes he has never needed a vacation more. The long commute in rush-hour traffic, the hectic nights with two young children, the pressure of contending each day with errant students, angry parents, and dissatisfied teachers—this punishing routine has worn him down. School has only been in session for a little more than three months, but it feels to him like three years. His mood turns melancholy when he recalls the students he has lost. He thinks of Toya and the scholarship to Cornell's summer program that she had to turn down. He called Toya recently—just to see how she was doing—and she told him she was thinking about enrolling in nursing school or joining the Air Force because it has a good child-care program. But the truth of the matter is, at this point she is a high school dropout.

He thinks of Sabreen and how she worked forty hours a week and struggled to stay in high school. How she made it a point to turn in her English paper the day she checked out. A student told him that after Sabreen moved to Riverside, she earned her high school equivalency degree instead of enrolling in a local school, and is considering attending community college next semester. Still, Braxton fears that Sabreen will marry and that the exigencies of married life will sidetrack her.

He thinks of Olivia and how she has missed exams in several classes and more than a week of school. He wonders if she will return to school after winter break or if she plans to go AWOL again, to avoid her trial.

He worries about Claudia and wonders if she will pass any of her courses this semester. He worries about Sadi, and wonders which Sadi will show up for the remainder of the year. The Sadi who was such an inspiring literature student during his sophomore and junior years, or the listless, apathetic Sadi?

In the past, even when Sadi had indolent stretches, he always was a dedicated member of the speech team. But a few weeks ago, Sadi, who is the captain of this year's team, arrived almost two hours late for a major speech tournament and was disqualified from competing. Neither Braxton, nor any of his teachers have an explanation for his desultory behavior. Braxton just hopes Sadi regains his focus, before it is too late. Braxton knows that middle-class kids might have the luxury of an off-year in school because their parents usually can find some college for them to attend. Sadi needs a scholarship to attend college, so his grades are of paramount importance.

Braxton's anxious rumination is interrupted by a secretary who walks into his office and asks him to sign a sheaf of documents. He stands up, grabs her by the elbow, and asks, wearily, "How am I ever going to make it through the rest of the year?"

FIFTEEN

CURT

STANFORD

During winter break, most of the class uses the time off to pick up extra hours at their jobs, including Miesha and Latisha, who work at a clothing store; Venola, who works at a convalescent hospital; Claudia, who works for a caterer; Princess, who works as a cashier; Willie, who works at a movie theater; LaCresha, who works at a fast-food restaurant; Kevin, who works in a bakery; Carroll, who works at a dry cleaner; Norma, who works at Sears . . .

Little transforms her garage into a library and then spends a few days visiting her sister, brother-in-law, and their two children in Ojai. The three-week vacation, however, does not improve her mood or her perspective on Crenshaw. She still feels persecuted and refuses to talk to Braxton, the principal, or Moultrie. She decides that for the rest of the year, she will only communicate with them by memo.

On a Monday morning in mid-January, the students trudge back into Little's class, grumbling about the end of vacation. It rained early this morning, and water still drips from the windowsills. The trees in the neighborhood surrounding the school are leafless, and their branches are silhouetted against the leaden sky, sharp and spare, like stick figures.

Little opens the class by talking about the *Portrait of the Artist* exams. "I've been reading your essays, and there's still a lot of work to be done. But I can see some progress. Your writing's starting to improve. I was extremely impressed with Curt's essay. It was incredible. I gave him 100 out of 100." Curt beams.

She points to the back of the room. "Sadi, your essay was decent. I gave you an 80. But I know you can do much better. You were my prize student two years ago. What happened to you? Who is corrupting you? Your essay met all the requirements, but it had no personality to it. There were some good ideas, but you didn't develop them." He stares sheepishly at his shoes.

"This year, you've got no real commitment to my class or to the literature." She walks over to his desk and waits until he looks up at her. "Don't you like me?"

"Yeah, I like you."

"Then what's with you?"

He shrugs and grins uneasily.

Little shakes her head, looking disappointed, and walks back to her desk. The rain kicks up again and the campus is enveloped in mist. This is a good morning to discuss *Wuthering Heights*, a novel with a bleak, atmospheric setting, where rain pelts the heath and the north wind howls across the lonely moors.

"Did you like the book?" she asks the students.

"Yeah," a girl calls out. "It was the best one yet."

Little opens the discussion: "What's a more powerful emotion: Love or hate?"

"Love," Curt says.

Little strolls over to his desk and pats him on the shoulder. She smiles beatifically. "He writes such great essays because he's such a sensitive guy."

"I think it's more like a constant war between love and hate," Miesha says.

The class engages in a heated discussion on the topic until Little asks,

"What formed Heathcliff's personality?" Latisha answers without bothering to raise her hand. "When Heathcliff first show up, everyone hated on him. He like, '*Dang,* everyone doin' me wrong.' Pops was the only one who showed Heathcliff any love. Everyone else in the family be doggin' him. Then Edgar steal his girl. That make him *all* torn up. He like an outsider. Everyone treat him like mess," she says, avoiding the other four-letter word in an effort to elevate the tone of her analysis.

"Heathcliff didn't feel love," a girl named Khaliah says. "Therefore he didn't get love. Isabella didn't love him. She was infatuated with him. And he jacked her around."

"Yeah," Miesha says. "They got into a wicked kind of love, and that's not cool. But for Heathcliff to do Isabella like that. Well, that ain't right."

"Do circumstances define you?" Little asks.

"My mom and dad never finished junior high school," says a girl named Brandi. "But I want to go to college, so I found other role models."

"It's like gangbangers," Sadi says. "They never had love, so they never give it. People go by the way they raised and the way they treated. It's a love thang."

"I could be a psycho, with what I been through," Latisha says. "But I chose not to. So I'd tell Heathcliff, 'Be strong, brutha.' Heathcliff felt love and the whole nine. He had the power to love. But the brutha just chilled. I still sympathized with him. I know what it's like to come into life when no one care about you. I'm not makin' excuses for the brutha. I'm just sayin' I can understand where he's comin' from."

"Where were *your* identities shaped?" Little asks. "Literature shaped me. Not my parents or the world around me."

"Did your parents buy you books?" Sadi asks.

"Yes," Little says.

"Well, what if your parents just shot dice and took dope all day," Sadi says. "Maybe you'd do that, too. So your parents *did* shape you."

"Right on, brutha," Latisha says.

Sadi is that rare student, an independent thinker bright enough to challenge his teachers. Little glances around uneasily and changes the subject. "Think of someone," she says, "who has a sullen exterior, but, underneath, is a good person."

"I can think of someone like that," Sadi says.

"What would you tell that person?"

"I'd tell her to chill out," Sadi says, smiling slyly. "I'd tell her to relax and go with the flow. Because all that stress and worry could lead to health problems. Because all that stuff she focusing on may not be that important, after all."

"I know you're talking about me," Little says, irritated.

"I'm only sayin' it 'cause I love you," he responds, laughing.

"Okay, let's talk about something that doesn't include *me*. Did you hate Heathcliff in the end?"

LaCresha nods. "I thought he was a punk."

"But he was vindicated in the end," Danielle says.

"I disagree," Curt says. "He never made amends for what he did."

"In each of us, is a little of all of us," Little says. "If my philosophy is true, then there's a little of Heathcliff in all of us."

The class nods somberly. "Isn't there choice in this world?" Little asks. "Isn't there free will? Catherine wouldn't marry Heathcliff because of their income disparity. But that was her decision, wasn't it? Didn't she have a choice?"

"Hey," Latisha says. "Romance without finance don't stand *no* chance. You know what I'm sayin'? I can see sister-girl's point of view. *I* don't want some brutha who's not accomplishing anything. *I* don't want to be takin' care of no brutha. I won't be gettin' my Land Cruiser that way," she says, grinning.

"What happens when nature conflicts with nurture?" Little asks.

Miesha says, "Some are like, 'I'm gonna do to you what my mama done to me.' I don't go along with that. For example, I'm never going to strike a child."

"Some girls," Latisha says, "they get themselves a rough neck-type nigga. They feel he hit them 'cause he care."

"Nigger?" asks a girl, who finds it distasteful to even repeat the word.

"Yeah, *nigga*!" Latisha says. "If he hit a girl, he a nigga!"

Little would prefer that Latisha discuss the literature in a more traditional manner. She wants to prepare her for college. But during the first few months of class, Latisha barely said a word, so Little is grateful that now, at least, she participates in class. *Portrait of the Artist* gave Latisha a voice. Now, for the first time, she freely expresses her opinions.

After class, Little stops Curt as he is leaving. Last month he infuriated her by chatting while she was lecturing, and she denounced him several times in front of the class. Little was so splenetic that Curt's mother called. She was worried that Little would refuse to write Curt a letter of recommendation for Stanford. But Little has forgotten the past acrimony and now, in her eyes, Curt can do no wrong.

"That was a terrific essay," Little tells him. "Your work can stack up with anyone's. I said that in my letter to Stanford. If they don't accept you, they're crazy."

In a class where many of the students are poor enough to qualify for the federal free meal program, live in rundown apartments, have a parent on welfare, work up to forty hours a week to support themselves, Curt is an anomaly. Both of his parents are college graduates. Both are professionals.

Curt's parents graduated from Crenshaw in the early 1970s. His father was a basketball star and received a scholarship to the University of Washington. His mother was a cheerleader. They later married and, when Curt was eleven, they divorced. But Curt's father, a sales representative for an electronics company, stayed involved in his son's life and always stressed education. He is a commanding presence—six feet seven, 250 pounds—so when he talked, Curt listened.

Curt and his younger brother live with their mother, Yvonne, a chiropractor who owns her own practice. They live in a spacious, well-appointed home in View Park, Los Angeles' wealthiest black neighborhood, known as "the golden ghetto." Set in the Baldwin Hills, just west of South-Central, but high above the grim poverty of the flatlands, View Park is composed of custom-built Spanish and ranch-style homes with manicured lawns and sweeping views of downtown Los Angeles. If the Huxtables moved to Los Angeles, they would live here.

When Curt was in elementary school, Yvonne demanded that he do his homework in the kitchen, right next to her, while she completed her medical paperwork. Every night when Curt had finished, she inspected his homework, to make sure it met her standards. Curt was never allowed to use street slang in the house, and if he ever spoke in a manner that his mother did not consider "proper English," she corrected him. She refused to allow him to wear baggy or hip hop clothes.

Curt has been classified by the school district as "highly gifted," and in the predominantly black elementary school he attended, he was enrolled in several gifted classes. But in the mainstream courses, he constantly was harassed by the other students. They did not like his precise manner of speaking, his preppy clothes, the way he would volunteer answers in class. He was called a "punk" and a "fag." He was accused of "acting white." In class he was teased constantly. In the schoolyard he was goaded into fights.

"Curt would get interested in a subject and during lunch he would read the encyclopedia," Yvonne recalls. "But he'd have to do it on the sly, hide what he was doing. He was afraid someone would see him and begin teasing him again. He was so confused. It's very tough for a young black male who wants to be a scholar. Curt wanted to be a scholar, but he didn't want to deal with kids telling him he was selling out his race. That's a heavy load for a child to deal with."

During junior high school, Curt finally succumbed to the peer pressure. He wanted to fit in, so he stopped raising his hand in class, stopped striving for As. His mother could see that his enthusiasm for learning was ebbing. When he was in the ninth grade, she enrolled him in a private, Catholic high school. But Curt was miserable. He did not like going to a predominantly white school so far from home where he felt teachers were condescending toward him because he was black. Some teachers awkwardly attempted to use street slang in an effort to—as they characterized it— "relate to him." Curt wanted to transfer to Crenshaw, partly because he had a few friends there, partly because of its basketball team, which is always one of the best in the state. Curt's father had been a star at Crenshaw, and Curt wanted to emulate him.

Curt's parents, however, were strongly opposed to his enrolling at

Crenshaw. They knew how much the school had changed since they had been high school students; they knew about all the gang problems and the shootings. But when Yvonne researched the school and discovered the gifted program, she decided to let Curt enroll on a trial basis. Even though Curt would be in an autonomous program, she knew that before and after school and during lunch he would be subjected to the same dangers and distractions as the other students.

By the end of Curt's freshman year, Yvonne was impressed. "In the gifted program, Curt found his niche," she says. "He found other kids just like him—African American kids who wanted to learn. Curt was able to excel and express himself in class and not get dragged down by other kids. He could act smart in class. He could be himself. Being in the program reinforced what I'd been telling him—there's nothing wrong with being black and being a scholar."

Shortly after Curt transferred to Crenshaw, he made the mistake of wearing a red shirt to school. Crenshaw is in a Crip neighborhood and red is a Blood color. After school, as he was leaving the campus, a car pulled up in front of him and the passenger yelled out a traditional gang challenge: "Hey, cuz, where you from?"

"I'm not banging," Curt told him. "I'm just wearing this today," he said, fingering the red shirt. "It's doesn't mean anything."

The passenger aimed a shotgun at Curt. Just as he was about to dive behind a tree, the passenger spotted a police patrol car in the distance. He nudged the driver and they sped off.

About ten minutes later, as Curt was walking home, two other gang members spotted his red shirt and chased him. He cut through an alley and sprinted home. He never told his mother. And he never again wore red to school.

At the end of Curt's sophomore year, Little discovered a summer program for high school students held at Stanford. Several hundred students from throughout the country participated in the program, about twenty of whom were black. Little pushed her sophomores to apply for scholarships, and she helped them with their applications. Curt and three other Crenshaw students were accepted and offered scholarships. But none of them wanted to go. One girl who had been accepted stopped by Braxton's office and told him she had decided to turn down the scholarship. When he pressed her, she began to sob. Finally, she blurted out, "I don't think I'm at the same level as all those white and Asian kids. I don't think I can compete." But the girl's father, Curt's mother, and the parents of the other Crenshaw students forced them to go.

In elementary school, when Curt excelled in class, he encountered animosity from other black students. At Stanford, when he excelled, he encountered animosity from white students. Shortly after he arrived, when a few students discovered that he received one of the highest grades in the class, they stared at him incredulously and said, "*You* got that grade?" Once, during lunch with a group of other students, one prep school boy from a wealthy family said, "These guys from the inner city wouldn't even *be here* if they hadn't of got scholarships and all kinds of special privileges."

These comments angered Curt and motivated him to study harder, to counter the other students' preconceived notions about black students. He often stayed up until three in the morning, poring over his homework and perfecting his papers. During class, he spoke up, expressing his opinions articulately. One of the reasons Curt succeeded, he felt, was because Little had prepared him so well in tenth-grade English. She had taught him the principles of essay writing and had pushed him and prodded him until his writing had acquired a level of sophistication that had impressed his teachers at Stanford. At the end of the summer, one of the Stanford administrators wrote Braxton, telling him how well the Crenshaw students had done. He singled out Curt and wrote that, by the end of the summer, he had become one of the most outstanding students in the program.

During Curt's first two years of high school, he had been a good student, but not an inspired one. He maintained a B-plus average, which is not up to Stanford standards. But when he returned from the summer program, he had an entirely different attitude. He no longer wanted to merely do well in his high school classes, he wanted to excel. He wanted to write the best essays, earn the highest grades, offer the most trenchant comments in class, win the most scholarships. And he had a new goal: He wanted to return to Stanford for college.

Curt knows that this year, if he is to have a chance for Stanford, he must make up for his first two years of high school. He cannot afford a single B. He must excel on his SATs. His teacher recommendations must be superlative.

After the first few months of his senior year, the teachers in all his classes are impressed by his motivation, his exam results, his polished essays. When a local television station wants to give an award called "Beating the Odds" to an inner-city scholar, they pick Curt. The reporter interviews Braxton and asks him how Curt has beat the odds. Braxton says that while Curt is a wonderful young man and a fine student, he had not really overcome great odds. His father is a businessman. His mother is a chiropractor. He lives in View Park. This, however, does not mesh with the story that the reporter wants to tell. Braxton, trying to be helpful, adds that Curt is a sensitive young man and it was very traumatic for him when his parents divorced. This still does not satisfy the reporter. She continues to press Braxton to tell her about some of the great privations Curt had endured and transcended.

In the end, Curt is given the award and profiled on the news. Braxton's taped comments are cut to only a few words: "Curt loves learning."

While Curt's academic career is flourishing, his basketball career is in the doldrums. It is now clear to Curt that he will never be able to emulate his father's success. Although Curt is six feet three, 205 pounds, he is not quick enough to play guard and he is several inches shorter than the dominating high school forwards. Curt practices hard every day with the team, but during games he sits on the bench.

His father, however, is encouraging. Too many young black males, he tells Curt, are obsessed with basketball and neglect their educations. Curt's dream of becoming an orthopedic surgeon, his father tells him, is a more worthy goal, and a more attainable one.

SIXTEEN

MAMA MOULTRIE

OUR BEST HOPE

As the semester draws to a close, Little is still consumed by the dispute with Moultrie, still grumbling about how she has been persecuted for merely speaking the truth. One morning, after class, she waves a memo the principal sent to her and says to me, "They're all lining up against me."

The memo states: "This . . . is my response to your requests for copies of statements from adults and students who were named as having heard you making derogatory statements about Anita Moultrie. I have received one written communication from one member of the English department . . . he alleged he heard you making such statements. . . . Mrs. Moultrie also gave me a list of the names of those students who have reported back to her some of the uncomplimentary statements that they allegedly heard you make . . . Each student with whom I spoke corroborated Mrs. Moultrie's allegations . . . Since I am not at this moment considering disciplinary action against you, I am not required to give you copies. However, I am admonishing you to refrain from discussing in the presence of students any individual . . . when the contents of that discussion can be construed as derogatory."

It is clear that the dispute is wearing down the principal; it is wearing down Braxton and it is wearing down Moultrie. They are seeking a way to finally end the exchange of accusatory memos, the battle of frozen glances in the hallway. Little, however, is energized by the increasingly contentious dispute.

Moultrie—who has five children, a business, a full-time teaching schedule, and is chairwoman of the English Department—does not have the energy for a protracted feud. She is hoping for a quick and a quiet detente.

In Moultrie's eleventh-grade English class, she spends almost the first three months of the semester on *The Scarlet Letter*. Little has criticized her for not assigning enough novels in the class, for devoting too much time to each work. Moultrie angrily defends her style of teaching and contends that her goals are greater than merely lecturing and giving exams. "I'm interested in dealing with the *whole* child, not just counting how many books they read and how many pages of notes they take," she says one afternoon, after class. "I want the kids to know *The Scarlet Letter* backward and forward. But I also want to teach them morals and to respect and take pride in themselves and their people. I want them to understand the social, political, and historical issues that impact their lives. Literature is the framework to teach them many things. And if it takes longer to get through *The Scarlet Letter*, so be it."

Four of her eleventh graders live with their grandparents; others live with impoverished single parents; a few are foster children. Many of them come to her with innumerable personal and family problems. Moultrie feels she does not have the luxury to simply teach literature and remain aloof from their lives.

During the next class, she writes an African proverb on the blackboard: "Rain beats on the leopard's spots, but it does not wash the spots off." This is the students' writing assignment for the day. "I don't want the literal meaning," she tells them. "For example, what does the rain represent? . . ."

Before they begin writing she tells them, "When I was in graduate school, I was often the only African American in class. Many times, people would approach me like I was this dumb little black girl. It was very demeaning. I let them know, in no uncertain terms, that I was an intelligent young woman. But if I couldn't write, this would just reinforce their preconceived notions. So all of you have to be excellent in everything you do. You have to be able to take notes and speak effectively. You have to be able to write effectively. Remember, some people will judge you before they know anything about you. You have to learn to play the game and play it well. And it is a game. So you better learn how to deal. You understand me? Hel-*lo*?''

In unison the class replies: "Yes, Mrs. Moultrie."

When they finish their writing assignment, Moultrie discusses *The Scarlet Letter* chapter in which Hester is confronted in her prison cell by her husband, Chillingworth. Hester has not seen him for several years, and he has just discovered she had a child and will not reveal the father.

Moultrie reads one of Chillingworth's statements to his wife: "It was my folly . . . I . . . a man of thought—the book-worm of great libraries— a man already in decay . . . what had I to do with youth and beauty like thine own!''

"Sisters," Moultrie says, "I know y'all are sayin', '*Dang,* he may be old and not much to look at, but he has money and a good job.' And what old man wouldn't want some *fine* tender girl like that.''

Moultrie continues reading: "And so, Hester, I drew thee into my heart, unto its innermost chamber, and sought to warm thee by the warmth which thy presence made there!'' She sets the book down. "The brutha is *deep*. All you bruthas out there, you got to tell these sisters, 'I want you to be in the innermost chamber of my heart.' Oooh. They'll love that.''

She reads Chillingworth's admonition to Hester: "Thou has kept the secret of thy paramour. Keep, likewise, mine! There are none in this land that know me. Breathe not, to any human soul, that thou didst ever call me husband!''

Moultrie puts the book down. "What Chillingworth is really saying to Hester is: 'You got this boom-boom body and you're so *fine* looking, but I'm just an old dude. And that's hard, baby. I know that. We got big problems. But for now, don't let on who I really am. You can't be sayin', 'Hey, wha's up?' Pretend you don't know me.''

Moultrie skips to the next chapter and reads: "If she entered a church, trusting to share the Sabbath smile of the Universal Father, it was often her mishap to find herself the text of the discourse. . . .''

Moultrie interprets the passage: "What Hawthorne is saying is that when Hester got out of jail and would go to church, everybody would dog her. They'd just run her down. That's cold. But it's all there in the book.''

On the next Monday morning, as Moultrie gathers *The Scarlet Letter* homework, several students tell her they did not have time to finish the assignment. She stares at them with an expression of righteous indignation. "I worked fifteen hours Saturday at my business and still got up early Sunday morning. I taught Sunday school, worked at the business, and put on a birthday party for my eight-year-old. Last night I fell asleep with *The Scarlet Letter* in my hands. If I can fulfill my commitments, you can fulfill yours. You all are in a gifted program. You should take that honor seriously.''

Moultrie opens *The Scarlet Letter* and reads a few sections from chapter six, a chapter entitled: "Pearl." Moultrie discusses the symbolism of the name Pearl—Hester's daughter—and how Hawthorne uses symbolism throughout the novel. Then Moultrie tells the class, "Some mothers will say, 'I'm not wit' yo' daddy, but you sure do remind me of him.' You all have heard that. Well that's what Hester is feeling. She's a single mother . . . She's on her own and she spoils Pearl. She backs up on that punishment gig. It's like when you're in church and some child acts up and the mother doesn't say anything. That gets on my *last* nerve. Everyone in church wants to say, '*Girl,* take care of your child.'

"It's different when one of you acts up in here. Then I *will* tell your parents. That's because I'm your second mother. Well, yang, yang, yang. You've all heard this before.

"Remember how Pearl would react when other children would tease her?''

"Yeah," a girl says, laughing. "She *fight* for her mama.''

"That's right," Moultrie says. She reads: "If the children gathered about her, as they sometimes did, Pearl would grow positively terrible in her puny wrath, snatching up stones to fling at them with shrill, incoherent exclamations that made her mother tremble, because they had so much the sound of a witch's anathemas in some unknown tongue."

"Pearl was tough," Moultrie says. "That girl was baaad."

She reads: "But Hester . . . remembered . . . the talk of the neighbouring townspeople; who, seeking vainly elsewhere for the child's paternity and observing some of her odd attributes, had given out that poor little Pearl was a demon offspring . . ."

Moultrie tells the class, "Hester, too, was thinking of her daughter in all these negative terms: evil, fiendlike, demonic. It's a self-fulfilling prophecy. And that's a lesson you see all around you with children. Today. Right here.

"Now in chapter seven, Hester sets out for the governor's mansion. He's a Puritan, don't forget, but he's got this plushed out house. And he's going to judge Hester. There's a contradiction there, and I'm going to ask you about this on your next test. So pay attention."

On another morning, before Moultrie's lecture on *The Scarlet Letter,* the daily writing dispatch is: "Interracial Marriage." The class discusses the issue before they start writing.

"I don't believe a woman from another race will understand me," a boy tells the class. "As a black man. What a black man goes through."

"I understand, my brutha," Moultrie says.

"My family is all mixed," a girl says. "I have black, white, and Japanese. I'm not confused. I love everyone."

"I just like black men better," another girl says. "There's just something about them I prefer. You put a black and a white man in front of me, I'll take the black man every time. The reason is white men just don't have no . . . no . . ." she halts in midsentence. She glances around the room self-consciously and lowers her eyes. She collects herself and says, "They just don't have no booty."

The girl explains that the white man's behind is simply too flat. The class breaks up laughing, but Moultrie holds up a hand and quiets them.

"This is a legitimate view," Moultrie says. "She simply prefers a man with more of a booty. And she feels black men have more booty. So she has clearly expressed her preference."

"My cousin lives in South Pasadena and he never even been out with a black woman," another girl says.

"That's like Clarence Thomas," Moultrie says. "He has a white wife and he lives in a white world. He's forgotten he's black . . . When I graduated from high school, I was looking at the world with rose-colored glasses. Then I got to college. I wasn't viewed as a student any longer. Now I was viewed as a *black* student. Racism is woven into the fabric of our country. Why did the Puritans have to steal from the Indians? Why did Americans have to go to Africa and get slaves?

"All of you have to realize what it's like out there. So think about these things. You all know what I'm talking about. So don't make this dispatch pretty. Be real."

During the next few classes, Moultrie guides her students through *The Scarlet Letter,* occasionally pausing to parlay one of Hawthorne's images into an impromptu lecture on life in South-Central. At the end of Chapter 14, Moultrie quotes Chillingworth telling Hester: "By thy first step awry, thou didst plant the germ of evil; but, since that moment, it has all been a dark necessity . . . Let the black flower blossom as it may." She taps the book with a forefinger and tells the class, "That black flower is sin and that sin has blossomed. Now listen to me, all of you. Nothing good can come of sin. Did everyone read in the paper about Freeway Ricky Ross?" (Ross, one of South-Central's most notorious crack dealers, was sentenced earlier in the week to life in prison.) "Freeway Ricky's sin germinated into that black flower in *our* community.

"He brought drugs into our community. This led to turf wars, and dependency, and stealing from your own mama, and knocking grandma over the head to get twenty dollars, and shooting someone at the automatic teller." She is preaching now, pacing back and forth, waving *The Scarlet Letter* above her head like a Bible. "Now sin begets sin. Because of these drugs we have the Three Strikes law. We have so many African American men in jail. We have so many African American women who can't find husbands because all their men are locked up."

She strides up and down an aisle. "None of you are an island. What you do—good or bad—will affect other people. Do you hear me?"

"Yes, ma'am," the class cries in unison.

"Remember, the good you do comes back to you. And the bad you do comes back to you, too. That's some free advice from Mama Moultrie."

When the students finish *The Scarlet Letter,* Moultrie assigns the next work the class will study—the novel *Jubilee* by Margaret Walker. *Jubilee,* which has been characterized as "the black *Gone With the Wind,*" portrays a black woman who lives through slavery, the Civil War, and reconstruction.

Little is strongly opposed to Moultrie assigning *Jubilee,* which was published in the mid-1960s and is located in the young adult sections of some libraries. She does not think the work is challenging enough for high school juniors in a gifted program.

Moultrie, however, feels it is important that her students are afforded the rare opportunity to learn about their country's history—and their own heritage—from a black perspective. She uses *Jubilee* to launch the next segment of the class. The segment will culminate in a term paper, due at the end of the semester, which she delineates on the blackboard:

Five Chapters:
1. Before Slavery
   —Describe African Civilizations
   —John Brown and Harpers Ferry
   —Harriet Tubman . . .
2. During Slavery
   —Slave ships
   —Auctions
   —Living Conditions
   —Treatment of slaves . . .
3. After Slavery
   —Emancipation Proclamation . . .

4. Looking Beyond
   —Civil Rights Movement . . .
5. Where Do We Go From Here?
   —What does the future look like for African American people?
   —Unemployment, poverty
   —Affirmative Action . . .

Moultrie tells the class, "It's okay to be African American, even though the media tells us it's not. We weren't always slaves. We weren't always impoverished and rundown and poor. We have wonderfully rich roots that exist in the very power of our beings. Young people don't know that. We were once kings and queens. We once constructed great tombs and underground cities and great civilizations. Too many of us don't feel connected to anything. If all of us knew we were a part of something important, there wouldn't be all these problems on our streets today."

At the end of the semester, when the class concludes the slavery segment, Moultrie tells them they will share a soul food lunch. "I know everyone loves ham hocks, pigs' feet, chitlins, okra, yams, and greens. Y'all be lickin' your fingers when we through. I know I will. When I was little, I'd see my mom washing, cleaning, and preparing the chitlins. I realize now that this is all part of a tradition, culture, and history that ties us together.

"Our people who lived during slavery had very meager portions. They'd see the slave owners, who kept pigs, eat the prime meat and discard the rest of the pig. They wouldn't be discardin' no bacon, either. It would be the pig's feet, tail, chitlins [intestines] and the rest. We would take those remains and they became a staple for us. That's what we call soul food today."

Moultrie tells the class that when Margaret Walker was in college she interviewed her grandmother extensively. The grandmother recounted the story of her own mother, who had been a slave. Walker wrote a paper in college based on those interviews, Moultrie says, and the paper evolved into *Jubilee*. "The book," she says, "all comes from asking questions. So that's what I'm going to ask you to do."

She writes on the blackboard another assignment for the class: "Inter-

e/female, 65 or older. Have them retell a memorable event
racism, discrimination, how they were treated differently because
of color, religion, culture. Write story of the event. Tell the story in the
first person. . . ."

When Little hears of this project, she is irate because she feels it has
nothing to do with literature and does not prepare the students for her
class, the AP exam, or college. But Moultrie emphasizes that she is not
merely preparing students for college, but for life. There are more ways
to prepare black students for college, Moultrie contends, than lecturing
about novels, symbolism, and literary imagery.

The students interview grandmothers, grandfathers, aunts, uncles, and
neighbors, most of whom were reared in the South. They tell moving
stories of enduring the humiliation and degradation of Jim Crow, before
migrating to Los Angeles and enduring a more subtle, but in some ways
more insidious, discrimination in South-Central Los Angeles.

Later, after the students hand in the papers and Moultrie grades them,
she tells the class, "They were great! I get goose bumps just thinking how
good they were. To put it in ebonics: 'Sho enuf, they fine.' " She laughs.
"I'm tickled pink, with them. Well, to be exact," she says, smiling, "I'm
tickled brown."

Steven, a tall, slender boy with braces, interviewed his sixty-six-year-
old grandfather, who told a chilling story:

*The year I first experienced racism was 1934. I was four years old, but . . .
this was one of those things you just can't forget.*

*Me and my family moved from Lockesburg, Arkansas, to Provo, Arkansas.
My daddy was a sharecropper, and we moved to Provo to work for a white
man on his land. The white man my daddy worked for went by the name of
Ruford Steele . . .*

*When word got out that Steele was moving us to Provo to work for him,
white folks all over the place got mad. Provo was an all-white town. There
were no blacks there and they wanted to keep it that way. . . .*

*Our problems started the first night we were in Provo. Mama and Daddy
heard some noise outside and looked out. They saw some white men behind*

bushes and trees. Me and my older brother, Arthur Lee, went to see what was going on. We saw the men and we heard them yelling, "Get out niggers."

Then they opened fire—they shot right through the house. Mama grabbed us and threw us down on the floor. Mama laid on top of me and my brother. Daddy also dropped down on the floor. I don't remember how long they shot at us. I just know that it seemed like a long time . . .

The shooting went on every night for two weeks. You had to know my daddy to understand the type of man he was. My daddy was not afraid of anything or anyone, and he was not going to let them run us off. Then, one night, Arthur Lee was lying down, and a bullet almost hit him. It was about an inch above his head. Then another bullet hit the window above, and the glass splattered in his face. It was a close call. My daddy finally decided to move after this. We loaded up the wagon the next day . . .

The day we left, me and Arthur Lee were playing around outside and we went under the house. We ran across two sticks of dynamite between the pillars . . . When we found that dynamite, we knew that we wouldn't have made it through another night.

Patricia, a soft-spoken girl who is one of the best students in the class, interviewed her sixty-seven-year-old next-door neighbor:

It was a gloomy, rainy day of 1949. I was twenty years old and lived in Poplar Bluff, Missouri. I had been trying to find a job for a long time. . . . I needed money fast to support my two growing sons . . . In those times, black people . . . were only expected to be cooks and maids . . .

But one day . . . I saw a sign on the window . . . of a dental office saying there was secretarial help wanted. I walked in to ask for an application. But before I could even ask, the white receptionist yelled at me, "Now, you know niggers are not allowed to have these jobs or even apply. Go across the street to the restaurant or something. Get your black ass out of here before I call security!"

I was completely shocked and did not know what to do. As I stood there staring, I felt a big hand go across my shoulder. The receptionist had called security anyway. The security guard had such a tight grip on my arm as he was pushing me out the door that I had to scream, "Lord, help me please."

All of a sudden I felt wet concrete against my cheek and then a sharp pain. He threw me in the middle of the street on a piece of glass that cut the side of my face. Blood was just oozing out of my nose and cheek . . . I looked up and saw the other white applicants standing outside the office, staring and laughing at me . . .

A young man finally came up to me to give me a hand. He put out his hand and pulled me up half way and . . . then let me go. I fell and hit my head on the hard cement. I can remember him laughing and telling his friends to look. He left and I remember hearing a crowd of male voices chanting, "N-I-G-G-E-R." I felt wet drops falling on my arms and legs . . . They were spitting on me . . . I felt so helpless.

I didn't find a job until ten months later. It was at a restaurant. Since then I have never desired to have a job as a secretary or anything pertaining to that field.

Moultrie grabs a book off her desk entitled: *Growing Up Black: From Slave Days to the Present: 25 African-Americans Reveal the Trials and Tribulations of Their Childhoods*. Moultrie searches for the story of Elizabeth Eckford, one of the first black pupils to integrate Little Rock's Central High School in 1957. She reads the painful, poignant account of Eckford's first day at school, when she was confronted by a racist mob screaming, "Lynch her!" and "No nigger bitch is going to get in our school." Moultrie's voice cracks and tears well up in her eyes. She faces the blackboard, so the class will not see her cry. She wipes her eyes and says, "Every time I read this passage I feel this girl's anguish. But this happened in 1957, so why do I get so upset? It's because this kind of thing is still going on. So we people of color better get our acts together. And fast. You hear me?"

Moultrie has an ebullient personality. She always is upbeat and enthusiastic in class, always intersperses her lectures with jokes and humorous asides. But there is a reservoir of anger beneath her placid exterior, an anger born of slights she has endured and bigotry she has observed over the years. Occasionally this anger erupts in class. "When I was a graduate student, I went to rent a cottage in a North Hollywood bungalow court," Moultrie tells the students. "None of these people who lived there had college degrees and I was a graduate student. But they looked at me like

I was dirt. I asked the guy who was renting the place, 'What's with these people?' He told me, 'Well, I promised that I wouldn't rent to any niggers . . .' "

She lowers her chin, and arches an eyebrow. "You see, some things haven't changed that much since 1957. There's still a lot of racism around. Some on the surface. Some beneath the surface.

"Look what's going on today. Look at Proposition 209 and how they took affirmative action away from us. And the way they justify it is pure hypocrisy. Don't tell me you care about equality and then make the playing field even more unequal. Unlike a lot of Crenshaw students before you, when you apply to colleges, you won't be getting any help from affirmative action. But at least all of you have a fighting chance. You're the *crème de la crème* in our community. You're the filet mignon. You'll be the doctors, dentists, lawyers, and accountants. You'll defy the media stereotype and movies like *Dangerous Minds*. You all aren't loud, boisterous, and raggedy. I know you aren't. Not all black men are in jail. Not all black women are Sapphires. Hel-*lo*!

"People say, 'Anita, you're too militant. You're too Afro-centric.' Yes, I'm militant. Yes, I'm Afro-centric. That's because I care about all of you. I got to watch out for my babies. Don't your mamas count on me for that? I love all of you." She places both palms over her heart, nods her head, and says softly, "I love you with the love of Christ. You know that.

"I care so much about teaching you for a lot of reasons, some of them selfish. Who else am I going to send to college? Not these boys who walk the halls all day, cutting class, scribbling their names on the walls. I want my children to go to black doctors, black dentists, black lawyers, and black accountants. *You* are the ones who are going to fill those professions. You are our community's best hope."

Gifted programs across the country are criticized because they are predominantly white; blacks and Latinos are dramatically underrepresented. These programs are, essentially, a bargaining chip, a way to persuade middle-class white parents to keep their children in public schools. Crenshaw's gifted program, of course, is quite different. Still, the practice of creating separate classes for gifted or high-achieving students—called tracking—is a controversial practice, even in minority schools.

Gifted is a subjective term, and the criteria for gifted programs across the country vary greatly. To qualify for Crenshaw's program, students must score at least 125 on an IQ exam. (The average IQ is about 100, and 120 to 129 is considered to be in the superior range.) Students can also qualify by scoring in the top 20th percentile in the nation on both the mathematics and verbal sections of a standardized exam. At some suburban schools, the minimum qualifying scores are much higher. But there is a great gap in standardized exam results between suburban and inner-city students. And students who can meet the criteria at Crenshaw's program have test scores that are considerably higher than the vast majority of South-Central students. For example, the tenth graders at Crenshaw who are not in the gifted program scored in the bottom twelfth percentile of the nation on a recent standardized reading exam.

In 1989, the Los Angeles Unified School Board planned to open a "highly gifted" magnet high school—for students with IQs over 150—in the San Fernando Valley. But several minority school-board members intimated that they might not support the program if a second "gifted" program was not created in a minority neighborhood.

In the past, promising students in South-Central who wanted to attend a highly ranked high school were bussed to the San Fernando Valley or West Los Angeles. Yet even after the creation of Crenshaw's gifted program, many top students in South-Central continued to participate in a voluntary bussing program because their parents still did not want to send their children to an inner-city high school. Recently, an increasing number of South-Central parents have grown disillusioned with bussing and have been won over by Crenshaw's gifted magnet.

Some South-Central teachers, however, do not like losing their best students to the gifted program. They complain that gifted programs are, inherently, antiegalitarian and elitist. They contend that Crenshaw's program excludes—and even stigmatizes—many bright students who do not make the cut. The program, they say, is a Band-Aid solution to an intractable problem, and merely diverts attention from the abysmal education that many nongifted inner-city students receive.

Supporters of Crenshaw's gifted program insist that it is the only way for talented minority students to get the preparation they need to succeed at top colleges, the only way they will be able to compete with their college classmates. Joseph Renzuli, the director of the National Research Center on the Gifted and Talented, wrote: "The middle class takes care of its own—SAT prep courses, reading material at home, summer computer classes. That's why we need programs that serve economically disadvantaged children who are gifted."

A landmark report by the U.S. Department of Education stated that many of the country's brightest students—particularly minority students— face a "quiet crisis" because they are not sufficiently challenged in school or encouraged to pursue rigorous course work. The report, the first comprehensive federal study on gifted students in twenty years, urges that the nation's school districts provide greater opportunity for gifted minority children.

"The talents of disadvantaged and minority children have been especially neglected," according to the report. "Almost one in four American children lives in poverty, representing an enormous pool of untapped talent. Yet most programs for these children focus on solving the problems they bring to school, rather than on challenging them to develop their strengths. It is sometimes assumed that children from unpromising backgrounds are not capable of outstanding accomplishment. Yet stories abound of disadvantaged children who achieve at high levels when nurtured sufficiently."

SEVENTEEN

OLIVIA

LEGAL LIMBO

On the first Friday following winter break, Little resumes her discussion of *Wuthering Heights*, but after about thirty minutes she stops midsentence and places her hands on her head. She staggers around the room in mock surprise.

"It's about time," she says, pointing to the door.

Olivia ambles through the classroom and takes her seat. She has just endured the worst Christmas vacation in her life. Her car would not run, she had no money to fix it and, since school was out, she could not ask her auto shop teacher for help. She was stuck at the foster home every day and, by the end of vacation, it felt more like a prison than a residence. She sat around the house watching soap operas, leafing through her custom Volkswagen magazines, worrying about her court date.

On Christmas day, there was only one other girl left at the foster home. Everyone else had gone to visit relatives. Olivia walked to the store, bought some brandy and egg nog, and she and the girl drank all afternoon. On Christmas night, she scoured the refrigerator for something to eat. She discovered some leftover gumbo, ate it in front of the television, had some more egg nog, and was grateful when she was inebriated enough to fall asleep and, mercifully, put an end to a wretched day.

Initially, Olivia was too depressed to return to school after winter break, but she finally decided to make up the exams and homework she missed. After Little resumes her lecture on *Wuthering Heights*, Olivia pulls a notebook and pen out of her purse. Venola fills her in on the assignments and exams she has missed in AP English and Government. Olivia jots it all down.

"Did you read *Wuthering Heights*?" Venola whispers.

Olivia shakes her head.

"Oh, it was goooood," Venola says.

"Actually I read the first chapter," Olivia says. "I just haven't had any time to read any more. It's been too crazy."

After class, Little walks over to her desk and asks her, "How'd it go in court?"

"I haven't gone to court yet," Olivia says. "It got delayed."

"To when?"

"Next Friday."

Early Friday morning, I stop by the foster home to give Olivia a ride to court because her car, once again, will not start. A series of roommates have trashed Olivia's bedroom. Someone punched several deep, jagged holes in a wall. On another wall, a few girls, using nail polish, printed their names in big block letters. Another wall is streaked with dirt and pencil slashes and hand prints. The tan curtains are so threadbare and torn they barely block the morning sun. On Olivia's small desk, she has neatly lined up her deodorant, hair spray, shampoo, and makeup.

She is dressed in a pool-table-green suit with a short, tight-fitting skirt—a questionable choice for court. She is wearing black patent leather high heels, large gold hoop earrings, and her hair is pulled back into a ponytail, with one long swirl sweeping across her forehead, down to the corner of an eye.

As we drive east along the Santa Monica Freeway, Olivia somberly stares out the window. It is a cool, wind-swept morning, one of those rare mornings in Los Angeles when the air, thinned of pollutants, is truly translucent, and the downtown skyline is sharply silhouetted against a powder blue sky. Beyond the skyline loom the San Gabriel Mountains, which usually are obscured by smog, with only a faint, vaporous outline visible. On this sparkling January morning, however, it is as if a scrim has been lifted and the mountains look majestic in the winter light, with sharply etched ridge lines, a purple escarpment, dappled shadows in the canyons, and a dusting of snow along the peaks.

"I'm not nervous," Olivia says, talking more to herself than to me, as if to psych herself up. "I figure the worst that can happen is that I get a few years' probation." She resumes staring dolefully out the window.

We arrive at Eastlake Juvenile Court, a low-slung, faded yellow-brick building on a winding side street in East Los Angeles. The entrance to this grim civic structure is flanked by a few arthritic palm trees with desiccated, brown fronds broken at the base and swaying in the wind. Olivia lines up by the metal detector at the door. She empties her purse on the luggage X-ray machine and walks through the metal detector. After she buys a cup of coffee and a sweet roll in the snack shop, she sits on a bench outside the courtroom where her case is scheduled to be tried.

Eastlake, the busiest juvenile court in the county, has a single long, dim, narrow hallway flanked by courtrooms with graffiti-scarred wooden benches outside. The linoleum floor is cracked and the low ceiling is lined with stained and chipped perforated tiles. The noisy hallway is crowded with attorneys—conferring with witnesses and clients or cutting deals with prosecutors—and Latino gangbangers, with spider-web tattoos on their necks and gang tattoos covering their arms, and the occasional hardened-looking gang girl with a tear drop tattooed under her eye, and black gangbangers with corn rows and pants worn so low that half of their boxers are showing. They look so menacing it is easy to forget that, according to the law, they are all children.

Most of them are accompanied by a single parent. Only one boy is with both parents. Olivia is alone. She sips her coffee and nibbles on her sweet roll, waiting for her foster mother to arrive. When she finishes breakfast, she slumps on the bench. She has an expression of weary resignation, like an elderly pensioner waiting at a bus stop.

Her court-appointed lawyer, Peter Weiss, rushes up to her, and leads her to a corner of the hallway, where they can confer. He has just had a brief conference with the judge about her case. His gray hair is disheveled, he is out of breath, and his briefcase is overflowing with a host of other juvenile cases he is handling.

"Apparently your probation officer was not impressed with you," Weiss says. "She thought you were arrogant. She thought you rationalized the whole thing. Why couldn't you have just said you were sorry?"

Before Olivia answers, he spots her foster mother, Gretchen Fairconnetue, ambling down the hallway. He motions her over. A few weeks ago, Weiss met with Olivia and Fairconnetue. She had threatened to kick Olivia out because of her arrest.

"Have you decided yet?" Weiss asks. "Can she continue to live with you?"

"I don't know," replies Fairconnetue, a small, taciturn black woman who works at the post office.

"If she can't stay with you, the judge has indicated she might sentence her to do time in a camp for juvenile offenders."

Olivia's eyes widen with fear. "You know the other girl who was arrested with me at the bank?" Olivia asks. "She went to court recently and only got probation. How come I'm facing camp?"

"How do you know she got that?"

"I go to the same school as her. So I know. I think we're being treated different 'cause she's got parents." Olivia stares at her shoes and says softly, "That's not fair."

Weiss shrugs. He turns to Fairconnetue and asks, "Do you want her?" Weiss asks.

"No," Fairconnetue says evenly.

"If you don't want her, where's she going to go?" Weiss asks.

"If she gonna stay with me, I want more money," Fairconnetue says.

"I don't know if you can get more money."

"Well, that's what I want. If she's on parole, I want more money."

The lawyer stares at Fairconnetue, exasperated. "How's Olivia doing at home?"

"She do what she want to do. She not an easy girl."

Olivia extends a hand toward Fairconnetue and pleads, "Will you keep me?"

"I don't know if I want to keep you. You have to learn you can't have your way all the time. You can't be doin' these criminal things."

"I stopped," Olivia says.

"Yeah. 'Cause you got caught."

The lawyer checks his watch. "I can't stay here all morning. I got to get out of here by 10:30 because I have another case." He asks Fairconnetue, "You going to tell the judge you're willing to keep Olivia?"

Fairconnetue glares at him. "I don't know *what* I'm going to say."

"Can't I just go to another foster home?" Olivia asks.

"It's getting too late for that," Weiss says. "Will you keep her?" he asks Fairconnetue.

"I don't think so."

"Look, she's not a bad girl," Weiss says. "She just got caught in this stupid check thing. But since you haven't entirely made up your mind about Olivia, let's put this thing off for a few weeks."

"I don't want to," Fairconnetue says. "I don't want to have to come back here."

"All we're doing is delaying your decision. At that point you can make up your mind."

Fairconnetue stares sullenly at him.

"In the meantime, we can talk to Olivia's social worker and see if we can get you some additional money."

Fairconnetue raises both eyebrows and nods enthusiastically.

"Frankly," Weiss says, "I don't understand why you think you deserve extra money if she's on probation. But I'll talk to the social worker about it, anyway. I can see that, today, we're not going to resolve whether Olivia can finish out the year with you. So let's come back in three weeks. I'll talk to the judge. By then you'll have made up your mind about Olivia. Remember, if you won't let her stay with you, the judge will probably just send her to camp. They'll pull her out of school and she'll be locked up."

Olivia stares intently at Fairconnetue, trying to glean some sign from her stony expression. Fairconnetue returns Olivia's stare and then emits a loud harrumph, lifts her chin, and marches down the hallway, out the door, and into the parking lot, leaving Weiss looking bewildered and Olivia chewing a cuticle, anxious and distressed.

It is Monday morning, January 27, the last AP English class before the final exam on Wednesday, which will conclude the first semester. Little opens the class by playing a tape recording of a teacher from England reading a chapter of *Wuthering Heights* in a strong, Yorkshire accent— where the novel is set. Olivia arrives midway through the recording, wearing faded jeans and a tattered sweatshirt. Her hair is unbrushed and she wears no makeup. She pays no attention to the recording and just stares disconsolately out the window.

After Little plays the recording, she asks the class, "What does Chapter 13 reveal?"

"How wicked love can be," Latisha says.

"Yeah," Miesha says. "I'd go to Heathcliff and me and that brutha would have a talk."

"Cathy should have given Heathcliff a chance," Venola says. "She should have given him a chance to make money and be a success."

"Even though he's not a nice person, like Edgar?" Little asks.

"Nice ain't all that," Latisha says. "If he just nice, it ain't gonna jump off. Let's say some brutha not so nice. But if I get that *warm* feelin' from him and my kids like him, well, all right then."

The class erupts in laughter and Little tries to quiet them. "Should Catherine have married Heathcliff, even if he couldn't provide for her financially in the way she wanted?"

"If my man ain't makin' no money and he just layin' up at home, well, that's no good," Miesha says. "I won't stand for that."

"Speak on it, girl," a student calls out.

"It wasn't just about the jack [money]," Latisha says. "Catherine thought the brutha was dirty and stanky, too."

"Are you impressed with the level of heart and soul that their love represented?" Little asks the class. "Or do you think their love was the height of indulgence? Don't forget, a lot of people were harmed because of their love. Doesn't that sound familiar?'' Little slips to one knee and says, in a quavering voice, '' 'I loved her *too* much. If I can't have her, *no one* can.' ''

"Othello," Curt calls out.

"No," Little says. "A more recent character.''

There is a long silence. The students glance at each other uneasily. A few students mutter, "Uh oh.''

Little nods. "That's right. O.J. Heathcliff has *that* level of love. Do all you girls want to be loved like Catherine?''

"No," Miesha says. "That's scary.''

"You're damn right it's scary," Little says. "But isn't this the kind of love that our society promotes? I see so many girls here at Crenshaw who are just floating, not getting their educations, mooning, and spending all their time with some guy. These girls don't have a clue.''

"Who are you to say I treat my man wrong," Miesha says, looking miffed. "It all depends on who you are and who you with.''

"Where do you learn about love?" Little asks the class. "From the record industry? From movies? If you're my age and you're not married, there's supposed to be something wrong with you. All you hear today is love, love, love.''

This prompts a spirited, rambling discussion on Heathcliff's love for Catherine, how black men treat black women, how black women treat black men. For a half hour, the students shout and pound on their desks and argue and laugh and stamp their feet. Little has managed, once again, to engage the class, showing them how the themes in a nineteenth-century English novel apply to their lives. The ringing bell halts the clamor, but as the students file out, many continue the discussion. Little bangs her coffee cup on her desk and calls out, "Remember, your *Wuthering Heights* essays are due this week.''

As Olivia walks out, Little stops her. "How'd it go in court on Friday?''

"It's been put off again," Olivia says, staring at the ground. "But they're talking about sending me to camp.''

"I heard you had a cavalier attitude and your probation officer didn't like that."

"What's cavalier?"

Little waves her hand impatiently. "Look, you got to be like: 'I'm sooo sorry. I won't do it again. I learned my lesson.' "

"Okay," Olivia says, without much enthusiasm.

She walks toward the door, but stops and looks over the shoulder of a girl who is studying a magazine that features dozens of pastel prom dresses. Olivia looks longingly at a few of the pictures.

"You going?" a boy asks her.

"I don't think so," Olivia says.

"That's what they all say."

"No, I mean it," she says. "I might be in jail."

He warily backs out the door.

As Olivia follows him into the hallway, Little calls out, "Look up cavalier in the dictionary."

EIGHTEEN

TONI LITTLE

THE RIDE OF THEIR LIVES

After weeks of rainy or overcast days, the clouds clear Wednesday morning. A glorious golden light washes across the campus and the classroom windows shimmer in the sunshine. It is one of those false spring days when the unseasonably warm weather and brilliant sunshine bake the ground and the subtropical plants and flowers bloom—in the middle of winter. A soft breeze carries across the campus the smell of orange blossoms.

When the eight o'clock bell rings, all the students are in their seats—except Olivia. Little wonders if Olivia is too distracted with her legal problems to show up for the final. She also wonders if Claudia will turn in her exam. This is her last chance. If she does well on the final, Little will pass her. If she does not submit her exam, she will flunk the class and might not graduate.

Little hands out copies of the three-part final. The first part is a twenty-five-question objective exam on *Wuthering Heights*. The second part lists four questions and the students are required to answer two. The first question is: "Describe the point of view that Brontë uses in *Wuthering*

Heights. Explain why this point of view is particularly effective for this novel . . .''

Little decides to give the students the opportunity to do something unconventional in the third part: ''. . . I believe that you have learned the most valuable lessons from authors who have presented characters of depth and insight . . . on your own, without my instruction . . . *Decide which work most impacted your mind.* After deciding, choose a character from that work whom you grew to understand. Write a letter to this character. In this letter, express the things about the character that you grew to understand . . . Express the lessons that you learned on a personal level from the character. . . . Write this letter from a stream-of-consciousness level. You do not need to present formal discourse on the subject; however, you may wish to offer scholarly ideas about the themes you wish to discuss.''

As soon as Little hands out the exams, the students—including Claudia—hunch over their desks and start to write. As Little wanders up and down the aisles, Claudia drapes her arm over her paper so Little cannot see her work.

At 8:30, Olivia shuffles into the classroom. Little stares at her irritably for a moment and then hands her the exam.

When the students finish their exams, Braxton stares out his office window, in a bittersweet mood. He has decided to take the school district's assistant-principal exam. If he passes, he knows he probably will be assigned to a new school next year.

About an hour after he received the news, Olivia's social worker calls. She tells him Olivia's probation officer is recommending that the judge send her to a juvenile detention camp because she has shown no remorse and because of her history of going AWOL. The social worker has not decided what to recommend to the judge and wants Braxton's opinion.

He certainly does not want Olivia consigned to a camp, he tells her, but he feels Olivia needs to learn a lesson, needs to understand the consequences of her actions. He tells the social worker that if it were up to him, he would delay sentencing until June. If Olivia graduates with perfect attendance and good grades and does not go AWOL again, he would put her on probation and allow her to attend college. If she screws up, he would send her to a camp.

The social worker thanks Braxton and tells him she will let him know when she makes a decision.

As the bell rings, the students hand in their final exams to the front of their rows and file out the door. Claudia grabs her backpack, which is stuffed with books—not school books, but books she is reading for enjoyment, including *A Brief History of Time* by Stephen Hawking. She tries to slip out of class, unobtrusively, but Little stops her.

"Did you turn it in?" Little asks.

Embarrassed, Claudia mutters, "No."

"Why not?" Little asks.

Claudia blushes and stammers, lowers her head and rushes into the hall. Little watches her and says, "Well, that's it for Claudia." (Students who flunk a semester of an AP class are dropped from the class.) Claudia will now have to transfer to a less challenging English class at Crenshaw. The only question remaining is if Claudia will have the gumption to make up this F at night school so she can graduate and be eligible for college.

After the classroom empties, Little walks to a corner of the room and basks for a moment in the sunshine streaming through the window. "The stream-of-consciousness part of the final is important to me," she says. "I wanted to see which of the characters touched them to the core, if the literature impacted who they are and who they will become. That's the whole premise of my instruction. That's why I became a teacher."

Little often tells her classes that there was a single "inciting moment" that compelled her to be a teacher. When President John F. Kennedy was murdered in Dallas, school was canceled, and Little's third-grade class was sent home. She huddled around the television set with her family, watching the newscasts and a montage of Kennedy's memorable speeches. When she saw the clip of Kennedy calling on Americans to "Ask not what your country can do for you, ask what you can do for your country," she was riveted. That speech, she tells her students, sparked her conviction and her social conscience; it impelled her to become a teacher.

When she is enthusiastic about teaching, this is her explanation. When she is drained by some personal battle at Crenshaw, and less sanguine about her career, she offers a different account. "I needed a job," she says one afternoon after school. "Teaching wasn't so much a calling as a way to make a living. I figured, I'd do it for awhile, then maybe try something else."

These two contradictory accounts are not mutually exclusive; both stories contain elements of truth. And they reflect much about her cyclonic personality, her alternating moods of idealism and cynicism, graciousness and pettiness. One day she might be inspired in class, passionate about teaching; the next day she might be peevish and uninterested in the literature. One day she might show great concern for a student; the next day she might be so self-absorbed that she ignores a half dozen troubled students.

Little grew up in Lomita, a working-class community south of Los Angeles. Her mother was a nurse and her father was a house painter who would put on his derby with the green shamrock every Friday night and join his Irish buddies at the neighborhood bar. Little has five brothers and sisters and she was always considered the intellectual of the family. She loved to read, and in the third grade she was classified by the school district as gifted. But she was an indifferent student, and during high school she spent more time in Hermosa Beach, surfing with her friends, than she spent studying.

Theater, however, captured her interest, and during her junior and senior year she worked backstage with a drama teacher during the student productions. When she enrolled at California State University, Long Beach, she began dating the drama teacher. When she was twenty she moved in with him.

During the next few years, Little, who had a double major of English and film, worked her way through college as a waitress and then earned her teaching credential. She obtained a job at a magnet high school for the performing arts in the San Fernando Valley—the same school where the man she lived with taught.

Little has such a spontaneous, theatrical manner that she was a natural drama teacher, and the students were drawn to her. She especially appreciated the freedom of putting on productions, running the shows, creating her own fiefdom at the high school, without any interference from administrators. This was an idyllic time for her. Her work was fulfilling. And she was living with a man she deeply loved, whom she envisioned marrying.

Her world was decimated one afternoon when she heard a rumor that he was having an affair with a woman who worked in a delicatessen near the school. The woman was a voluptuous blonde who bore such an uncanny resemblance to Marilyn Monroe that she was sometimes hired to impersonate the actress at parties.

When Little returned home that night, she confronted him.

"I'm not having an affair with her, but I'd like to," he told Little. "I want to pursue a relationship with this woman."

As Little stood there, stunned, he asked her to move out. He then said matter-of-factly, "Some things just come to an end."

He owned the house, but Little refused to leave. She was so adamant, her refusal so implacable, that he did now know what to do. So he told her she could move into his guest cottage on the property. Little agreed because she was convinced that his affair was just a fling; she simply would not accept that their relationship was over. Eventually, she believed, he would come back to her. He did not.

She lived in the guest house for two years before she finally abandoned all hope. Bitter and defeated, she found her own apartment.

She still has not completely recovered from the breakup. It was so devastating to her, she believes, because this was her first serious relationship, and the man was much more than just a boyfriend. She met him when she was just a high school girl. She idolized him. He guided her through high school and college and the first few years of her career. He influenced what she studied in college, what career she chose. He was such a significant part of her past that she could not imagine the future without him. Then he abruptly terminated the relationship, as if he were canceling a Saturday night date, casually dismissing their years together, which had meant so much to her. The relationship consumed almost a decade of her life—almost five years with him and several more years of therapy. She has not had a long-term relationship with a man since then.

"It was very damaging," she says, stubbing out a cigarette. She stares into the ashtray and says, "It created a bitterness in me. I'd been really passionate about life . . . When it was over, I lost some of that passion."

Little survived the breakup by sublimating all of her grief into her student plays. She often spent more than twelve hours a day at school, directing the plays, helping to build the sets and design the costumes. After three years of working late in the evenings with her students, her career was almost destroyed. She was forced to leave the school, in a firestorm of controversy. She had been accused of having sex with students.

During the school's investigation, the principal wrote in a memo to Little: "I brought to your attention that I was investigating rumors and allegations that had been verbally made by students and parents to . . . staff members . . . These allegations and rumors were that you had sexual relations with male students, had hugged and kissed them during class . . . and that you had in the presence of students, talked openly of your personal life implying sexual connotations . . . I told you I had talked with the male students allegedly involved and that they had denied any involvement outside of the teacher/student relationship."

At the conclusion of the investigation—after she left the school—the district superintendent wrote a letter to Little, informing her that she had been exonerated. "I can assure you," the superintendent wrote, "that . . . the principal's investigation of the matter has resulted in your total vindication, and that you were so notified . . . and [the principal's] memo . . . includes the following statement: '. . . my investigation to date had produced no evidence to support the allegation of sexual relations between you and the male students.' "

The rumors began, Little says, after a student's father asked her to house-sit for a week while he was on vacation. Although his son stayed at his grandmother's during this time, some students, and later some misinformed parents, Little says, gossiped about the arrangement. The speculation and innuendo persisted, she says, because several boys had crushes on her, and because she was young, worked closely with the students on productions—sometimes until midnight—and talked to students like peers.

Little was traumatized when she was forced to leave the school and forced to fight for her job and her reputation. This is one reason why she is now so distrustful of authority, why administrators find her so defensive and fractious.

She found a job the next fall at another San Fernando Valley high school. Putting on big productions, working long hours, directing the young, aspiring actors and actresses, helped her forget the ordeal at her previous job. Once again she realized how much she enjoyed teaching. But after a few years, she decided to see if she could earn a living producing drama instead of teaching it. Little took a sabbatical from the school district, and she and a friend produced a play that chronicled Bob Dylan's life and his music. Little enjoyed the experience immensely. The play, however, was a bust. It closed after a two-week run at a San Francisco theater.

When Little returned to Los Angeles, school was already in session so she could not land a teaching job that semester. She eventually found a job at an entertainment public-relations firm, which hired her because of her experience drumming up publicity for the Dylan play.

Little decided to try a career change, and she stayed at the firm for several years. Los Angeles teachers are allowed to take up to thirty-nine months off without losing their seniority. At the end of Little's thirty-nine months she decided to return to teaching. She was bored with setting up press interviews for celebrity clients—in addition to arranging their hair salon appointments and limousine pickups. She missed the intellectual stimulation of the classroom.

Little taught for a year at a Watts high school, and her complaints—then—are almost identical to her complaints—now—at Crenshaw. "The administrators were total fascists," she says with contempt. "The principal was a district henchman who was put in place to get rid of someone like me, someone inclined to teach ideas. The assistant principal always hassled me. They weren't interested in instruction. It was an anti-teacher environment. They tried to turn the teachers into factory workers. I liked the kids—I always like the kids—and they liked me. But I didn't feel welcome by the teachers. Most of them were black. I don't think they wanted me there. It was a racist environment.''

She obtained a temporary, one-year position at another school. The following year there was an opening at Crenshaw's gifted magnet program, and the school district sent her there to interview for the job because she had experience teaching at another magnet school—the drama magnet. After an interview, the Crenshaw principal hired her. A week later, the principal transferred to another school and a new principal, Yvonne Noble, was hired. Noble asked an administrator at a school where Little had previously taught what he thought of her. ''She's a fool,'' the administrator told Noble. ''But she can teach.''

During Little's first few years at Crenshaw, she impressed both Noble and Braxton. Little, who had more experience teaching drama than English, dedicated herself to learning as much as she could about Advanced Placement classes, interpreting literature, and teaching gifted children. She attended conferences every month, enrolled in summer workshops, and read extensively. She was a martinet when it came to essay writing, and marked up almost every sentence on students' papers. By the end of the year, however, Noble and Braxton were amazed at how her students' writing had improved. During her first year at Crenshaw, about half of Little's students passed the AP English exam, an extremely high ratio for an inner-city high school.

But during the past two years, Little has devoted an increasing amount of class time on tangents, railing about her battles with the administration, her many irritations at the school, and other topics that take time away from instruction. She is more short-tempered with students, more sensitive to slights, more irascible with administrators. Last year only three out of the seventeen students in her class passed the AP exam. Braxton and Noble are concerned that, if Little does not regain her focus, the pass rate will be even lower this year.

Little owns a duplex in Culver City, down the street from the Culver Studios movie lot, about five miles northwest of Crenshaw. She rents out one of the units and lives in the other, a small one-bedroom apartment. While Little can be intimidating at school, at home she caters to the whims and moods of her three yapping Papillons—toy spaniels that look like long-hair Chihuahuas. She talks to them in a high-pitched, sing-song voice, frequently interrupting a conversation to hug and cuddle them.

Little often spends Saturday nights with a girlfriend at a karaoke bar near the airport, singing '60s standards. She is close with her sisters—they are married and have children—and visits them on vacations. On week nights, her house is a gathering spot for a group of friends, who frequently stop by to sip wine and smoke cigarettes. Sometimes, students show up on weekends to use her computer. And Olivia, on occasion, will help her organize her files on Sunday mornings, and Little will treat her to breakfast at a local diner.

Little has a part-time job—twice a week, after school—teaching juvenile offenders at a halfway house how to use computers. The house, a way station from juvenile hall to the streets, is a frenzied place, where the halls echo with shouts and screams and altercations. Little is a surprisingly calm presence amid the furor. She is happy because there are no school administrators here, and she is in complete control of her classroom. Little rarely has problems with her students. And these students are no exception, even if they are thieves and muggers and hard-core gangbangers. She enjoys teaching them, and they respond to her.

Because Little does not have a husband or a family, because she is not involved in a serious relationship, her job—or the peripheries of her job—is the focus for all of her intensity and volatility. For better or for worse. She is easily ensnared by office politics and takes every slight at school personally. She elevates each skirmish into a war.

"If I were married with children, maybe I wouldn't care so much," she says, shrugging. "I'd probably be out the door every day at three o'clock . . . and I wouldn't look back."

While Little can be snappish in English class, most of the students are entertained by her flamboyant personality, the melodramatic way she characterizes every conflict. Some worry about her, and wonder if she will stick it out at Crenshaw until the end of the year.

One morning, Latisha says to Little in class, "You seem so riled up all the time. Don't you like us?"

"Yes, I like you," Little says. "It's the administrators and a few of the teachers I can't deal with."

"Would you leave us?" Latisha asks. "I don't want you to leave."

Little shrugs. "If the working conditions don't improve, I can't make you any promises."

On the last day of the semester, Little fumes in her classroom during a free period after reading a memo the principal sent to all the teachers: "Please submit a copy of each of the final examinations that you administered and place them in the administration box by two o'clock Friday." Most of the teachers do not mind the request, but Little views it as a challenge to her authority.

"I'm outraged," Little says, pacing in her empty classroom. "Like I don't have enough to do. I've had it. This is a factory. I'm a widget maker on an assembly line here."

Her rant is interrupted when she hears loud voices in the hall. She rushes out the door and confronts two menacing, tattooed gangbangers with shaved heads, who are cutting class. Little, however, is not intimidated. She marches up to them and says, "Get out of this hall. You're disturbing me."

"Who are *you*?" one asks, staring at her sullenly.

Little jabs a finger in his face and shouts, "*Never* talk to me like that again! You got that? I'm going to call security and they're going to drag your ass out of here. What do you think of *that*?"

The two boys exchange an uneasy glance. They are not afraid of security. But they do not know what to make of this woman with the wild eyes and disheveled hair who is screaming at them. The students jog down the hall, eager to get away from her, but she sprints after them, shouting, "Stop! Come back here!" When a teacher sticks his head out of his classrooms, Little yells, "Call security!"

Two school policemen arrive and Little offers a physical description of the students. She returns to her classroom and tells me that earlier in the day, two Latino students, who were sitting in the bleachers, were robbed by six black gangbangers. The victims refused to identify the robbers, Little says, because they were afraid of retaliation. They have decided to transfer next semester to a high school with a larger Latino population.

"Isn't that typical of this place," Little says. "The semester ends with a robbery."

Little grouses about the final exam Moultrie gave to her eleventh graders. Moultrie showed a segment of the television series *Roots,* and then the students wrote essays comparing and contrasting how Margaret Walker in *Jubilee* and Hollywood depict slavery.

"Moultrie's teaching *self-esteem,*" Little says with disdain. "I'm teaching James Joyce and Emily Brontë. Yet I'm the one who's called into meetings and gets disciplined. I'm the one who has to defend myself."

She stands up and resumes pacing. "I don't know how much longer I can stand this place. There are people here who hate me. Well, if that's the way they feel, I'll *really* give them a reason to hate me. I'm pulling out all the stops. Next semester I'm going to give these students the ride of their lives."

PART THREE

SECOND SEMESTER

NINETEEN

WILLIE

WISHING IT WAS JUST A DREAM

Little spends the brief break between semesters reflecting on the past few months. She realizes that the distractions of the first semester prevented her from properly preparing her students for the AP exam. The exam is in only three months, and she is acutely aware of how much there is still to do. She decides that she has to stop obsessing about her squabbles and grudges, that she must regain her focus in the classroom. She feels she owes it to her students.

On the first Monday in February—the first day of the second semester—Little addresses the class the moment the 8 A.M. bell rings. "Write down on a piece of paper what you think the literary term 'theme' means," she tells the class. After the students finish, Little writes on the blackboard: "In literature, the theme is the central or dominating idea . . . The message that's implicit in a work . . . The subject of a poem may be a flower; its theme may be . . . the fleeting nature of existence . . ."

Little introduces the next work the class will read, the play: *The Elephant Man*. After *The Elephant Man*, the class will study *Hamlet*. Little assigns more plays than most English teachers, partly because of her drama background. She also believes that, because the students play the parts in class, they can fully "inhabit the roles," easily identify with the characters, and quickly grasp the literary concepts she is trying to teach them. Another advantage to assigning plays is that while students are reading their parts, Little can sometimes slip into a corner of the room and catch up on paperwork.

"Some of you are familiar with the movie version of *The Elephant Man*," Little says. "What do you think the theme is?"

Latisha raises her hand. "Ain't this the same Elephant Man that Michael Jackson's interested in? Didn't he want to buy the brutha's bones?"

Little ignores her, and says, "The theme of *The Elephant Man* is man's inhumanity to man."

After Little passes out copies of the play to the class, the students fight for all the roles—except one. Everyone agrees that it would be appropriate if Princess portrays the part of the princess in the play. Little assigns the other roles, and the students begin reading their parts.

A few minutes before the end of class, Little stops the reading and tells the students, "The AP test will be here in only a few months. So let's make the most of the time we have left. I want everybody here on time from now on. I'm going to start locking the door at eight o'clock, sharp, and I'm not going to let anyone in who's late." Then she adds, more to herself, it seems, than to the students, "We need to stay focused. We've got a lot of work to do in here. So let's not get sidetracked."

It does not take long for Little to get sidetracked again. The next day, a civil jury finds O.J. Simpson responsible for the deaths of his ex-wife and Ronald Goldman and orders him to pay $8.5 million in compensatory damages. Two years ago—when the students were in Little's tenth-grade English class—she frequently interrupted class to inveigh against Simpson and a society insensitive to the plight of women. Whenever the students were bored in class, or wanted to goad Little for amusement, they would bring up the case. But this year, the students were so tired of listening to her diatribes that whenever the subject of O.J. emerged during class discussion, they often exchanged uneasy glances and attempted to change the subject.

On the morning after the verdict, Little struts into the classroom, grinning. As soon as the bell rings, she tells the students, "I'm so happy. I'm jubilant. Eight point five million bucks, baby."

"They wanted it to be equal," Latisha says. "They gave the black folks a verdict. So now they gave the white folks a verdict. Anyway, fuck O.J. He never did nothin' for me or my folks. But I wouldn't mind, at least, some respect from the brutha."

"O.J. Simpson is *never* going to give you respect," Little says. "He's a murderer."

"You don't know that," a girl says. "You don't know if he did it."

Little tries to respond, but the students shout her down.

"Nicole was sleeping around," a girl says. "She took drugs. She was a junkie."

"She wasn't a junkie—because she had money," Miesha says. "If you're white and take drugs, you're a recreational drug user. But when we take drugs, we're crackheads."

"What's O.J. favorite drink?" a boy calls out.

"Slice," a few students answer in unison, laughing.

After forty-five minutes of arguing and wrangling about the case, Little finally quiets the students and they resume reading the play. At the end of the class, she writes their essay assignment on the blackboard: "Part I: The central character of a novel or play often encounters moral, physical, or psychological danger. Select a situation . . . in which either John Merrick or Dr. Treves encounters danger . . .

"Part II: Recall an incident or situation in your life, when you encountered moral, physical, or psychological danger. Describe how you reacted to the situation and how your reaction demonstrated strength or weakness of character."

When the students hand in their essays the following week, Little is surprised—and moved—by Willie's essay. Willie, who is six feet four, with a full beard and a diamond stud earring, has the appearance and self-assurance of a man in his mid-twenties. He is outgoing and popular, active in student government and enrolled in several honors classes. Little has known Willie for three years, but it is only after she reads his essay that she learns, for the first time, about his grim childhood.

"I didn't grow up with any of my brothers and sisters," Willie wrote. *We all lived in our own homes and had our own families and our own lives. . . .*

"I lived with an aunt. Two of my brothers lived with a grandmother, 365 miles away. My sister lived with another grandmother, 30 minutes away. And my other brother lived with an aunt, just 10 minutes away. The last time we lived together as a family was twelve years ago, when I was just five years old . . .

"We had what one would consider to be a stable family. That is until my mother became addicted to crack cocaine.

"Her dependency on the drug destroyed our lives completely. One night the police came and arrested my mother. We didn't know what to do, until an officer came and told us to follow him. We were going to McClaren Hall [the county shelter for abandoned and abused children]. We stayed there for weeks while my mother was on trial. We waited for the social worker to find us placement for the duration of the time my mother would be in jail.

"A vivid memory of mine is standing on one side of a gate staring at my sister, as she stood on the other side. We were happy to see each other, but yet we wouldn't hug, speak, or even wave to one another. We could only smile.

"As time passed, I began to forget what happened. I kind of pushed it to the back of my head, wishing and hoping that it was just a dream and would go away. But it didn't.

"On holidays, I would long to be with my mother and brothers and sisters, but that was impossible. Some nights I would lie awake, crying and praying for the ones I truly loved. I felt I had no one to turn to. Not my teachers, friends, or even God, Himself, because, to me, He, too, had let me down.

"So I began to work harder in school. Trying to get everyone to like me, especially the adults, so I could feel loved. I always joined a lot of clubs and organizations, so I could stay after school late because I didn't want to go home . . .

"In high school, I began to realize that I was not just another person

*that attended the school. I was an individual. I didn't like followin[g]
all the other kids did. I liked to lead the other kids. So I began a career in
school politics. My ninth grade year, I ran for student body president and
won. That one day was one of the most joyous days of my life.*

*"I joined a lot of new clubs and organizations during my first years in
high school, such as speech and debate, and stayed active in student government. I also joined varsity football and ran track. I even worked Saturdays
and Sundays, eight hours a day, at the local McDonald's . . .*

*"Now I'm a senior, getting ready for graduation and a new life. Some
might say I've encountered a lot at a very young age. This is true. But it
has only made me a stronger and better person."*

Before his mother was arrested, she often left Willie and his brother
and sisters alone for long stretches of time. When she returned, Willie
recalls feeling perplexed, as he watched her fire up a glass pipe and smoke
a little white rock. One afternoon, after she had been gone for several
days, Willie's aunt stopped by and noticed that all the children were alone
and the electricity had been shut off. She called the police.

After his mother was arrested, Willie, who was the youngest child,
lived with his aunt. His parents were divorced, his father worked the
swing shift at the post office and did not think he could properly supervise
a young child. But after Willie lived with his aunt for a few months,
Willie Sr. changed his mind and brought his son home. He arranged for
Willie's cousin to take care of him at night, while he was at work.

Every day, he picked Willie up after elementary school and they had
an early dinner at a fast-food restaurant. They talked about what Willie
learned in school that day. His father, a Vietnam veteran, always encouraged Willie, emphasizing the importance of education. He always told
Willie, "Don't do what I did. Get an education. Follow your dreams."

After dinner, Willie's father dropped him off at his cousin's house and
drove him home after work. But Willie did not like sleeping at his cousin's,
waking up at midnight, when his dad arrived, and then trying to fall asleep
again when they reached home. When he was ten, his father let him stay
home alone. And he was on his own every night, through elementary
school, junior high school, and high school. One afternoon, he was watch-

ing an *Oprah* segment on latchkey kids, and after the show he recalls thinking: "Hey, that's me."

For much of Willie's childhood he was lonely. By the time he started junior high school, he saw his father even less. They no longer had dinner together because school was not out until midafternoon and Willie participated in so many extracurricular activities. It was only on weekends that Willie was able to spend time with his father.

In an autobiographical essay, Willie wrote how forlorn he felt after receiving his first poor grade in high school. "I wanted to cry," he wrote. "Actually I just needed someone to talk to about it. Then I remembered, once again, there was no one."

Still, Willie never hung out on the street, was never tempted to join a gang or do drugs. He spent his evenings finishing homework and, during his senior year, putting in thirty to forty hours a week as an usher at a movie theater. Willie saw how hard his father labored at the post office, how concerned his father was with his grades. He did not want to disappoint him.

In elementary school and junior high school, if Willie's grades slipped, his father would withhold his allowance, or refuse to let him use the telephone, or curtail some other privilege. All of Willie's teachers knew his father because he never missed a parent-teacher conference and he frequently called to check on his son's progress.

Willie was one of only three tenth graders on the varsity football team, but his father persuaded him to quit. "You'll be too tired to do your homework," his father told him. "Sports, ultimately, isn't going to get you anywhere. They're just going to use you."

His father is always giving him advice, always lecturing him, always warning him about the dangers a young black male faces in inner-city America. His friends, many of whom rarely see their fathers, envy Willie. They tell him that the relationship reminds them of the movie, *Boyz N the Hood*, and the close relationship between the father—a strong, caring, opinionated black man—and his son.

After Willie's mother was arrested, she moved to San Jose. But the summer before his senior year, he spotted her passed out on the front yard of a house in the neighborhood. She had just been released from jail and was back on drugs. He called his brother, who lived in San Jose, and asked him to drive down, pick her up, and take her home. Willie cried often that summer, thinking about how much he loved his mother and how he missed her, thinking about her on that front lawn, disheveled and disoriented.

Later that summer, Willie attended a program for high school students at Pepperdine University in Malibu. He was dazzled by the beauty of the campus, the sweeping ocean views and bucolic foothill setting. At home, he could hear the police helicopters hovering overhead, the occasional fusillade of gunfire in the distance. At Pepperdine, he listened to the crash of the surf and the wind rustling through the eucalyptus trees.

Willie was assured of receiving a scholarship to Pepperdine and planned to enroll there in the fall. His father was elated with the choice. He liked the idea of Willie attending a private Christian college, only an hour away from home. He is so close to his son, he wants to remain involved in his life, even during college.

At the beginning of Willie's senior year, he was almost certain he would attend Pepperdine. But in October, when he had the opportunity to join a group of students on a tour of black colleges in the South, he decided to go. "Visiting these schools changed my mind," Willie says. "At Pepperdine, the only black students I saw were the basketball players. But when I got to Morehouse College, I looked around and felt something deep within me. It was like a religious calling. In L.A., black people are portrayed negatively. But in Atlanta, I saw so many successful black professional people. I felt like this is where I was supposed to be."

When Willie told his father about his decision, they argued. Atlanta was too far from home, his father felt. And, he told Willie, an all-black college was too insular, too removed from reality. Willie grew up in a black neighborhood and attended predominantly black schools. His father felt that Willie should attend a school that reflected the reality of America, that would prepare him to interact with different races, that would prepare him for a future in the corporate world.

Willie was torn between his desire to please his father and his need to assert his independence. After a few stressful days, his father called him one night from work and said, "I just wanted to tell you that whatever your decision, I'm behind you 100 percent.'' Willie was relieved. Now he could apply to Morehouse—with his father's blessing.

A month after Willie returned from the black college tour, Crenshaw students voted him homecoming king. Few students knew that Willie and the homecoming queen—Latisha—both had lived through and suffered grievously from their mothers' cocaine addiction. That is why the vote was so important to Willie—and to Latisha—and why being named homecoming king was a powerful symbol to him that his past had not defined him nor deterred him from success.

TWENTY

NAILA

ALL-AMERICAN

Olivia peers into a broken mirror that is leaning against a wall in her room, and hurriedly puts on her makeup. She is running late, as usual. It is 7:30 A.M., and her court hearing is scheduled for eight. Her foster mother, Gretchen Fairconnetue, is fuming. "I tried to get you up, but you just laid in bed," Fairconnetue says, shaking her head in disgust. "Now you're gonna be late. I'm sick of this. Well, I ain't keepin' you. And I'm tellin' the judge that."

"I've got a half hour, so don't worry about it," Olivia says. "I'll be there on time."

"I got to drive a girl to school, so I'm leaving," Fairconnetue says, dashing down the stairs. She opens the front door, yells, "You better get started for court—right now," and then slams the door. Olivia spends a few more minutes on her makeup, grabs her purse and a copy of her high school transcripts, and heads out the door. I am giving Olivia a ride to court again and as we drive toward the freeway, she lights up a cigarette. She takes a drag and says, "For the past two weeks I've been kissing her butt. Every night I've been cooking, making her favorite meals. Last night I made shrimp enchiladas for her. Every night I sit by her bed and talk to her. Yesterday she said she was going to keep me. This morning she said she wasn't." Olivia takes another drag, exhales sharply, and says, "Who knows?"

On the freeway, Olivia stares out the window and lights another cigarette. It is warm and still and the high-rises downtown glitter in the early morning sun. In the distance, the San Gabriel Mountains, which are well over a mile high, are almost completely obscured by a soupy, white haze, the outline of the escarpment barely visible, like a faint, one-dimensional pencil sketch.

"I'll tell you one thing, I'm not going to any camp. Nobody's locking me up," she says with a bit of bravado. "If the judge won't give me probation and she sets a trial date, I'm not going to risk it. I'm heading for Vegas."

We arrive at the juvenile court about thirty minutes late. Olivia does not seem to care, but Fairconnetue is spitting mad. She sits on a bench, arms crossed, scowling. She stands up and studies Olivia's outfit for a moment and then shakes her head. Olivia is wearing a lavender suit, with a short skirt, lavender nail polish, and white patent leather high heels.

"*Girl,* you don't wear a skirt this short to court," Fairconnetue says. "It's disrespectful. You look like a prostitute."

Before Olivia can reply, her lawyer, Peter Weiss, who always seems harried and overloaded with cases, rushes up to her, out of breath. He snatches the transcripts from her and hurries into the courtroom.

Olivia sits beside Fairconnetue on a bench outside the courtroom and waits to be called. She has been back to Eastlake Juvenile Court several times during the past few months and the surroundings are familiar to her now. With its echoing babble of voices, its low ceiling, and dim lighting, the narrow hallway resembles the hold of a ship. Olivia feels claustrophobic as she waits for her case to be called.

Fairconnetue, who is wearing an aquamarine pantsuit with a Western-style top adorned with fringes, says to Olivia, "You not home when you should be. You not in bed when you should be. You supposed to be a school girl. But you always late." Olivia ignores her, stares at her coffee, and swirls it around the cup. About fifteen minutes later, Weiss returns and crouches beside Olivia. "Okay, here's the deal. If you admit to the check thing, I think you can get probation with a camp stay. If you won't admit it, you have the right to a trial. But I don't think you'll beat it. The odds are against you. The camp stay means you avoid camp, as long as you don't get in trouble again."

He turns to Fairconnetue. "Now this is crucial. She's got to stay with you. Will you agree to that?"

Fairconnetue stares at Olivia for a moment. "Okay. But she better not do anything wrong."

"Do you wish to waive the right to a trial and the right to subpoena and cross-examine witnesses?" he asks Olivia.

She nods.

"Because of your report cards, because the judge sees that you have college potential, she's indicated she'll keep you where you are. But on a camp stay. Now that's just the judge's inclination. She hasn't made up her mind completely. They haven't found your file yet. That's why the thing's still a bit up in the air right now. But when this is settled, it means you can't mess up."

"What's mess up mean?" Olivia asks.

"Breaking the law in any way. Going AWOL. If you so much as jaywalk, they can revoke your probation and send you to camp."

"Can I still go to college?" she asks.

He walks back toward the courtroom and without turning around calls out, "Yes."

Fairconnetue wags her finger at Olivia. "If you do anything wrong, and I mean *any*thing . . . If you are five minutes late . . . You're going to camp."

Olivia is too distracted and jittery to listen to her. She knows her whole future could be decided this morning. The judge's decision will determine whether she faces juvenile jail and flees to Las Vegas or whether she finishes high school and attends college. Each time a bailiff walks into the hall to call the name of a case, Olivia swivels her head toward him and listens intently.

When Fairconnetue sees that Olivia is not listening to her, she faces me. "The other girls don't like her," she tells me. "They don't like the way she come and go as she please. They got to knock on the door to get in. They not allowed to have a key. Olivia got herself a key. Somehow. So she do what she want. I decided to keep her because I don't want to be blamed if she don't get her college education. I want her to go to college. I pray about things. I'm a Christian. So I gave her a chance."

Fairconnetue strolls down the hall for a drink of water. Olivia whispers to me that if Fairconnetue's motivation was Christian charity, why did she tell Weiss last month that she would only keep Olivia if the county provided her with more money? The only reason Fairconnetue has agreed to keep her, Olivia whispers, is because she thinks she can squeeze a few more bucks from the system.

A few minutes later, Weiss emerges from the courtroom. He shakes his head. "The judge thinks this is a sophisticated crime."

Olivia groans.

"Hold on," Weiss says. "She couldn't make a final decision today because she still hasn't found your file. It looks pretty good for you, but I can't say for sure. I can't read the judge's mind on this. You'll have to come back next Friday."

"I can't be coming back here every week," Fairconnetue complains. "You said we'd be through today. I work, you know."

"This will be the last time," Weiss says. "I promise you that. This was a freak thing today. Next Friday the judge will have Olivia's file. The judge will make her decision then. It'll be final."

The following week, the students receive in the mail their grades from the first semester. In Little's class, only six students earned As, including Olivia, Curt, Miesha, and Danielle. Most of the other gifted magnet students received Bs. Before English class, the students discuss their grades, and a few students congratulate Olivia. For a moment she appears pleased, but then she frowns and says, "It might not make any difference. It depends on what happens Friday in court."

When the bell rings, Little waves a newspaper article from the *Los Angeles Times*. She beams with pride. The article is a profile of Naila, a tall, quiet girl who sits in the front row and always wears sweat suits and sneakers to class. Naila is the first student in the class to receive a college admission letter. She has been awarded a full scholarship to Stanford.

But Naila has a distinct advantage over the other students in AP English. She is a high school all-American basketball player and has received recruiting letters from more than fifty colleges. An excellent student, she has a 3.52 grade point average and is ranked sixteenth in the class.

Little reads the newspaper story aloud to the students:

At a high school with one of the richest traditions in boys' and girls' basketball in the Southland, Naila Mosely has earned a special place among Crenshaw's elite athletes.

The . . . senior forward is the first to receive a basketball scholarship to Stanford, one of the country's most prestigious academic universities. It also has arguably the premier women's basketball program . . .

The achievement didn't come as a surprise to Mosely, who entered Crenshaw in the ninth grade with the dream of making the varsity team and earning a scholarship to Stanford.

She accomplished both, also becoming the first girl at the school to start four consecutive seasons. She's a favorite to be selected the section's player of the year . . .

To reach her goals, Mosely mapped out a strategy before starting high school. She wanted to take as many college preparatory classes as possible . . .

"Naila has been incredibly focused since she started here," Crenshaw coach Greg Cobbs said. "That's why I didn't hesitate to start her as a freshman. It's a lot of pressure for a young girl, especially at a school with high expectations."

Mosely's parents, Isaac and Margie, said they never had to motivate their daughter to do the right thing.

"Naila knew what she wanted, and she really never swayed from that," Margie said. "She just understood that she wasn't going to get too far in sports without the academics. She always wanted to be the first in our family to graduate from college . . . ."

Naila joined a T-ball team when she was six years old, and when she swung the bat for the first time, her father knew she was a natural.

She had a sweet swing, a rare combination of power, quickness, fluidity, and timing.

She was an even better basketball player, and when she enrolled in ninth grade at Crenshaw, she was a major college prospect. She was a starter as a freshman, a city co-player of the year as a sophomore, and, at the end of her junior year, an all-American. This year she is the star of a team that is a contender for the state championship. She is nearly six feet tall, weighs about 175 pounds, and has a deadly jump shot from fifteen to eighteen feet. She is quick enough to run with the guards and tall and strong enough to rebound with the forwards.

Her father, Isaac, never had a doubt that Naila would succeed athletically, but when she started kindergarten he harbored misgivings about her academic future. He was familiar with the limitations of inner-city elementary schools and was concerned that she would not have a proper foundation for college. So he enrolled her in a private Christian school and scraped up the $300 in tuition every month for Naila and her younger brother.

Isaac is a clerical worker for a South-Central elementary school and his wife is a sales representative for the telephone company. They knew how the lack of a college education had held them back in their own careers. They wanted to make sure that Naila would be prepared for college.

In the fifth grade, Naila wanted to transfer to a public school so she could attend classes with her neighborhood friends. Her parents relented, partly because they found a good public elementary school for her, partly because they were having a hard time paying private school tuition for two children.

Naila, who grew up in the Oakwood section of Venice, is one of the few students in the school who does not live in South-Central. Oakwood is an anomalous Westside neighborhood, a kind of reverse oasis—a mini ghetto surrounded by affluence. Oakwood has a large black and Latino population, a number of warring gang factions, a thriving tar heroin trade, and fifteen federally subsidized housing projects. There are pockets of gentrification here, but Naila's house—where her father was raised—is far removed from the renovated beach bungalows. It is a narrow strip of a house with a roof that has seen better days—an occasional shingle curls up at the edges—and a rickety carport out front that shelters an old station wagon. The house is located across the street from a Baptist church and next door to a run-down, low-income, government-subsidized apartment building. The neighborhood is indistinguishable from countless South-Central neighborhoods. The only difference is its proximity to the ocean.

When searching for the right high school for Naila, she and her parents picked Crenshaw. Although she did not qualify for the gifted program, she was accepted to the teacher-training magnet. Isaac felt Naila would receive more individual attention at one of the magnet schools, which are open to students from throughout the city. And he knew that college coaches would see her play often because Crenshaw always had a highly ranked team.

Naila had always been motivated and competitive—in both sports and school. In elementary school, on the rare occasions when she received Cs, she would cry, Isaac recalls. When she was a ninth grader, numerous colleges were heavily recruiting a teammate, but because her grades were poor she never qualified for a scholarship. Naila knew that a full scholarship to a top private college was worth well over $100,000. She saw how hard her parents worked, how much they cared about her education. She vowed that when she was a senior, she would be in a position to sift through the scholarship offers. And she was.

Naila is one of a handful of students in AP English who are not in the gifted magnet program, but were accepted into the class because their grades were good and their counselors recommended them. Although she has performed much better on the writing assignments than the other outsiders, she knows her writing needs improvement. She knows that when she enrolls at Stanford in the fall, the competition—both on the court and in the classroom—will be onerous. She wants to be ready.

After Little passes around the newspaper article about Naila, the class finishes reading *The Elephant Man*. Little discusses a few themes of the play, and the discussion soon segues to the topic of trust. Little asks the class, "How do we test people's trustworthiness?"

"I have lots of associates, but no true friends," Sadi says. "I believe my mom is my only true friend. She's the only person I really trust."

Miesha points to Little and says, "I trust you, education-wise. I trust that you'll teach us what we need to make it in college. I know you're trying to give us the tools to succeed. A lot of teachers don't do that."

Latisha raises her hand. "Miss Little, I trust you in the classroom and on the street. I let you in on some things I usually keep inside. You helped me through a rough time."

Little is in an upbeat mood all morning. She was excited after reading the article about Naila, and she was moved by Latisha's and Miesha's testimonials to her. After class, Braxton stops by to see a student. Little greets him, for the first time in months. He has noticed that since the beginning of the second semester she seems more even-tempered. Students have told him that with the exception of the day following the Simpson verdict, she has been more focused in class. They have told him that she seems to have put her dispute with Moultrie behind her.

Can she, Braxton wonders, finally transcend academic politics and simply focus on teaching? Can she avoid outside distractions for the rest of the semester?

Later in the week, Braxton gets his answer. She can't. An incident takes place that shatters her fragile equanimity.

Little orders a pizza during lunch and sends a student to the administration office to pick it up. The student is stopped by two parent advisors because her short skirt violates the dress code. Parent advisors are mothers of current or former Crenshaw students, and they monitor the halls looking for students who cut class or violate the dress code.

The student explains that she has to pick up a pizza for a teacher. When the women find out which teacher ordered the pizza, the student says, they denounce Little.

Little tells the student to write an account of the incident. One of the women, the student writes, "began saying that Miss Little didn't give a rat's ass about us black kids . . . She then called her a fucking white bitch . . . they went on and started saying that I should not trust that white lady because she acts friendly at school and then goes back to her white people and bad-mouths us . . ."

Little is using the Xerox machine in the gifted magnet office when the student reports what the women said. Later in the afternoon, Little marches into Braxton's office. She relates the story to him. But she does not appear insulted or angry. She seems energized by this new conflict. The battle with Moultrie has dragged on for so long, with so few new developments, that Little appeared almost bored with the dispute. Now she is presented with a new skirmish, and she is roused to action.

"I'm going to the board of education right now," she says, standing in the doorway to Braxton's office. "This is a clear case of racism. They can't get away with this. I'm filing a racial discrimination complaint this afternoon. This thing isn't over. It's just beginning."

She marches down the hallway and heads off to the board of education. Braxton slumps in his chair. He stares into the hallway with an expression of shock and horror, looking like a man watching his house burn down.

The next morning, Little is still scurrying about in a manic mood of high alert. She decides to buttress her racial-discrimination complaint with student testimonials. She tells the students that two women have made outrageous comments about her, but she does not give them the details. As a result of the comments, she tells the class, she wants them to write an essay answering two questions. She writes on the blackboard:

1. Does Ms. Little meet the expected student learning results for Advanced Placement English literature?

2. Does gender or race affect her ability to deliver meaningful instruction?

The entire class on Friday is consumed by the assignment.

Little stews about the incident during the long Presidents' Day weekend. By the time she arrives for class on Wednesday, her initial excitement has transmogrified into rage. After the bell rings, several students trickle in. A handful of students have been wandering in late since September, and most of the time Little responds by threatening to lock the door at eight o'clock. But this morning she is in such an angry mood, she will not let it slide.

"I'm sick of all these tardies," Little says. "The casual attitude in this class is outrageous. Getting to school on time doesn't seem to matter to a lot of you."

At this point, Olivia saunters through the door.

Little throws up both hands and says, "See what I mean? Doesn't anyone in here give a damn?"

"It ain't like that," Latisha says. "People here ain't got no dip."

"What?" Little asks, irritably.

"No car, no ride," Latisha explains. "This ain't Beverly Hills, Miss Little. Nobody's got a car in this class. We all got to rely on someone else to get to school. Sometimes these buses run late. What we supposed to do?"

"I'm tired of you kids running me," Little says. "I'm tired of how you regard this class. I'm tired of being insulted at my own school." She pounds a fist on the blackboard and screams, "I'm SICK, SICK, SICK, SICK of this!"

"You *losing* it, girl," Latisha tells her. "I thought you'd be in a good mood after O.J. But you flipping out."

"I'm perfectly fine," Little says.

"No," Latisha says. "You not."

"Don't tell me that."

"You flipping out."

"Nobody's flipping out here."

Latisha is about to respond, but Little cuts her off. "This conversation is finished." She walks over to the television, slips the movie version of *The Elephant Man* in the VCR, and dims the lights.

As the students watch the movie, Little tells me she is still outraged by the parent advisors' comments. And she is deeply hurt. "I've put my heart and soul into teaching these kids. I give up weekend after weekend so I have time for their essays. I go over and over their essays, to make sure they become better writers. I spend hundreds of dollars every year, out of my own money, Xeroxing things, because I can't get a textbook for the class. I've invested so much of myself—emotionally, financially, and academically—to bring a strong academic program to this school. And after all that, I get called a fucking white bitch?'' She exhales loudly. ''Let me tell you, that's hard to take. This is a hostile work environment. Why should I be subjected to this? I'm sick of people just thinking I'm a disgruntled employee.

''I'm ready to walk out. I'm going to start making calls and see if I can transfer to another school before the year is out. I'm going to put my application in to some other places. Right now.''

She pulls a teacher transfer form out of a desk drawer, walks down the hall to the Xerox machine, and makes a copy. She plans to spend the afternoon filling it out.

TWENTY-ONE

OLIVIA

SENTENCING

On the morning Olivia's fate will be determined—when she finally finds out if she will graduate from high school or if she will be sentenced to a detention camp—she is hobbling down the juvenile court hallway, on crutches.

After her arrest, she quit her job as a taxi dancer because she was afraid that if the judge found out about the work, it might hinder her chance for probation. She recently landed a job in a flower shop, and a few days ago she slipped on a scattering of wet rose petals and sprained her ankle.

Olivia gives me her crutches and slowly eases onto a court bench. I hand her a Bible and a folder—which she had asked me to carry—with an acceptance letter from California State University, San Diego, which she just received. During the tumult following her arrest, she almost missed the college application deadlines. Her application to Babson College in Massachusetts—her first choice—was due February 1, and she faxed her application that morning. She also barely made the deadline for a few California state colleges that she applied to as backups.

She brought her college acceptance letter to show to the judge. The Bible is Little's, and Olivia spotted it on her bookshelf last week and asked to borrow it. Olivia has decided to read the Bible from beginning to end, Old and New Testaments, all 1,313 pages. She was raised a Catholic, but after the years of abuse at home, she abandoned the religion. She never entirely lost her faith in God, however, and her arrest precipitated a spiritual crisis. Olivia decides the best way to determine exactly what she believes—or if she believes—is to read the entire Bible.

For many defendants, a Bible is a handy prop to brandish before a judge, a hustle for clemency. But Olivia has read chapter after chapter during the past week, and truly seems absorbed by the contents. As she waits almost two hours for her case to be called, she reads intently, barely looking up, engrossed in the stories of Deuteronomy.

When her lawyer, Peter Weiss, and her foster mother, Gretchen Fairconnetue, arrive, Olivia glances up briefly and returns to her reading. Weiss taps Fairconnetue on the shoulder. "Can I talk to you for a moment? In private?" She shrugs. He motions for her to follow him. Since there is no private place for them to meet, he talks to her in the crowded hallway, far enough away from Olivia so she cannot hear. "What's your decision about Olivia? Can she stay with you?"

"I think she need to go to camp," Fairconnetue says. "She need to learn her lesson. She involved in a lot of funny business. I don't think I want to keep her."

Fairconnetue had been under the misimpression that a foster mother could obtain more money from the county if she housed a foster child who was on probation. Olivia is convinced that Fairconnetue decided to oust her when she discovered she was not entitled to additional funds. But neither Weiss nor Olivia are too concerned about Fairconnetue's decision because they discovered, during the past week, that Olivia has other options.

Weiss walks back down the hall and motions for Olivia to join him for a brief conference. "Since all Gretchen talked about the last time we were in court was money, it's clearly evident that you're in an unstable placement," Weiss says. "So I get the impression from the court that you can be placed in another foster home."

"I'm afraid," Olivia says, "that my social worker will put me in the worst possible place because she's mad about the arrest."

"It won't be like that," Weiss says. "The court will monitor the placement."

Olivia tells him that last spring and summer she lived with the parents of a Crenshaw classmate, and although she eventually went AWOL the mother has agreed to give her a second chance and let her live there for the rest of the school year. Olivia talked to the student's mother earlier in the week, she tells Weiss.

"Is she here today?" Weiss asks.

"No."

"Do you have a letter from her?"

"No. I've been trying to call you all week about this. But you're never there," Olivia says, looking exasperated.

"Anyway," Weiss says, "it's good to know about the other foster mother." He tells her that her case will not be called until later in the morning and then rushes off to meet with another client.

Olivia sees that all the benches are filled, so she reluctantly sits beside Fairconnetue, and resumes reading her Bible.

"I have a lot of doubt about you," Fairconnetue tells Olivia.

"That's understandable," Olivia says, not glancing up.

"You have all this money. How you have that?"

"I work."

"Don't you have to be eighteen to work?"

Olivia enunciates very slowly, as if she is talking to a child: "When you're sixteen years old, the law says you can obtain a job."

A few minutes later, Fairconnetue says, "Your social worker thinks your earrings are too big. She don't like 'em."

"Well, I like them," Olivia says. "That's all that counts."

She returns to her reading. Fairconnetue is bored and keeps trying to engage Olivia in conversation. "Is Crenshaw like these other schools the girls in the house go to? Where they holler so much you can't even hear the teacher?"

"That's regular school," Olivia says. "I'm in gifted classes. They're different."

Fairconnetue heads off to the court's snack bar and Olivia says to me, "Now I know why I like to talk to adults like Miss Little. At least she's smart. I have no tolerance for stupid people. I just don't. They should give these foster mothers psychiatric examinations. Lots of them are head cases."

At eleven o'clock, Weiss returns, sits beside Olivia and prepares her for court. "Because you've gone AWOL so many times, the judge thinks you're a bit of a risk. That's why she was considering sending you to camp, even though this is your first offense. So you have to convince the judge that you'll accept responsibility. Convince her that you shouldn't go to camp. Another thing. Even if you're able to avoid camp, the judge might want you to spend the weekend in juvenile hall, just to teach you a lesson."

"I understand," Olivia says. "But I do want you to know that San Diego State is having an open house this weekend and I really think I should go."

"With your ankle, how can you go?"

"A friend's taking me. I don't care if I need a wheelchair, I really think it's important that I go."

He nods. "Okay."

When he walks off, I ask Olivia if she is truly planning to visit San Diego State this weekend.

She flashes me a skeptical—*What do you think?*—look.

At 11:07, the bailiff calls out Olivia's name. She grabs her crutches and hobbles into the courtroom.

Half an hour later, Olivia hobbles out of the courtroom, accompanied by a bailiff. She looks as if she has just been punched in the stomach.

A few minutes later Weiss wanders into the hallway. "They're locking her up," he says, collapsing against a wall. Juvenile court proceedings are closed to the public, so Weiss fills me in. "Everything was going great. The judge had read all the letters from Olivia's teachers. She was very impressed by them. She was also impressed by how bright Olivia is and how focused she is on college. That's one of the reasons the judge was about to give her probation. She was about to send her to another foster home. Olivia was virtually out the door. She was home free.

"But at the last minute, Olivia's foster mother stepped in. She crucified Olivia."

He shakes his head in disgust. "I wish to hell she'd never come today. Without her, Olivia would be in class this afternoon."

Just as the hearing was ending, Weiss says, Fairconnetue jumped up and denounced Olivia. She told the judge that Olivia has a fake ID and has recently been getting food stamps and county aid checks, under false pretenses.

The judge asked Olivia if this was true. Frightened, she denied it. So the judge asked the bailiff to search Olivia's purse. He found the fake ID and a check from the county.

Olivia had planned to flee to Las Vegas if she did not get probation. But the judge was a step ahead of her and ordered that she be arrested immediately. She will be sentenced this afternoon. Olivia is now awaiting the afternoon hearing in a courthouse holding cell, under the watchful eye of a deputy sheriff. She sits at a table, with her sprained ankle elevated on a chair, staring glumly at a plate of beef Stroganoff with gray gravy, her first exposure to juvenile-hall food.

"What's with this fake ID business?" Weiss asks her.

"The DMV must have put the wrong date on my driver's license," Olivia says in a monotone, not even making the effort to sound convincing.

He dismisses her with a wave of the hand. "Don't give me that. You tell the judge that this afternoon and she'll go through the roof."

"Okay," Olivia says. "I have a fake ID."

"So you're getting aid from the county?"

"I got it for two months."

"How?"

"You can get it at seventeen," she says.

"Not if you're living in a county foster home. So you told them you live on your own?"

She sighs and, in a weak, high-pitched, little-girl voice, says, "Yeah." Weiss nods and heads out the door. Olivia wants me to pass a message to a friend at school, but before she can finish a sentence, the deputy guides me out of the holding cell and slams the door.

Before the afternoon hearing, Weiss and I grab a quick lunch at a nearby Chinese restaurant. He is angry with the foster mother and he is angry with Olivia for not telling him about the fake ID and the county checks. "Damn," he says. "If I knew the foster mom was going to be so derogatory, I'd have just sent her home. And I'm disappointed with Olivia for not leveling with me. But that's typical in juvenile court.

"This whole thing is a very unusual situation. I've been in this business for twenty years and I've never represented a kid like Olivia. I never had a kid this bright, with such a strong academic record. If somebody like her—with no juvenile record—had parents at home and had a stable family life, there's no way she'd be getting locked up. In crimes like this, with no priors, 99 percent of the time they get probation. But Olivia's got no home. It's unfair. But that's the way it is.

"It's a shame she has no one to talk to. No mother. No father. No counseling. That would cause anyone to be screwed up."

Weiss finishes his fried rice, wipes his mouth with a napkin, and heads back to court.

There is no question that Olivia will be incarcerated. The question is where. She could be sentenced to a juvenile detention camp—a locked facility that is basically a prison for teenagers. Weiss is hoping that Olivia will be sentenced, instead, to the Dorothy Kirby Center. Although a locked facility, it is designed for nonviolent offenders, and offers daily group therapy, weekly individual therapy sessions, and close supervision. The center emphasizes rehabilitation, not punishment. At a camp, Weiss fears, Olivia will simply be warehoused. The problem is that there are only one hundred beds at Dorothy Kirby. And each year, thousands of juveniles, who are eventually locked up elsewhere, could benefit from the program.

Fortunately, the judge was intrigued by Olivia's academic background and impressed with her potential. She sentenced her to six months at Dorothy Kirby. Weiss is relieved. Olivia can finish high school at Dorothy Kirby, and the judge will review her case in August. If the judge determines that Olivia has made satisfactory progress, she will be released in time for college. Because this is a juvenile offense, it will be expunged from her record when she is eighteen.

But if Olivia is not cooperative at Dorothy Kirby, if she defies the staff or resists the therapy, the judge will extend her sentence. And in the fall, instead of enrolling in college, she will remain locked up.

"I think the judge was concerned that Olivia has never received much therapy," Weiss says. "Any kid who grew up in a home like Olivia's, who was physically abused like that, obviously needs a lot of therapy. But Olivia didn't get it because when she was placed into the system, she was a dependant child, not a delinquent child."

Olivia's case illustrates a tragic flaw in the juvenile system. Like so many other children who have been abused, who have been made wards of the county, who have been psychically scarred, Olivia was drifting, inexorably, toward a criminal offense. She could not get the kind of extensive counseling she needed—the kind of counseling that might have deterred her from committing a crime—until she had actually committed a crime.

So Olivia committed the crime. Now she will receive the help she has needed for so long.

TWENTY-TWO

TOYA

I'M REALLY HERE

On Friday afternoon, Braxton is sitting in his office, frowning and frustrated, elbows on his desk, one hand covering an eye, the other hand massaging a temple. He has just heard the news about Olivia.

During the past four years, Braxton has spent countless afternoons encouraging Olivia, pushing her to succeed, helping her through various crises. When she rented her own apartment and planned to drop out of school, Braxton talked her out of it. When she was in danger of flunking several afternoon classes, because she worked every afternoon at the mall, he assigned her all morning classes. When she was AWOL, he often negotiated her return with her social worker. And now, midway through her senior year, only four months away from graduation and a college scholarship, she is pulled out of high school and locked up. To see Olivia's senior year end this way is agonizing for Braxton.

"Four years," he says wistfully to a teacher in his office. "I've been with Olivia for four years. I've been through so much with her. And now she's gone. Just like that.''

Braxton is interrupted when Little barges into his office, shouting about a tenth grader in the gifted program who treated her disrespectfully in the hallway. Little tells Braxton she just called the administration office, demanding that the student be suspended, but nobody took her complaint seriously.

"I was treated disdainfully,'' she says, her voice trembling with outrage. "I made a complaint and was met with complete indifference. That little girl is *horrible*. But everyone treats her with more respect than me. At this school they're mean to the people with integrity and nice to the people who're evil.''

Braxton ignores her complaint. He tells her that Olivia is now in custody and will not return to Crenshaw. Little forgets about her irritant du jour for a moment. She raps her knuckles on his desk and says angrily, "The system ignores her all these years, and now, all of a sudden, people are paying attention to her. Where was the system when she was getting robbed blind and beaten up? Where was the system when she needed someone to talk to? That whole social service system is totally reactive. If it was proactive, maybe Olivia wouldn't be in jail now.

"I think it was all over for her when the probation officer classified her as arrogant and not having any remorse. That was a bullshit call. These gifted kids are smart and look people in the eye and tell them what's what. They don't kiss butt. These probation officers aren't used to kids like this. That's why she was screwed from the beginning.

"The other girl involved in the scam with Olivia got treated much differently. She went to court once. It was slam, bam, you're on probation, and just don't do it again, little girl. But because Olivia doesn't have any parents, she had to go back to court over and over, kept getting jacked around, and then gets thrown in jail.''

Little's eyes tear up. She grabs a Kleenex off Braxton's desk, wipes her eyes, and says, "It's so damn sad.''

The next week, Braxton gets some unexpectedly good news that ameliorates, for him, the loss of Olivia. On Tuesday morning, he receives a call from Toya, the student who had a baby and dropped out in September. His last conversation with her, in the fall, l[e]... foundly discouraged. She seemed destined to be another casualty of South-Central—a teenage girl with a baby, and without a high school diploma. Now he discovers she will return to Crenshaw this week and enroll for the second semester.

Braxton is elated because Toya has been through so much in her life. When she was nine, she discovered her mother's body, shortly after she had been murdered. For several months, she lived in a Georgia foster home. An aunt, who lived in a crime-ridden Watts neighborhood, finally agreed to take her in. Toya had been one of Crenshaw's best students, but at the end of her junior year, she became pregnant and had to turn down a scholarship to a summer program at Cornell University. She enrolled at Crenshaw for her senior year, but was forced to drop out because she could not afford child care.

This news about Toya's return buoys Braxton's spirits tremendously. And he is amazed at the timing, at the synchronicity of events, at the return of a favorite student with a troubled past, within a few days of losing another favorite student with a troubled past.

When Toya left Crenshaw last September, she was living with her baby, Kaelen, and her cousin in a ramshackle, one-bedroom Watts apartment. Kaelen's father—who was not a Crenshaw student—has had very little contact with Toya or his son. She attempted to enroll in an unwed-mother program at a nearby Watts high school, but her legal guardian—her aunt—lived in one school district and the program was located in another. Toya could never negotiate the bureaucratic maze and obtain permission to attend the school.

Toya then decided to enroll in a program that provides a stipend and trains teenaged mothers to be registered nurses. If she had completed the program, she could have been able to properly support herself and her son. And as a nurse, she would have had flexible enough hours so she could have returned to college one day. Toya had excelled in honors science classes at Crenshaw, and she planned to major in chemistry in college. This program would have enabled her to merely delay, not abandon, her dream of becoming a doctor.

But because Toya was only seventeen, she needed a parent's or guardian's signature for the program. Still angry over her pregnancy, her aunt refused to sign the application. "You got yourself into this mess," she told Toya. "You're going to have to get yourself out of it. Without my help."

By the end of November, Toya was despondent. And destitute. When she returned home one afternoon she discovered that her cousin, who had been splitting the $400-a-month rent with her, had disappeared. She had pilfered every scrap of food in the refrigerator and the cupboards, in addition to every towel, sheet, and pillow. Toya could not pay the rent, which was due in a few days. She could not buy food for Kaelen. Down to her last five dollars, Toya knew that within a few days she and Kaelen would be homeless.

On Thanksgiving morning she appealed to the one person she believed might be able to help her—Alta Ray, her best friend's mother. "I've always been independent and a little proud," Toya told Ray. "But I've got to swallow my pride now. For Kaelen. I've got to make sure I can properly take care of him. But I've hit rock bottom. I don't have any food. I don't have any money. I can't pay next month's rent. I need a place to stay."

Ray, whose daughter Kemit is also a student at Crenshaw's gifted program, has known Toya since she was a seventh grader. Ray always respected her because she knew how difficult her life was. She was amazed at how she remained motivated in school and focused on her future. When she became pregnant and dropped out of high school, Ray was enormously saddened.

Ray and her husband and their four children live in a modest two-bedroom, one-bathroom Watts bungalow that is already cramped. But when Toya asked for a place to stay, Ray immediately said yes. She knew Toya had no place else to go. Toya had Thanksgiving dinner with the Ray family and moved in two days later.

Ray helped Toya explore and then apply to a number of academic programs for teenaged mothers. Finally, in early February, Toya was accepted to a program, sponsored by a nonprofit social service agency. The program will pay for child care and enable her to enroll in any high school in Los Angeles. She called Braxton. He told her that he had to obtain permission from the school district to reinstate a student who has dropped out, but he intended to get it immediately. She could enroll, he told her, later in the week.

During Toya's first week back at Crenshaw, her daunting schedule does not faze her. She is too excited about her return to school.

She arises at 5:30 in the morning, dresses, and feeds Kaelen. She packs his day-care bag with lunch, snacks, juice, three milk bottles, ten diapers, wipes, diaper-rash ointment, and extra clothing.

Kemit drops Kaelen off at day care and drives them to school. After school, Toya takes several late-afternoon classes at Crenshaw's night school—to make up for the last semester she missed—walks a half mile to the day-care center, picks up Kaelen, and walks another half mile to the bus stop.

When she returns home at about 7 P.M., she feeds Kaelen, plays with him, reads to him, and puts him to bed. Then Toya tries to squeeze in a few hours of homework. At midnight, she slips into the living room, which is cluttered with the belongings of seven people and a baby. She opens up the convertible sofa and falls asleep next to Kaelen's portable crib.

When Toya was holed up in her grim Watts apartment, she was always worried about money and frightened about her future. Now, during school hours, she can be a seventeen-year-old girl again. During lunch, she is ebullient as she gambols across the quad with Kemit, greeting old friends, laughing, gossiping, talking about the upcoming prom.

Toya was always a favorite of her teachers because, unlike some students who were more concerned with their grades than the subject matter, she had a reverence for knowledge. During her months away from school, what she missed most was the intellectual stimulation. Sometimes, when Kaelen was napping, she would read the dictionary—searching for unfamiliar words—or a grammar or anatomy book, just to savor the sensation of learning. Now, after almost a year away from school, Toya is excited to be in a classroom again. Because she missed the first semester, she cannot enroll in any AP classes. Still, she is enrolled in a number of challenging classes, including Little's honors English class. She is taking economics and physics at night school.

At the end of the week, when the three o'clock bell rings, she dashes into the quad. She falls onto a cement bench, out of breath, and grins. "Man, it was great today. I missed school sooooo much," she says, drawing out the word. "The whole beauty of learning was incredible. I forgot how much I missed just being in class. In chemistry today we did an experiment to determine the acidity in vinegar. It was such an exciting adventure. The thrill of discovery was wonderful." She pauses, eyes shining at the memory.

"Being back in school really makes me happy. I look around, and I see so many students who don't want to be here. They don't appreciate learning. I can't relate to that. Because I was forced to drop out, I appreciate every day I'm here."

She stands up, scans the quad, and extends both arms. "Wow," she says, shaking her head in wonderment. "I'm really here."

TWENTY-THREE

DANIELLE

EDUCATION BEFORE ATHLETICS

The students will finish discussing *The Elephant Man* this morning and then move on to *Hamlet*. Little tells the students that Dr. Frederick Treves, the surgeon who educated John Merrick—the Elephant Man—and introduced him to London society, showed "moral courage" for challenging the preconceived notions and prejudices of the time. She asks the class who else they can think of who has shown moral courage.

The students call out a number of names:

"Dr. King."

"Malcolm."

"Medgar Evers."

"How about Tommie Smith?" Latisha says. "I saw a show on TV about what he did in the '68 Olympics. When I saw the brutha put his fist up on that victory stand, that motivated and inspired me. He's one of my biggest heroes. He risked everything to take a stand for us folks."

A few students chuckle.

"Don't you know who that is?" a girl asks.

Latisha looks puzzled.

"That's Danielle's daddy."

Latisha swivels around and stares at Danielle. "*Damn,* girl. Is that yo daddy?"

Danielle smiles shyly and nods her head.

Little walks over to Danielle. "You know, it would be really great if your dad could come to class and talk about what he did. It would fit into the theme we're discussing. He could talk about what it takes to show moral courage."

"Okay," Danielle says. "I'll ask him."

The next Friday, Tommie Smith arrives at eight o'clock and his presence creates a stir at the school. Several teachers and counselors show up to see a man who was a hero to them when they were students. There are not enough seats, so the teachers and counselors line up along the blackboard and in front of the windows, waiting for Smith to address the class.

Smith is fifty-two years old, balding, and wears wire-rimmed glasses and a black sweat suit with purple streaks. He is about thirty pounds heavier than his running weight, but he is tall and broad-shouldered enough to carry the weight. Smith now has the heavy grace of an NFL middle linebacker, not the lithe form of an Olympic sprinter.

Little thanks Smith for visiting the class, and then she asks Sadi to recite his poem, "Tell Me Why," which won the city speech championship last year in the original poetry category. Little thinks this will be an appropriate way to open the class because Sadi pays homage to Smith and John Carlos, who won the bronze medal in the race, and also raised his fist and bowed his head on the victory stand.

Sadi walks to the front of the class. He closes his eyes for several seconds, summoning up his powers of concentration. He then delivers an impassioned reading and ends the poem with these lines:

> . . . *Tell me why there are more black men in prisons than college . . .*
> *Tell me why . . . with all this in my midst*
> *I'm so proudly able to throw up my black fist*

The same as those brothers in the '68 Olympics.
Tell me why?

Sadi bows his head. He clenches his right hand into a fist and raises it, an exact pose of Smith on the medal stand at the Mexico City Olympics. After his reading, Sadi explains that he wrote the poem during the 1996 Olympics when he saw, for the first time, news footage of Smith at Mexico City. The class cheers, and Smith smiles broadly, pleased that a younger generation has not forgotten.

Little asks Latisha to introduce Smith. She walks to the front of the class, unfolds a piece of paper, and reads the introduction she has written: "Often, we wonder what we would do if we were thrust into a situation that required great moral, physical, or psychological courage. In literature, we experience characters who often are forced to make such choices.

"We recently read *The Elephant Man* and learned a lot about the strength and weakness of a person's moral character. In our class discussions we named . . . individuals that showed strong moral character in risky or important situations, and Mr. Tommie Smith's name came up.

"In my eyes . . . this man is an inspiration. He stood up for what he believed in and he dealt with the consequences. He took a major risk for the rights of his people. And . . . he did it where it counted: The Olympics. A place where the whole world could see. A place where he could make a lasting impact on society."

Smith strides to the front of the class and delivers an inspirational address in a staccato, disjointed speaking style. Although he rambles from topic to topic, the students follow him all the way, raptly listening to his every word, watching him with obvious admiration.

Smith leans over, places his hands on a desk and says, "Two black athletes put their lives on the line for something they believed in. I'm Tommie Smith. I'm from the South.

"A person is only real if he's true to himself. The problem us ethnic folks have is we usually live someone else's dreams. There was a time when if we had a big ol' Cadillac and a big lean, that meant we had money.

"Listen y'all. Don't try to live someone else's dream. Live your own dream. How are you going to succeed if you don't believe in yourself?

"It's not about: What do you wear? How do you dress? What do you drive? It's about: Who are you, inside? . . .

"Tommie Smith and John Carlos were twenty-two years old. But they put their life on the line for a belief. We did it on the world's platform."

In a mock-white voice he says, " 'You shouldn't have done it there, where everyone could see you.' But that's what we believed. So that's where we did it . . .

"Black athletes are pushed into jumping high, dunking basketballs, running fast." He pauses and says, "Money isn't everything. It's something. But don't take that dollar bill and say, 'I'm a man now because I got a lot of it.' Do something real! . . .

"Before the Olympics, we had to sit down and make a plan. We had to put up or shut up. We organized a national group of black athletes. We called it the Olympic Project for Human Rights. Ever heard of it?"

The students shake their heads.

In a mock-white voice, Smith says, " 'These black athletes are going to boycott.' " He shakes his head. "We weren't going to boycott—if a number of our conditions were met. Remember, you have to fight for what you believe in. All right, now.

"This was the Olympic Project for Human Rights, not a black boycott. We were able to ensure that South Africa didn't participate in the Olympics. We were able to get black coaches hired. We were able to get housing for black San Jose State athletes—where I went to school—because we were being discriminated against. People wouldn't rent to us.

"We stood up and stated what we believed in. And we paid a price. A very big price. But there were a lot of lies going around after it. They said we were kicked out of the games. That's false. They said they took my medal away. That's false. They said we were kicked out of Mexico City. It didn't happen, folks. It's all propaganda. They said we were kicked out of the Olympic Village. We weren't. We were smart enough to leave. After the race, we got out of Dodge . . .

"Me and John were two of the baddest black athletes in the world. I had eleven world records . . .

"The year before I could have signed with the Rams. I didn't because I wanted my education." He pauses, smiles, and gestures to his daughter.

She is wearing a T-shirt with a picture of her father on the victory stand in Mexico. Beneath the picture is emblazoned: WINNING A RACE IN ORDER NOT TO LOSE ONE.

"Danielle knows I'm scattered," Smith says. "So bear with me. After Mexico City, we were looked on as outcasts. They put us on a plane to San Jose. They let us out the back door. I was afraid to return to school. I'm serious. I returned to San Jose, broke.

"We all paid a price . . . But I kept jamming. I eventually got my master's degree . . .

"Education is the key. Don't look at yourself as second-class citizens. Walk with pride. And ask yourselves, 'Who am I?' 'What am I doing?' 'Where am I going?' "

He points to Sadi and says, "A lot of our people look at sports as the way to get us there. But if you have a chance to use that brain of yours to get there, then use it. Use your gift."

He holds a hand out to the class and asks, "Any questions?"

Latisha asks, "What would you have done differently?"

"I did what I thought was necessary," he says. "We didn't throw a rock or scream at anyone. It was a silent gesture heard round the world. Negativity is in the eye of the beholder."

"Did you know you were going to win?" Curt asks.

"I couldn't waste the energy to think otherwise," Smith says.

"What was going through your mind when you gave the Black Power salute?" Andriana asks.

"That I was dead. I realized I was a dead man, even though there were no bullet holes. I knew my life would never be the same. Here in Los Angeles, I ran in the Olympic-torch relay before the Atlanta Olympics and I had to have security—in front of me, and behind me. I was the only runner who had security . . .

"In Mexico City, while I was on the victory stand, the whole time they were playing the national anthem, I was praying. I always reach back to my religion. I need something bigger than me. There is redemption in prayer . . . I asked the other black athletes why they didn't help us. Why they didn't do something. They told me they were afraid."

"Do you regret it?" Miesha asks.

"No," he says. "I never felt regret. I've felt mad, though. I've felt a controlled rage."

Smith walks over to the desk in the back of the room where he had been sitting and holds up a stained, dusty green box, mended with tape. Inside is his Olympic gold medal.

"I keep it like this because I like it in the original state," he tells the class. "I keep it in a trophy case that I built in high school."

He hands the medal to a student to pass around. After the students examine the medal, Braxton and a group of teachers and parents study it. "When I see the picture of Smith on the victory stand, I still get chills," Braxton tells another teacher. "I was in the eighth grade at the time, and it still amazes me that the brother did that."

Tommie Smith has placed so much emphasis on Danielle's education because education played such a crucial part in his own life. Education— and the promise of better schools—prompted his family's move to California. Education freed him from dawn-to-dusk work as a field hand, like his father. And years after the Olympics, after he was cut by a professional football team and shunned by the track-and-field establishment and much of white America, education was, as he recalls, "all I had left."

One of eleven children, Smith was born in a small Texas town near the Oklahoma border, the son of a cotton sharecropper. When he was in the second grade, Smith's father decided his children would receive a better education in California than in segregated Texas. So the family piled into what was known at the time as a "labor bus," with a number of other farm workers. Little Tommie was given a bottle to urinate in— because the bus would not be stopping. Four days later they were deposited in a migrant labor camp in the San Joaquin Valley, about forty miles south of Fresno. The family moved into an unheated wooden cabin.

On weekends, after school, and during the summers, Smith and his brothers and sisters labored in the fields alongside his father, chopping cotton, cutting grapes, picking melons. Sometimes the entire family earned only twenty dollars for a full weekend of work.

Smith attended a small country school, and he struggled in class. His reading comprehension was limited and his writing was barely literate. He was extremely self-conscious and afraid to speak out in class because his grammar was so poor. Although bright, he had missed a lot of school working in the fields, and the white teachers did not give him the extra attention he needed to catch up. The black children of farm laborers were a low priority, and failing in school proved a self-fulfilling prophecy.

Still, he never lost his desire to succeed. For Smith, the alternative, the image that pushed and prodded and motivated him was right outside his front door: the fields. This is where Smith knew he would end up if he did not learn. So he studied. He paid attention in class. He never abandoned hope, like so many other farm-worker children. The steely determination that transformed him into the finest 200-meter man in history—according to many track historians—sustained him in school.

At Lemoore High School, the fields were a great incentive to Smith athletically, as well as academically. "I went to my daddy and asked him if I could miss a day of picking on a Saturday because I had a track meet in Bakersfield," Smith recalls. "He said, 'Okay. But if you take second place, don't ask to go running in the next meet. You're going to be back in the fields, working with us.' "

Smith won the Bakersfield meet and countless others in high school. He never had to return to the fields on a Saturday when there was a track meet in the San Joaquin Valley. By the time he graduated, he was a football and basketball star and one of the best high school sprinters in the nation. He accepted a scholarship to San Jose State, which later became known as Speed City because of its remarkable collection of world-class sprinters.

Unlike so many of the gifted athletes in San Jose, Smith never missed class. At night, after workout, while some of his teammates were carousing, Smith tucked his improbably long legs beneath a small desk in the library stacks and finished his homework. During his freshman year, he was placed on academic probation for a semester and finished the year with barely a C average. He knew he had a lot of catching up to do.

He played freshman basketball and was the team's leading scorer with a fourteen-point average. The football coach watched him on the track, and tried to recruit him as a wide receiver. But during Smith's sophomore year, he quit basketball and refused to play football because he wanted to devote his time to his school work, and wanted to focus on track. His hard work in the classroom paid off. His grades improved and he gained confidence that he was slowly, inexorably making progress.

On the track, it quickly became apparent to the coaches that Smith was a rare talent, a runner with the blazing speed of a sprinter and the strength of a quarter-miler. By the end of his senior year, he had tied or broken eleven world records for individual and relay events. The dominant sprinter of his era, he set world records in the 200 and 400 meters indoors and outdoors and came within one-tenth of a second of tying the 100 record.

Unlike some sprinters, who had hurly-burly form, Smith exploded out of a curve and down the straightaway with a silky stride that was wondrous to behold, an awesome mélange of grace and power. He floated around a track wearing his omnipresent black sunglasses, his face devoid of expression, his stride looking effortless. A jazzman in flight. Smith was one of the progenitors of the ultracool athletes who brought élan and individualism to their sports.

When a San Jose State sociology professor, Harry Edwards, began organizing black athletes and exploring the possibility of boycotting the 1968 Olympics to protest racism in America and the country's social policies, Smith reluctantly participated. He desperately wanted to achieve his childhood dream of winning an Olympic gold medal, but he felt he must follow his conscience. He later joined the group of black athletes who created the Olympic Project for Human Rights. They submitted a list of demands to the U.S. Olympic Committee, including the ban of South Africa from the Olympics, the hiring of black coaches and administrators, the resignation of International Olympic Committee president Avery Brundage, whom they considered a racist.

Because of Smith's participation, his reserve, his omnipresent sunglasses, he was labeled by some a surly, black radical. But he was not surly, merely shy. And he was far from a dangerous radical. Smith, who always considered himself a patriot, was a member of the Army Reserve Officers Training Corps. But he grew up in the 1950s and 1960s, during the white-hot years of the civil rights movement, and his outrage and his activism had been slowly building. He finally was galvanized into action by what he had learned and experienced during four years of college. In the classroom, he studied America's legacy of slavery and racism and segregation and inequality. On the streets, just blocks from the track where he brought international renown to San Jose, apartment owners refused to rent to him because he was black. When he returned home, he recalled the many indignities and humiliations his father had endured and how he had been cheated by white field bosses.

Before the 1968 Olympics, the boycott was called off. Instead, an amorphous plan was put into place. The athletes decided that they would make a gesture—if they were moved to do so—on the victory stand that would embody the ideals they had discussed during the past turbulent year.

During the semifinal of the 200 meters in Mexico City, Smith pulled a muscle in his upper thigh and had to slow down at the end of the race. He had qualified for the finals, which would be held in two hours, but he did not know if his leg would hold up. He iced his thigh and then warmed up. As he waited for the finals to be called, he said to himself, "No, Lord. You ain't going to do this to me. I have to win so I can portray my message."

In the final, Smith came out of the turn trailing his teammate John Carlos by a yard and a half, and then, shifting into a gear no one else in the world had, he blew by Carlos on the straightaway and built such a big lead he was able to thrust his arms into the air and smile and wave, well short of the finish line. He set a world record that stood for eleven years.

Smith enjoyed a moment of supreme exultation, but it was only a moment, because when the race was over, after the medalists picked up their sweat suits and athletic bags and were on their way to the victory stand, Smith prepared for another moment—the moment that would define his life. He told Carlos he had a pair of black gloves in his bag and explained to him his plan and the symbolism of the act. Their clenched fists in the black gloves would signify black unity and black strength. They would not wear shoes, and their stocking feet would symbolize black poverty. Smith's black scarf and Carlos's beads would represent black lynchings. Smith wanted to convey to the world that America's constitutional promise of equality for all was not being fulfilled in black America.

He asked Carlos if he would join him. Carlos agreed. Smith kept the right glove and gave Carlos the left.

As the national anthem played, and the American flag was hoisted to the top of the mast, Smith bowed his head and raised his clenched, black-gloved fist. The stadium, holding about 80,000 fans, rocked with catcalls and boos. Smith repeated the Lord's Prayer to himself, over and over. He knew a daunting ordeal would await him the moment he stepped off the victory stand and his life would be immutably transformed.

The gesture, by today's standards, is a mild form of demonstration, a truly nonviolent protest. Smith and Carlos did not set anything on fire. They did not throw a punch. They did not unfurl a banner. They did not shout or chant. Their gesture was silent, but eloquent. Yet it created a firestorm of outrage and animus in white America, which considered the athletes dangerous revolutionaries. Ronald Reagan, who was then governor of California, and Vice President Spiro Agnew vilified the athletes for what they considered to be a traitorous act. The Associated Press described their raised fists as "a Nazi-like salute." Brent Musburger, then a sports columnist in Chicago, called them "black-skinned storm troopers." Countless sports fans sent them death threats and hate letters.

In the small California farm town where Smith had been raised, instead of being lauded for his Olympic accomplishment, residents dumped cow manure and dead snakes on his parents' front porch. He attributes the death of his mother—two years later at the age of fifty-seven from a heart attack—to the unending stress she endured following the Olympics.

He received so many death threats that he was afraid to attend class and finish his final semester of college. He decided to attend night school, where he would be less conspicuous. Smith had a wife and a young son and desperately needed money, but he was fired from several jobs as soon as his employers discovered who he was and what he had done.

Smith had the courage to make his gesture, but not the temperament to withstand the controversy. He had an earnest, forthright manner that reflected his rural roots, and he was not prepared for the criticism. Carlos, who had grown up in Harlem, had the savvy, street-smart demeanor,

the glib carapace that enabled him initially, at least, to better ᴄ.̣
what ensued.

After Smith graduated from college, his fortunes continued to sour.
The Los Angeles Rams, who had drafted him the previous year in the
ninth round, backed out because he was too controversial. No other team
would take a chance on him, until a young assistant coach for the Cincinnati
Bengals by the name of Bill Walsh had the moxie to give him an opportunity. Smith's brilliance on the track, however, did not carry over to the
football field, and his career was undistinguished. He played on the Bengals'
taxi squad for three years—making $300 a week—until he was cut. The
years of financial struggle since the Olympics, the pressure of the controversy, and constant death threats had taken a toll on his marriage. His
wife left him.

Carlos's marriage also was a casualty of those few minutes on the
victory stand in Mexico City. He attributed his wife's suicide to his struggle
to find his way after the Olympics, to their struggle to survive. The only
jobs he could land were menial ones, such as bar bouncer. He occasionally
gave speeches at college campuses and would pass the hat afterward. Years
after the Olympics he was arrested for cocaine possession.

Smith never descended to those depths of desperation because he had
one significant advantage—an education. While Carlos dropped out of
college, Smith graduated and eventually earned a master's degree in sociology. Carlos, a proud man who was one of the great athletes of his time,
had to scuffle for jobs, but Smith could always fall back on his degree.
After Smith was cut by the Bengals, he taught and coached at a Bay Area
high school.

In the early 1970s, Oberlin College in Ohio hired as its athletic director, Jack Scott, an activist who was best known for harboring Patty Hearst
while she was a bank robbery fugitive. Scott then hired Smith to coach
track and teach sociology. Six years later, when Smith believed the administration was intent on purging all of Scott's hires, he was denied tenure.

Smith had married an Oberlin graduate, had one child from his previous marriage, and now had another child to support—Danielle. But he
could not find another job in Ohio, so he returned to California. Proposition 13 had decimated school budgets, and there were few openings for

track coaches. Desperate, he borrowed money from relatives to pay the bills, but once again his education saved him. Santa Monica College had an opening for a track coach and had two prerequisites for candidates— an extensive track background and a master's degree, which ruled out many former track stars. Smith had the master's degree, but there was a lot of competition for the job. A stigma still surrounded his name. Smith, however, had one resplendent credential no other candidate could match— an Olympic gold medal. He was hired in 1978 and is still coaching there.

A decade after the Olympics, Carlos sought to put into practice the idealism and activism that embodied his Olympic gesture. He founded an organization in Los Angeles to work with impoverished children, but could not garner the funding to keep it going. He worked as an aide to a city councilman. About two years prior to the 1984 Olympics, he was hired to promote the games and work as a liaison with the black community. When the Olympics ended, so did his job. Finally, after years of hard times, Carlos, like Smith, eventually found stability and peace of mind and his place in the world. In the early 1990s, he was hired as the track coach at a high school in the California desert.

Smith's small office at Santa Monica College—a two-year community college—located in a portable classroom not far from the track, is filled with mementos from his remarkable career. All four walls are covered with photographs, trophies, and *Life* magazine and *Sports Illustrated* covers featuring him, in midstride, setting world records. One of his most treasured mementos—a reminder that the gesture that cost him so much is still venerated by another generation of athletes—is a picture of Edwin Moses with the inscription: "To Tommie . . . National Hero. From a protégé . . . Edwin Moses."

As he walks about the office, reminiscing about his life and his career, he is interrupted by a call from a Bay Area television reporter who wants to interview him. He still receives several requests a month for interviews, and he turns almost all of them down.

"What's the gratuity?" Smith barks into the phone. "Well, if you can't pay, I can't talk. I have a responsibility to spend my time on my runners and my kids."

He slams the phone down. Smith is acutely aware of the multimillion-dollar shoe contracts world-record holders receive today. When he was running at San Jose State, he received an eighty-five-dollar-a month scholarship, with an additional twenty-five dollars for books. Summers he mopped floors at the Lemoore Naval Air Station. When he returned from the Olympics, with a gold medal and a world record, he was two months behind in his rent. Since so many people are now making fortunes from track, he is reluctant to discuss his career, unless there is a payoff, or unless there is some educational or philanthropic purpose for the interview.

Because Smith sacrificed so much during his career, with such minimal financial reward, he refuses to allow his athletes to focus entirely on running, to the detriment of their education. He is as concerned about his runners' work in the classroom as their workouts on the track. On Smith's team, if you do not go to class, you do not run in meets. He tells his runners the same thing he tells his children: Education before athletics.

Smith's emphasis on education sometimes frustrates Danielle. During grade school, she was a gifted runner who rarely lost a race. When she enrolled at Crenshaw, she wanted to be a track star. She joined the team and frequently went to her father for encouragement and guidance. He gave her neither.

Smith is a reticent man and sometimes his children can discern what he thinks by what he does *not* say, rather than what he does. He never discouraged Danielle from pursuing track, but since he scrupulously avoided discussing running with her, she quickly got the point. And she could see his irritation whenever anyone asked him if she was on the track team. When she decided to quit track to concentrate on her studies, she suspected he was pleased.

Although Danielle never thought her father paid attention to her running form, when she is not around he says, "That right foot of hers was flared out. It slowed her down." Although Smith never told Danielle, he believed she was a born runner, a potential world-class track star. "Just take a look at her," Smith says matter-of-factly. Danielle is a female model of her father when he was her age—tall and slender with long legs and natural grace. Smith also noticed that Danielle, from an early age, shared another characteristic with him—she had a burning desire to be the best.

He saw how hard she studied every night, how she always wanted the highest grade in class; how intense she was before an exam. Smith decided that Danielle was too competitive to excel in both school and track. He was afraid her academics would suffer.

"I made it a point never to encourage her to pursue track," he says, sitting in the stands at Santa Monica College, watching his runners warm up. "It wasn't that important to me. I'd been there and done that. I was the best in the world. And after it all, I damn near starved to death. You can be the fastest in the world and end up without a dime. You can be the slowest in the world and be a millionaire. People are making big money now in track, but that only lasts so long. What are they going to do when they can't run anymore? Danielle is gifted in both school and track, but the percentage of people who can do both at a high level is very low. Maybe Danielle could have done it. But I wasn't willing to take that chance."

Smith is still angry about the lack of attention he received in elementary school from uncaring white teachers. He still recalls how difficult it was for him to learn to read after missing weeks of class because he was working in the fields. He never wanted Danielle to be in that position. So he and his wife Denise—who works for the city housing department—always read to her at an early age, always expressed interest in her school work. In elementary school, Danielle's IQ was above 150, and she was classified "highly gifted" by the school district. But unlike some extremely bright children, who grow bored and restless in class, she remained attentive and motivated.

When it came time to choose a high school, Smith and his wife decided Crenshaw would be a good compromise. The gifted magnet program offered smaller classes and a more competitive academic environment than the typical Los Angeles high school. And it was located in the neighborhood, which was important to Smith. He did not want Danielle to be bussed to a Westside or Valley school. He did not want to send her to a private school where he felt she would be cut off from her neighborhood and her race.

When he explains why he felt a social responsibility to send Danielle to a neighborhood school, he pulls out a pen and a piece of paper and sketches two large circles. Under one circle he writes, HOMIES. Under the other circle he writes, RITZ. These are two disparate worlds, he explains. One represents South-Central, the other represents a wealthy, all-white world. He did not want Danielle living in one world and attending high school in another. It is extremely important to him that his daughter know who she is and where she is from, and is proud of who she is and where she is from.

"I know who I am, too," Smith says. "Some people may say, 'That Tommie Smith once had eleven world records and now he's living in the 'hood, south of 75th Street. Isn't that too bad.' But that doesn't bother me. I know in my heart that I'm a successful person. I don't worry about what people say."

Smith now takes more pride in his daughter than he ever did in his athletic accomplishments. Danielle is unquestionably the star of Crenshaw's senior class. She has a straight-A average, is ranked number one in the class, and is the clear front-runner for valedictorian. And last year, on her AP Art History exam, Danielle scored a stunning success. A grade of three, four, or five on an AP exam is a passing mark—and earns the student college credit. Danielle scored a five, one of the few students in the history of Crenshaw ever to score that high.

Extremely shy, Danielle always sits in the back of the class and rarely participates in discussions. But she has earned the respect of all her teachers because she is so conscientious about her classes, so committed to learning. Her essays are beautifully written and show an insight and intellectual maturity rare for a high school senior. One Friday afternoon, at the end of an arduous week of trying to convince students to pursue their studies more seriously, her art history teacher wandered into Braxton's office and said, "What I wouldn't give for an entire class of Danielles. That would be teacher heaven."

At the end of February, Danielle is the second student in AP English to receive a full college scholarship. But unlike Naila, Danielle's scholarship is for academics, not athletics.

Pitzer College, which is about thirty miles east of Los Angeles, has offered her about $22,000 a year. Danielle recently visited Pitzer and she was enthralled by the campus and inspired by the professors. She is reluctant to commit to the college, however, because she is still waiting to hear from Stanford. But even if she is accepted by Stanford, she knows the decision will come down to money. If Stanford offers her a full scholarship, she will accept it. If Stanford offers her a partial scholarship, she knows her parents do not earn enough money to make up the difference. All she can do now is wait.

After Tommie Smith's lecture to the class, after he passes around his Olympic gold medal and signs autographs for the students, he walks out the door, but Little stops him in the hallway. Still riled up about being called a fucking white bitch, she tries to tell Smith about the incident and tries—in a bit of a stretch, to say the least—to draw a parallel between his experiences and her alleged victimization at Crenshaw.

Smith looks bemused as he listens to her for a minute or two and then, as she is in midsentence, he pats her on the shoulder and quickly walks down the hallway.

Braxton watches this exchange and shakes his head ruefully. This morning's class, he thinks, encapsulates the mixed blessing of Little's teaching style. Tying in Smith's Olympic experience with *The Elephant Man* and then inviting him to class is typical of the inspired, imaginative teaching she brings to Crenshaw. Captivated, the students grasped the theme of the play in a profound and meaningful way. As a former English teacher, Braxton is amazed at how Little is able to devise creative approaches that engage her students.

But watching Little harangue Smith after class also reminds Braxton of Little's volatility, how she becomes consumed by personal slights and private battles, and how these distractions often interfere with what she teaches on a particular day, how she teaches, or if she teaches.

TWENTY-FOUR

PRINCESS

A HAPPY ENDING

On a brisk, overcast morning, just as the sun peeks through the clouds, Little hands out copies of *Hamlet* and tells the students, without much enthusiasm, "We're entering the world of William Shakespeare now. So pay attention." She is too distracted to give a spirited introduction to *Hamlet*. Instead, she hands out several study sheets entitled: "Critical Responses to *Hamlet*," "Plot Synopsis and Literary Focus," and "Hamlet's Place in Intellectual History." She then asks the students to pick parts and begin reading the play.

As the students read, Little sits at her desk, unable to concentrate on the play. She is still indignant that no one at the school district or at Crenshaw seems concerned about the "fucking white bitch" incident. After she filed a complaint with the school district, an official called her.

"I have a question for you," he asked Little. "*Are* you a fucking white bitch?"

Little was infuriated, but the official, who is white, said he was only kidding. He didn't take her seriously, he told her, since he is inundated with so many frivolous complaints.

Another teacher with a more tranquil temperament might have ignored the parent advisors' comments. After all, the women did not even make the comment directly to Little. Another teacher might rationalize that since the parent advisors are not full-time school employees, are not teachers, are not academic peers, the best approach would be to concentrate on teaching, and slough off the incident.

But Little does not slough off anything. She remembers slights, major and minor, and analyzes, deconstructs, and stews about them. After class, Little tells me she plans to file a lawsuit against Crenshaw and the school district, claiming racial discrimination. She plans to push her complaint to the limit, and damn the consequences.

Instead of teaching *Hamlet* at the beginning of the next class, Little rips the students and she rips their parents for not standing up for her, for not protesting to the school about the way she has been treated.

"The Tommie Smiths of the world are not at Crenshaw," she tells them. "I'd like the people in my classes to stand up for something and act on it. I'm looking for radicals. I'm not interested in kiss butts. The kiss butts don't succeed in the end. There's a force here that's so evil I can't tolerate it any longer. I have to go at it alone. You aren't advocates. Your parents aren't advocates. Why don't they step in and root out the corruption?"

Miesha says that her mother puts in more than sixty hours a week as a bus driver. "Half the time, I don't see my mom," she says. "She goes to work at four o'clock in the morning at gets home at seven at night. I take care of all the school stuff. She's working so hard to make sure I have a decent place to live and food on the table. To me, that shows she cares. She doesn't have time to come to school. She's too tired."

"My mama lives in Alabama," Latisha says. "My pops works at night, so I hardly ever see him. If he wants to tell me something, he leaves a message on the answering machine. He pays the rent, but I work and pay the rest of my bills. You know what I'm sayin'."

Miesha, a gifted mimic, impersonates a white suburban mother and says, " 'Bye, Becky. Have a nice day at school. Here's your lunch. I'll have milk and cookies for you when you get home.' " She shakes her head. "Get real, Miss Little. It ain't like that around here."

Another girl says, "My mom works at night and sleeps a[l...] she suppose to come to school?"

"People can at least make a phone call," Little says. "No paren[ts] ever help me out or come to my support. Let me tell you, I'm sick of it. I'm out of here. I'm leaving this dive. I'm going to transfer to another school. But at least you can say you got an education in room 310 . . ."

As Little continues to bellow, the students lose interest in her tirade. Miesha and Latisha pass notes. Curt works on his economics homework. Sadi reads the sports page. Finally, Venola calls out a question to Little— which she ignores—"What about *Hamlet*?"

A few minutes later, the students resume reading the play—but without any help from Little. She sits at her desk and finishes up paperwork for other classes, while the students struggle with the play. Little tells me, "I'm just not into Shakespeare right now."

Most of the students read their parts in a bored monotone, without comprehension. At the end of Act 1, half the class is frustrated because it does not understand the play. The other half has already given up and stares out the window or doodles in notebooks. Latisha closes her book angrily and shouts, "I don't understand a motherfucking thing."

With great reluctance, I decide to step in and, relying on a fading memory of my college Shakespeare class, try to provide them with a rudimentary understanding of Act 1. I explain sections of Hamlet's soliloquies and offer some insight into his actions and ambivalence. As I talk, to my great surprise, the students listen.

"You broke it *down*," Latisha says. "You laid it *out,* brutha."

After class, a few other students, looking amused, thank me for my inaugural effort at teaching. I ask Little if she minded my abbreviated lecture. She shrugs and shakes her head. While I am gratified that the students responded to my comments, I hope that Little regains her interest in the class soon. This is not a role that I want to sustain.

On Friday morning, before class, Little smiles at the students as they take their seats and she enthusiastically greets them. The students whisper to each other, "What's with *her?*" As Little brews a pot of coffee, she tells me that she had an epiphany yesterday.

"I finally realized that the kids are on *my* side, that they truly love me and care about me. When I realized that, it was like a great weight was lifted from my shoulders. There may be all these other forces that are opposing me. But when I realized that the vast majority of the kids weren't on the other side, that they were on *my* side, it helped enormously.

"I talked to Danielle yesterday, and she helped me figure things out. I talked to her about everything, and I cried my eyes out. I was so upset. But it was like a cleansing for me. It was very cathartic."

She shakes her head in wonderment as she thinks about how caring, concerned, and mature Danielle was, how easily seventeen-year-old Danielle slipped into the role of the teacher, while she felt like the frightened, overwhelmed student.

"Talking to Danielle made me realize how fabulous these kids are. I love them with my heart and soul. It's the dictators here who I have problems with. But I shouldn't let them tweak my brain out. I realize I'm not delivering the literature to these kids 100 percent. I should apologize for that. But I'm only human. I get so damn incensed. Maybe I just need therapy. I know I've got to get my fucking head together and just teach."

Little realizes it is March now and she has only two more months to prepare for the AP exam. She knows she must regain her focus in class. After the bell rings, she rubs her hands together, surveys the class, and smiles placidly. "Okay, everyone," she says, "we're going to have a good class today."

A girl in the front row studies Little for a moment and asks, solicitously, "You *okay,* Miss Little?"

"I'm doing fine."

"You look like you're in a different mood," Curt says.

"I am."

"You look mellow today," another girl says.

"I'm going to be mellow from now on," Little says.

"Why do you say you're going to be mellow from now on?" Curt asks, looking skeptical.

"Because I've had an epiphany. You remember epiphany from *Portrait of the Artist,* don't you?"

Most of the students nod.

"Let's get started," Little says. "Describe the political situation in Denmark as it's revealed in the conversation between Horatio and the guard in Scene 1."

Naila, the basketball star who has won a full scholarship to Stanford, answers the question. When she finishes, Little walks over to her and studies her right eye. It is swollen and discolored.

"What happened to you?" Little asks.

"We had a playoff game," Naila says. "I got hit in the eye."

Little pats her on the shoulder and then discusses the play for a few minutes. The class resumes reading *Hamlet,* but this time Little does not sit at her desk and ignore the class. She opens her copy of *Hamlet,* follows along as the students read, and occasionally interjects a point, poses a question, or helps the students interpret a line.

"What's the ghost saying to Hamlet?" Little asks the class.

"One thing he's saying," Miesha says, "is to leave moms alone. He's saying, 'Don't mess with mama.' This ghost had it goin' *on*. That's how I learned what the real deal was, what was *really* happen' in the play."

Little launches into a discussion of "exposition," and "conflict." She tells the class that if a tale has exposition without conflict it is not literature. "There is so much conflict going on in Hamlet in the first act," Little says. "Would it be interesting enough to read *Hamlet* just for plot? I don't think so. It's the conflict—external and internal—that makes a play great. And it's the character of Hamlet that makes the play great."

She pulls out a rubber band and stretches it. "Conflict creates tension." She continues to stretch the rubber band. "Rising action leads to?" She lets go of one end and the rubber band snaps loudly. "Climax."

When the students first began reading *Hamlet,* they seemed to take their lead from Little. She seemed uninterested in teaching the play. They seemed uninterested in reading it. But today, Little stays on track during the entire two hours and teaches with enthusiasm. The students, in turn, are riveted by the play, by her interpretation, by the discussion.

After class, Little stops Sadi as he gathers his backpack. "Why didn't you try to get a part in *Hamlet* to read today?"

He shrugs.

"You're a poet. This is great poetry. You're not giving it the dignity it deserves. You should be reading a part in this play. Come on, Sadi. You need to take a greater position in class. You're not into it the way you should be."

He looks contrite and says, "You're right. I'm not going to argue with you."

"You were a different English student in the tenth grade. I thought you'd be a great AP student. But you're still just floating. Why?"

"I don't know. But I know I got to get it together."

"You better. There's not much time left."

Fifteen minutes before the next class, Little is at the blackboard, furiously writing: "1. Ghost Story. 2. Moment of Accusation. 3. Moment of Truth. . . ." She then sketches out "the rising action" of the play and writes, "Ghost Story. . . . Detective Story. . . . Revenge Story."

When the class starts, she asks them, "Why doesn't Hamlet act? Why does he delay?"

"Instead of showing moral courage, he debates too much," Curt says.

Latisha tries to draw a parallel between the drive-by murder of gangsta rapper Notorious B.I.G.——who was shot to death in Los Angeles a few days ago——and the murder of Hamlet's father.

"Oh, please," Little says, exasperated.

"My homie was at the party and he heard the shots," Latisha says. "He said they were shooting at the ambulance. They wanted to make sure his fat ass was dead."

As students chatter about the murder, Little sighs impatiently and rolls her eyes. Princess glances uneasily at Little and shouts to the class, "Y'all be quiet. Miss Little is nice today and I don't want her to start screaming again."

When the class quiets down, Little says to Latisha, "Can we get back to Hamlet?"

"People like Notorious are *our* voices," Latisha says. "And it was an act of revenge. So there *are* parallels between his murder and the play."

Little, eager to change the subject, asks the class, "Why is it so hard for Hamlet to kill?" She writes on the blackboard:

1. Hamlet is too pure and noble and the thought of rever
   gusts him.
2. Hamlet is overly reflective; because he thinks too much, he does
   little.
3. Hamlet debates the morality of revenge since he will then become
   a murderer.
4. Hamlet believes the ghost, but his mind still questions . . .
5. Hamlet is so disillusioned by life that he believes nothing has value,
   not even revenge.
6. Hamlet does NOT delay and does as much as he can, as quickly
   as he can.

For the remainder of the class, Little skillfully guides the students as they excitedly discuss the various theories. When the bell rings, a student calls out, "Hey, Miss Little, how about you? Could *you* kill anyone?"

"Yes," she says nodding. "I could kill anyone who was going to harm my dogs."

March is the month when the college acceptance letters begin to trickle in, and before class the students gather in the hallway and talk excitedly about the first few colleges they have heard from. A cheerleader named Nikia, who just received acceptance letters from the University of California at Irvine and San Diego and University of Southern California, is sharing her good news with a few other students.

"My mom was more excited than me," Nikia says. "After I got the letter from USC, she called my auntie, my uncle, my great uncle, and about ten other relatives. She told me how proud she was. Then I called my daddy. He told me it was a big accomplishment."

Curt tells Nikia he was accepted at UCLA and is still waiting to hear from Stanford. Danielle was accepted at Pitzer and UC Santa Cruz and is also waiting to hear from Stanford. Miesha was accepted at UC Santa Barbara and USC. Along with a number of other students, she is waiting to hear from UC Berkeley—her first choice.

Venola has just returned from a weekend at Colby College in Maine— which the school paid for—and before class she tells the other students about her trip. She loved the bucolic setting of the school, the beauty of the Maine woods, the remove from the congestion and crime of South-Central.

Two years ago, Venola decided to major in English in college because she developed a love of literature in Little's tenth-grade class. At Colby, she sat in on an English class and met with several English professors. She particularly liked the small classes, the way everyone on campus seemed to know each other.

"It was what I'd always dreamed college would be like," she tells the other students.

At the end of the weekend, Venola decided to apply to Colby. And school officials assured her she would be accepted. But for Venola and most of the other students, getting accepted is only half the battle. Scholarships are the key variable in their final decision. Last year a Crenshaw student was accepted by Yale, but because the school did not offer her a full scholarship, she ended up attending California State University, Long Beach.

Colby College costs about $30,000 a year. The scholarship Venola has applied for—awarded to a few minority students a year—pays $28,000 a year. Venola and the other students will not receive the final scholarship data for at least another month. They cannot make any plans until then.

Still, the acceptance letters generate much excitement. And on this March morning, it is all the students talk about before class. When Princess ambles down the hallway, a friend runs up and tells her about the letters she has received.

"What's happening with you?" the friend asks.

"So much," Princess says, looking dazed. "So much's been happening, I can't even believe it."

Princess was two and a half when her mother and father, who had never married, split up. Princess's grandparents invited her and her mother to live with them in their spacious four-bedroom home near 108th and Western. The house was pink, with white trim, had an enclosed front porch and a huge backyard, where her grandmother had planted collard and turnip greens and fruit trees. These were the happiest years of Princess's life, the only time when money was not a constant, nagging worry, when she truly felt secure.

Her grandfather, who owned a janitorial business, drove her to school every morning. She spent her afternoons at a dance studio, learning ballet and tap, or taking piano lessons. Each month the family attended one of her recitals.

Her grandparents were country people from Louisiana. Her grandfather, the eldest of thirteen children, could not read or write because he had to leave school and work in the fields. Her grandmother, the oldest girl in the family, dropped out of school in the eighth grade to care for her seven brothers and sisters. When she moved to Los Angeles, she worked as a maid. Because neither of them had the opportunity for education, they stressed the importance of education to their granddaughter. Education is not a right, they would tell her. Our own lives are proof of that. Education is a privilege that should be honored.

Princess's mother, Marie, attended community college for a few semesters, before dropping out. Her parents viewed Princess as a second chance, a final opportunity to see a family member attend a university. When Princess was in elementary school, and the school district classified her as gifted, her grandparents grew more interested in her education. God has given you so many talents, her grandmother would tell her. Be sure to use them.

Marie had great expectations for her daughter—whom she named Princess Rashaunda Tralesha—and that is one of the reasons she gave her such a regal name, in addition to two distinctive middle names. "I named her Princess because I believe God is sovereign over everything," Marie says, extending both arms. "If God is King of Kings, that makes all of us princes and princesses. If I had a boy, I'd have named him Prince."

Marie pulls out a thick scrapbook—with photographs and newspaper articles neatly clipped and pasted to the pages—that chronicles Princess's accomplishments. There are pictures of Princess winning beauty contests when she was in elementary school; pictures of Princess playing the piano in recitals; articles—clipped from the local black newspaper—of Princess winning various academic awards.

Princess's life was idyllic during those years she lived with her grandparents. They even had a housekeeper, Marie says with a sigh. An only child and an only grandchild, Princess was the cynosure of everyone's love. But when Princess was twelve, and her grandfather died of cancer, their lives changed, suddenly and dramatically. Marie and her mother assumed that he had left them financially secure. Instead, the family was confronted with a tangled skein of bills and debts. The bank foreclosed on their house. They were forced to file for bankruptcy.

Princess and her mother eventually relocated to a dingy one-bedroom apartment south of Century and Vermont, a neighborhood of hot-sheet motels, 99-cent burger stands, liquor stores, and derelict bungalow courts with old sofas and mattresses abandoned in the courtyards. Their new apartment was above a garage, with an unobstructed view of the alley. There were jagged cracks in the stucco facade and the entryway was crawling with water bugs. On their first night in the apartment, Princess examined the cracked walls, the chipped linoleum in the bathroom, the shabby kitchen, and turned to her mother.

"Are we poor now, Mama?"

"I'm afraid we are, honey," Marie said, stifling a sob.

The only job Marie could find was part-time, minimum-wage work as a nurse's aide for a home health-care company, a job she would hold— on and off—for the next few years. Eventually, she fell behind in the rent. As Princess was preparing for graduation from junior high school— where she was class president—they were evicted. Marie eventually borrowed money from some friends and they found an apartment a few blocks away.

This apartment was even worse. On their first night there, Princess refused to go to bed. She stood in the corner of the living room all night, crying and gripping a can of Raid, dousing roaches as they scurried past her. When she discovered that a roach had crawled into a neighbor's ear while she was sleeping, Princess was terrified every night, frequently waking up in a panic and examining her bed for roaches.

A group of drug addicts lived in the upstairs apartment, and one night the police kicked down their door and arrested everyone—while a camera crew filmed the bust. A few nights later, Marie was mortified when she watched a television show that featured the arrest on television, with the front of their apartment building prominently displayed. The apartment was in the cross-fire of several warring gangs, and when Marie heard the tattoo of automatic gunfire outside the window, she threw Princess to the ground and shielded her with her body until the shooting subsided.

One night, when Princess was ready for bed, she pulled her covers back and discovered mice droppings on the sheets. She screamed and tossed the sheets in the garbage. At the time, dozens of people had died from a virus spread by the droppings of deer mice in the Southwest. Princess was afraid she might have been exposed to the virus and talked to a science teacher at the school, who reassured her she was not in danger.

During Princess's sophomore year at Crenshaw, they were evicted again and found an apartment a few miles away. Instead of drug addicts upstairs, there were Jamaican drug dealers across the street. Princess could see customers pull up to the curb, peel off a few bills, grab the drugs, and drive off. Police cruised by all night, rousting the drug dealers and making busts. Instead of roaches, they were plagued once again by mice.

"One night it was raining and more and more mice came scurrying into the house," Princess recalls. "My mom bought those sticky traps and put them all over the house. I tried to go to sleep, but I could hear a mouse who was partially stuck to the trap drag himself across the room. He stopped by my bed. Then, over and over, he kept banging the trap against my bed. I started screaming. Finally, my mom got up, picked up the trap and threw it out the door. The rest of the night I just sat there with the lights on."

Right before midterms, their electricity was shut off because her mother could not pay the utility bill. Undeterred, Princess bought a dozen candles, lined them up on the kitchen table, and resolutely studied for her midterms by candlelight.

During her junior year, her mother found steady work as a nurse's aide. They moved to a better neighborhood, west of the high school, and rented a modest, gray stucco house with a bottlebrush tree in front and a small backyard. For the first time since Princess's grandfather had died, she felt comfortable enough to invite school friends over to her house. Before, she had always been ashamed of where she lived, had always concocted an excuse when a friend wanted to visit.

At the end of Princess's junior year, her mother's blood pressure became dangerously high and she had to take time off from work. The bills mounted and, eventually, the lights were shut off again. Princess had just received a $500 scholarship from Top Teens of America. The savings bond was supposed to be used for Princess's college education. Instead, she cashed it in and paid the electricity, gas, and other bills.

A few months later, during the fall of Princess's senior year, they were evicted again. Marie eventually found a less expensive apartment in a two-story building—painted several sickly shades of yellow—with a sagging roof and a rusty antenna that swayed in the wind like a weather vane. Their apartment had ripped and stained carpeting and a large, jagged hole in the bathroom wall, just above the tub. When Princess examined the bathroom and noticed the dead roaches, she burst into tears. All she wanted at that moment was to, somehow, get enough money so she and her mother could move into a clean, roach-free apartment. Princess, who already worked weekends as an usher at a theater, considered quitting school and finding a full-time job. But she thought of how hard she had worked in school over the years. She thought of her grandmother—who had recently died—and all the lectures she had given her about the importance of school. She realized that if she did not want to be living like this in ten years, she needed to attend college. She vowed to hang on until the end of the year.

Princess is striking-looking, with almond eyes and the high cheekbones and perfect features of a model. Some of her teachers dismiss her as vapid, another pretty airhead. Some question whether she belongs in a gifted program because she sometimes does not keep up in class, and stares off into space with a vacant expression. But none of them know that her expression is not vacant; it is worried. None of them know she recently was diagnosed with an ulcer because she had been under so much stress. And when she is lost in class, it is not because she cannot keep up with the other students. It is often because the searing pain from her ulcer makes it difficult for her to concentrate or because she is preoccupied with overdue bills and impending evictions.

Despite Princess's problems, she always has been conscientious about her homework and always maintained her grades. She is ranked in the top 10 percent of her class with a 3.5 grade point average. She was one of a few Crenshaw seniors who were named to a national academic honor society.

In February of Princess's senior year, Marie was out of work, yet again. And they were evicted, yet again. A friend of Marie's is putting them up, until she can find work, in a small house behind a house that she owns. The place isn't much—a squat shotgun shack, surrounded by fissured asphalt, with rusted strips of sheet metal for a fence, down the street from a pawn shop and a thrift store. But it is free.

The people who rent the front house have blocked off the driveway and front lawn with abandoned cars and garbage cans, and their snarling German shepherd roams the yard, so Princess can only get to the back house through an alley, where homeless drug addicts gather and smoke crack. Princess was despondent after moving in, and it was only the promise of high school graduation that sustained her. This would be the payoff for all the hard times she endured. But just a few months before June, she discovered that she would be denied the spoils of graduation, which she had dreamed about and aspired to for so long. Marie told Princess that they did not have enough money to buy her a school ring, to pay for her senior picture, or to reserve her cap and gown. They barely had enough money to buy food. And even though Princess was voted queen of the senior prom by the students, she could not afford to buy a dress.

"I felt so bad for her," Marie says. "The other students would ask her why she hadn't taken her senior picture yet and she'd get real embarrassed. I felt so small because I just didn't have the money to give her. She looked forward to graduation so much. She spent so many years working so hard for it. And now she couldn't even enjoy any of the benefits. After everything we'd been through, it was like this was too much for her. It was the final straw and it seemed to break her.

"She figured if we didn't have enough money for graduation, how could we pay for even a small part of college? She thought all her college goals were going down the drain. She was so negative about everything.

She was going to drop out of school. Her teachers knew something was wrong. They asked me what was the matter with her. She was so down. She told me, 'Mama, I just can't take it anymore. If I didn't know I'd go to hell, I'd kill myself.'

"I told her, 'Hang on and God will help us.' Then I began to do some serious praying."

This time was the nadir for Princess. She was living as a charity case, in another hovel. Her mother was out of work again. And after years of contending with roaches and mice and gunshots and gangbangers and drug dealers and evictions, now she felt it all amounted to nothing. She would not be able to participate in graduation; she could not afford college.

Princess was so depressed she stopped doing her homework, stopped coming to school. But just as she was about to drop out and look for work, Marie received a job offer—a full-time, well-paying job in Malibu to care for a handicapped man. "Hallelujah," she shouted. "Thank you, Jesus." She had to take two buses and a cab to reach work, but she was so happy that she could buy Princess the things she needed for graduation that she did not care. Marie used her first paycheck to pay for Princess's senior picture, her school ring, and her prom dress.

This was the affirmative portent Princess needed to get her back on track. It revivified her, shook her out of her poisonous depression, renewed her faith in her own future. She returned to class.

A few weeks later, in early March, Marie runs to the door when she hears Princess walking down the alley.

"Look! Look!" she shouts to Princess, waving a letter in her hand.

It is an acceptance letter from UC Santa Barbara. When Marie saw the letter in the mailbox, she was too excited to wait for Princess to get home. She ripped it open.

She saved the second letter—from UC Riverside—so they could open it together. It, too, was an acceptance letter. Marie hugs Princess and they both cry. Marie tells Princess that she has called several financial-aid officials at University of California campuses. She assures Princess that, because their family income is so low and because Princess's grades are good, she will receive enough scholarships and financial aid so she will be able to afford college.

"I'm so proud of you," Marie tells her. "After everything you've been through, you deserve to have a happy ending to your story."

TWENTY-FIVE

TONI LITTLE

THE BRINK OF MADNESS

Toni Little's seven days of serenity are shattered when she discovers Principal Yvonne Noble is considering filing a disciplinary action against her. She forgets all about the insights she gained the previous week during her conversation with Danielle.

During the past few weeks, when Little was grousing about the "white bitch" comments, she made a number of statements to her tenth-grade class, criticizing the school and the administrators, which angered some of the students and their parents. They complained to Noble, and she has scheduled a meeting with Little to discuss the complaints.

Little is enraged. She feels she is the victim, yet she is now being victimized. During her tenth-grade literature class—which immediately follows AP English—she is so angry at the administration, and complains so vehemently, that a student approaches her after class. Although a gifted student, the boy is also a hard-core gangbanger and a drug runner who was pulled out of class one day by detectives who were investigating a South-Central narcotics ring.

"If you ever want something done," he tells Little, "I know who to go to to get it done."

"What?" she asks, confused.

"You know," he says, nodding knowingly. "These people who are bothering you. I can make it stop."

When she finally understands what he is saying, she is horrified. "Look," she says. "I don't need anybody to use any *other* means to solve this thing. I can take care of it by myself."

"Okay," he says. "But remember, if you ever need *anything* done, let me know."

Before the next class, when the AP students see Little's angry, censorious expression, the tightness around her mouth, the nervous squint, they stay clear of her. One student, who is not as perceptive as the others, sallies to the front of the room and informs Little that it is a classmate's birthday today.

"Can we sing happy birthday to him?" she chirps.

Little fixes her with a withering stare and growls, "No!"

The student studies Little for a moment and thinks better of appealing her request. She slinks back to her desk.

After the bell rings, a student asks Little, "Are you really leaving Crenshaw, Miss Little?"

"Yeah."

"When?"

"As soon as possible."

"Where?"

"I'm looking at a school near my home."

Latisha says, "That's why you have to go out with a bang, homegirl."

"I intend to," Little says.

She walks to the window and stares at the quad for a moment. It is early spring, warm and so smoggy that the Hollywood Hills, to the north of the school, are only a faint silhouette, and the HOLLYWOOD sign is completely obscured. The trees on the streets surrounding the school are beginning to bud, tiny fists of green, and the bottlebrush trees on campus are blooming and sprouting spiky splashes of red.

When Little returns to the front of the class, the students expect her to resume discussing *Hamlet*. Instead she says, "In five years at this school, I've never been praised. Not once. Before I got here, no one ever passed an AP English test. Then a long list of students in my class passed. What do I get for that? I get these memos criticizing me, telling me to come to these meetings where I'm attacked . . ."

After Little fulminates about the school for another twenty minutes, a girl in the front row, Tashana, interrupts her.

"Why do we have to come to class and listen to your problems every day?" Tashana asks. "If you want to fix your problems, then *fix* them."

A small, feisty girl with close-cropped hair, Tashana is wearing orange pants and a top with a bare midriff—both violations of the school dress code. She is one of the most disruptive students in the class, frequently chatters while Little is trying to lecture, and often turns her papers in late—always with an inventive excuse. Although she does not have much credibility left, in this instance, most of the students agree with her.

"If I was interested in your opinion, I would have asked for it," Little yells.

"Why you yelling?" Tashana asks calmly.

Little suspects that Tashana and a few tenth graders have informed on her to the principal and their comments were the basis for the upcoming disciplinary hearing. Tashana has denied this.

"You're just one of those ass kissers," Little says.

Incensed by the comment, Tashana stands up and shouts, "You just mad 'cause I talkin' the truth. I don't come to class just to hear about your problems."

Little points to the door. "Go to Mr. Braxton's office. Right now! I don't want to teach you. Find someone else who'll teach you."

Tashana walks across the class and halts at the door. "You talk so much shit. I'm sick of it. I've heard so much of your bitchin'. I don't give a fuck about your shit." She storms out and slams the door.

After Tashana leaves, Little says, "I find all this despicable. I find all of these students who are reporting on me despicable. I'm sick of this place . . ."

By the time Little finishes her diatribe, it is almost 9:45 A.M. She has only fifteen minutes left to discuss *Hamlet*. Little emphasizes a few points about the play and then the bell rings. The students leave the class, they whisper about how they think Tashana is right, how the AP test is less than two months away, how they do not feel prepared for the exam, how they would rather spend the class time they have left discussing *Hamlet*, how they are tired of hearing about Little's private battles.

There are only a few AP English classes left in March, then the students are off for spring break. They will not return to Little's class until April 2. These final classes are more productive, but Little still is highly agitated, still wrapped up in preparing her defense for the upcoming meeting with the principal, still pushing her discrimination lawsuit against the high school. Only about half of the class time is devoted to *Hamlet*. Tashana has not been back since her spat with Little. Although it is midsemester, Braxton decides the only resolution is to transfer Tashana to another class.

On the morning of the last class before spring break, Little is in an excited, manic mood. She is preparing for the disciplinary hearing with the principal, assistant principal, and her union representative. Before class, she shows me a small tape recorder and microphone.

"Isn't this great," she says, admiring the tiny microphone. Little tells me she is considering slipping the tape recorder and mike beneath her blouse and surreptitiously taping the meeting, in order to impeach the principal.

When the students resume reading *Hamlet,* she grabs a pile of study sheets and tries to quickly devise a plan for the day's class. The students are back to reading in a monotone, oblivious to the meaning of the lines.

A student calls out, "What's 'wormwood' mean, Miss Little."

"Uh, where are you?" she asks.

She riffles through her copy of the play, finds the scene and says, "It means bitterness. Now are you all hearing it or just reading it?"

"I'm just reading it," Latisha says, " 'cause I don't have a motherfucking clue."

Little spots a newspaper on a student's desk and reads the headline about the aftermath of the O.J. Simpson civil trial. She raises a clenched fist and says, "Yeah! O.J. is going to lose his house. He's behind in his payments."

The students exchange uneasy glances. They fear another angry O.J. disquisition. Fortunately, Little returns to *Hamlet*. When the class ends, she tells the students, "For spring break, do all the Act 3 study questions and read all the background material."

After the students file out, Little remembers that she had planned to assign the class the novel *Jane Eyre* to read during spring break. She was so consumed by her upcoming meeting with the principal, however, that she never got around to it.

She surveys her empty classroom, shrugs, and says, "I just couldn't get it together."

An hour later, Little meets with the principal, the assistant principal, and her union representative. Later, in a memo to Little, the principal summed up the meeting:

> *The purpose of this memorandum is to provide a written summary of the . . . conference I held with you in my office on Friday, March 21. I opened the conference by giving . . . you . . . unsigned typed copies of handwritten statements of students enrolled in the class . . . whence the initial complaint emanated.*
>
> *[The statements from the tenth-graders included: "Miss Little said that she was leaving this school and we should leave because we could get a better education somewhere else . . ." "She was talking about how . . . this school is a bad environment to work in. . . ." "She gave the number out if you wanted to complain and move the [Gifted Magnet program] somewhere else . . ." "She began yelling and screaming . . . The harshest words . . . expressed was when Ms. Little said that there was a problem with the way our parents raised us . . ."]*
>
> *I am considering taking disciplinary action against you, either a Written Reprimand or a Notice of Unsatisfactory Act or Acts . . .*

Little seethes about the meeting all day. By afternoon she is apoplectic. She paces, muttering imprecations about the school and the administrators.

"I hate this place," she tells me. "I'll try to hang on until June. I owe it to the kids. But I don't know if I can make it. I just don't think I can hang on."

She begins to hyperventilate. She resumes pacing. She stops, whirls around, narrows her eyes, grits her teeth, and throws back her head: Little Agonistes. She shouts, "This place is driving me to the brink of madness!"

PART FOUR

SPRING

TWENTY-SIX

OLIVIA

LOCKED UP

For AP students around the country, spring break is a time for intensive study, the last stretch of days, free from the burden of class, when they can concentrate on the upcoming exams. Some teachers load their students down with books to read and assignments to complete. Others hold study sessions at their homes. Little, however, is so consumed with extraneous issues, she does not hand out any novels for the class to read, or any study sheets to finish, or any homework whatsoever. Most of the students will now use their spring break to put in some extra shifts at work.

For Olivia, spring break means just another week of incarceration. A few days after she was locked up, Olivia wrote to her best friend, Julia: "I'm very depressed, although I've found the desire to live. I'm not sure exactly why. I suppose it's the fact that I have to focus on the positive future that I envision for myself and how dearly I wish it to manifest in order to make it in here."

After she was transferred from juvenile hall to the Dorothy Kirby Center, she sounded less despondent. Unlike many other juvenile facilities,

ıates are merely warehoused, the emphasis at the center is on
on. After a few weeks at the center, Olivia wrote me: "Don't
worry about my well-being. I guess I'm doing as well as anyone could in
this predicament . . . In regards to attending college, I'm not sure if
they'll let me. My counselor said I might not be able to, but we haven't
really discussed it in detail yet. And I haven't pressed the issue since I've
only been here a few weeks. I'll know more next month. But I don't
know what I'll do if they won't let me go to college. The mere thought
of it sends me into tears."

Despite being confined to a locked facility, Olivia is still playing the
angles, still trying to work the system. She continues to correspond with
colleges and apply for scholarships. She has convinced administrators at
the center to let her use the office phone so she can call college financial-
aid officials. She has even written to all of her teachers at Crenshaw,
asking them to mail her class assignments and textbooks.

"I'm going to try to see if they'll let me take my AP tests in May,"
Olivia recently wrote Little. "I don't care if they take me up to Crenshaw
with my hands shackled to my feet, I want to take my tests. Also, if you
come across any scholarships, please mail me the applications. It's not as
though I can research any while I'm in here . . . Also, mail me some
good books." A few weeks later, Olivia wrote Little again, expressing
disappointment that she has not written back or visited. Olivia wrote:
". . . As you know, I don't have a family. I think of you, Miles, Mr.
Braxton, and Julia as the only people who really care, and I think of you
guys as my family. As you see, that isn't a lot of people. It really hurts
me to think that one of you guys don't really care . . ."

Little has been consumed by her feud with school administrators.
Braxton is overwhelmed by the crush of work at Crenshaw, his long daily
commute, and the care of his two small children. And Julia does not have
a car. Olivia feels forsaken because they have not visited her during her
six weeks in custody.

County authorities have finally granted my request for an interview. I
pick up a few novels for Olivia and drive down for the visit on a smoggy
Wednesday morning.

The Dorothy Kirby Center is an unimposing facility, a low-slung brick building at the edge of the freeway in a working-class Latino neighborhood just east of Los Angeles. The center, with its stand of palm trees by the front entrance and small park next door, resembles a weathered elementary school, not a locked juvenile facility.

But inside, it is apparent that extensive security measures are in place. Visitors pass their identification to a staffer in a kiosk enclosed by clear, bulletproof, security sheeting. They are then buzzed through the sally port. The juvenile inmates are kept in single-story housing units scattered about the facility. Each unit contains ten small cells that have metal desks and metal cots with thin mattresses. Inmates leave their cells for school, meals, and therapy and are given about five minutes for a shower and an hour of recreation each day. At 8 P.M., they are locked down for the night. Inmates have to ask permission to use the bathroom and are escorted there and back.

Olivia is brought to a visiting room where I am waiting, and I am surprised by her appearance. Without a stylish, color-coordinated outfit, an elaborate hairdo, makeup, or high heels, she appears smaller and younger than I remember her. She is wearing jeans, a white T-shirt, and tennis shoes. In school, she had always seemed so energetic and had such an indefatigable spirit. Now she looks tired and sad and vulnerable.

"You're my first visitor," she says, fighting back tears. "Hardly anyone's even *written*. Miss Little hasn't written. Julia only wrote me once."

I ask her about school and she swats the air. "What a *joke*. I can't believe they can even call what they've got in here a school. In English today we had a spelling test." She rolls her eyes. "I learned how to spell *those* words in the sixth grade. Last week we were going over what's a verb and what's a noun. I knew *that* in the third grade. It's nothing like Miss Little's class. In the back of the room, I saw a copy of *Death of a Salesman*. That's the kind of thing we read in AP English, so I asked the teacher if I could borrow it. It was pretty interesting.

"In math, it's *so* boring for me that the teacher has me tutor the other students. I've been trying to teach a girl algebra, but she can't understand *any*thing." Olivia looks disgusted. "Algebra's *so* easy."

Olivia is still hoping to attend Babson College in the fall. "I got a letter from Babson telling me I was eligible for a $7,000 scholarship if I mailed in an essay within a few weeks. I wrote the essay, but had to go through hell and high water to get it typed up in this place. But I made the deadline, so we'll see. I'm going along now on the assumption that I get to go to college in September. If I don't think like that, and start thinking about what I'll do if they keep me in here, I'll go crazy. So," she says, without much conviction, "I'm trying to think positive."

I fill Olivia in on what has been going on at Crenshaw, what the students are doing, and how Little is faring. We talk about a few of the novels that I had mailed her, and then a staff member tells us that the interview is over. She escorts Olivia back to class.

Olivia will earn her high school degree while in custody. In August, the judge will review her case. If she determines that Olivia has progressed sufficiently at the Kirby Center, Olivia will be released in time for college. But the judge will rely on an assessment made by Olivia's therapist at the center, Susanne Dunne.

After Olivia is led away, I talk with Dunne, a psychiatric social worker, in her office. Dunne, thirty-two, is English and attended graduate school at UCLA. She is both exasperated and amused by Olivia. She seems to enjoy talking about her because Olivia is such a novelty at the facility. Dunne first met Olivia when she was in Juvenile Hall, shortly after she was locked up.

"I'll never forget my first interview with Olivia," says Dunne, in a clipped British accent. "She was so out of place, so different from all the other girls. She wasn't into drugs; she wasn't into gangbanging; she wasn't into hanging with the homeboys. All she talked about was getting out so she could go to college. She was one of the rare kids we see who is focused on the future. It was her intellect, though, that really distinguished her. She was so articulate and such a smart cookie."

At the time Dunne interviewed Olivia, there was a four-month wait for the Dorothy Kirby Center. Dunne was so impressed with Olivia, and it was so evident that Olivia could benefit enormously from the center's therapy program, that she managed to facilitate her admission immediately. During their first counseling session, Dunne told Olivia she needed a year of therapy at the center.

"That's impossible," Olivia told her curtly. "I have to be out in six months so I can attend college."

Dunne smiles at the memory of Olivia's chutzpah. Because Olivia is different from the other girls, Dunne says, she is frequently teased. They refer to her, sarcastically, as "Brain" or "Miss Gifted Magnet." But for the teachers, who have a number of students who cannot even read, Olivia is a delight, and they use her in their classes as a teaching assistant. She has a better rapport with the teachers than with the girls in her locked unit.

I ask Dunne if there is a chance Olivia will be released in time for college.

"She's got to make a lot of progress if she's going to be released early," Dunne says. "In the group therapy, for example, she participates, but in a superficial way. She tries, but she's so disconnected from her emotions. Her intellect has been a godsend for her. It's saved her. But everything's so external with Olivia. Eventually, she's got to face some of her demons. I admire and respect her desire to attend college. But she really needs a full year here.

"I wish I could have started with her when she was twelve or thirteen. Olivia was bounced around from place to place so much. She's built up such a tremendous defense system. But with what she's been through, that's understandable.

"The kids we get usually have criminal histories that are a lot longer than Olivia's. This is her first arrest. I think she's here because of her runaway history. If she was living at home, the judge probably would have given her probation. The problem now is that Olivia still won't take responsibility for her actions. She says, 'So what. It didn't hurt the bank.' I want her to take responsibility for what she did.

"At this point, I'll just have to see how she approaches the therapy, how she progresses over the next few months. Then I can have a better idea about whether Olivia is ready to be released and can attend college in the fall."

TWENTY-SEVEN

SCOTT BRAXTON

DRAINED

On the first day back from spring break, Toni Little calls in sick. The substitute is a bald, slow-moving, elderly black man who seems half-asleep.

"What's wrong with Miss Little?" a student asks the substitute.

"She's disturbed," he says. "It's something between her and the principal."

"She better be back in time soon so she can prepare us for our AP test," another girl says.

"She'll be back," Latisha says. "She wouldn't dog us like that."

The substitute ambles to the front of the class and says, "Being a guest teacher, I'm *guest*ing what you're supposed to be doing today?"

A few students stare at him with bored expressions. Others shrug. Finally, the substitute turns to me. I suggest that the students finish reading Act 3 of *Hamlet*. The students divvy up the parts and read for a short time, but are interrupted by Cassandra Roy, the school's college counselor. She is here to tell students she can obtain funds for anyone who cannot afford the sixty-three dollar AP exam fee. Roy, who grew up not far from

Crenshaw, prides herself on staying one step ahead of the student scammers.

"If you're on the school lunch program, Chapter I funds are available so you get to take the AP test for free," Roy says. "If not, I'll meet you halfway. But no one pimps Mrs. Roy. I don't want you telling me you can't afford to pay for the test and then see you renting a stretch limo for the prom."

She glances around the room. "Who lives in Watts?" Several students raise their hands. "There's a scholarship available."

"Do we have to write an essay?" a girl asks.

Roy scowls at the girl. "As an African American woman, I'm insulted," she says angrily. While Roy lectures the girl, the classroom phone rings and I pick it up.

"Who's that I hear in my classroom?" Little asks.

I tell her.

"I don't want any *administrators,*" she says, spitting out the word, "in *my* classroom."

I tell her Roy is simply giving the students information about the AP exam.

"They already know it," she barks. "They're supposed to read *Hamlet* . . ."

After Little hangs up and Roy leaves, the class resumes reading the play. A number of students, however, take advantage of Little's absence. A few slip out the door when the substitute turns his back. Others read magazines or gossip about the upcoming prom. The substitute halfheartedly attempts to control the class, but the students ignore him. Those who are interested in the play forge on amid the chatter. A student named Larrin— a tall boy who plays on the baseball team and writes for the school newspaper—is confused by a passage in Act 3 Scene 4 in which Hamlet rebukes his mother:

> *Look here upon this picture, and on this,*
> *The counterfeit presentment of two brothers.*
> *See what a grace was seated on this brow—*
> *Hyperion's curls, the front of Jove himself . . .*
> *New lighted on a heaven-kissing hill;*

A combination and a form indeed
Where every god did seem to set his seal
To give the world assurance of a man.
This was your husband. Look you now what follows.
Here is your husband, like a mildewed ear . . .
Have you eyes? . . .

Larrin faces me and asks, "What does that Hamlet speech mean?" Like many of the students, I was distracted and had not been paying attention. The substitute is not interested in the play. Little is gone. The students are relying on me to fill the void. I quickly read the lines and explain the passage as best as I can. I tell Larrin that when Hamlet admonishes his mother he is pointing to a portrait of his slain father, whom he eulogizes as peerless, a husband nonpareil. Then he points to a portrait of his uncle, her new husband, a malevolent man whom he despises. "Have you eyes?" he angrily asks his mother. He then denounces her and accuses her of lustfulness for marrying her brother-in-law so soon after she became a widow. "Oh, shame," he tells her. "Where is thy blush."

When I finish my explanation, I scan the classroom nervously unsure if what I had said made any sense.

Finally, a boy in the back calls out, "There it is."

Larrin nods and the students continue reading. When they finish Act 3, they close their books. There are about twenty-five minutes left in the class. The substitute asks them, "What do you want to do?"

They tell him there is not enough time left to read Act 4, so they will finish their Act 3 study questions. After a few minutes, however, it is clear few students are willing to do any work. Instead, they pass around candy, tell jokes, argue about the Lakers' playoff chances, and listen to rap on their portable CD players.

The substitute sits at Little's desk, a bewildered expression on his face. He stares out the window, occasionally checking the clock, anxiously waiting for the bell to ring.

With about five minutes left in the class, he shouts above the clamor, "Anyone want to review the study questions for the benefit of the class?"

Several students shout in unison: "No!"

* * *

On Friday, Little still has not returned, so many of the students take their cue from her. Only about half the class shows up.

A different substitute arrives today, a tall black man wearing a sweat suit and sneakers, who usually fills in for physical education teachers. A few students recognize him and call him "coach."

"What are they supposed to be doing?" he asks me shortly before class. I tell him the students should read the Act 4 section from their "Plot Synopsis and Literary Focus" study sheets—out loud—and then pick parts and read the play. This is Little's format.

The substitute is more of a disciplinarian than the previous one, so the gossiping, note passing, and giggling is reduced to a minimum. Still, there is a mood of enervation in the class, a dispirited languor since Little has been gone. The students know that Little's absence is connected to her battle with school administrators. They are hurt that she is missing class when the AP test is fast approaching. They feel if she does not care about the class, why should they?

The students read Act 4 with scant interest. A few sneak out the door. One girl flips open a compact and applies makeup. Another girl brushes her hair. A boy lays his head on his desk and closes his eyes. Another boy reads the sports page. There are only two students in the class who are concentrating on *Hamlet*—Venola and Carol, a shy, soft-spoken girl who is sitting next to her.

When the students muddle through Act 4, Scene 6, the substitute tells the class that he wants to read the part of Claudius, the king of Denmark, in the next scene. This is a powerful scene that opens with Claudius reiterating to Laertes that Hamlet has slain "your noble father" and "pursued my life." Laertes then asks Claudius why he has not yet punished Hamlet. Claudius explains the reason for the delay and then engages Laertes in an elaborate scheme to kill Hamlet.

The scene includes a number of long speeches by Claudius. When the substitute begins the first speech, the students are stunned. A boy drops the sports page. A girl snaps shut her compact. Two girls, who had been chatting, stop midsentence. A dozing boy jerks his head up.

The substitute has a deep sonorous voice, a trained voice, a voice that can be easily heard in the back row. He reads the lines with complete command. He stands up, book in one hand, gesturing with the other, acting out the part, his voice rising and falling, shouting and wheedling, capturing the drama of the scene, the Machiavellian essence of the treacherous king.

The students have spent weeks listening to their classmates stammer and struggle and butcher the lines. This is the first time they have heard anyone read Shakespeare the way Shakespeare was meant to be read, the first time they have heard the poetry of the language. They are riveted by the substitute's reading and listen intently, gazing at him, eyes wide, in awe. When he finishes the scene, they give him a standing ovation, the boys whistling and rolling their fists.

He reads another scene, with the same mastery. When the bell rings, the students remain in their seats for a minute or two, like an audience reluctant to leave the theater after a remarkable performance. When they finally file out, a girl shyly approaches the substitute. "That was *incredible*," she says. "It was *amazing*. Before, the play just seemed like words, like it was just some book. Then *you* read it." She pauses, shaking her head in amazement. "You made it come *alive*."

After the class files out, I ask the substitute where he learned to read Shakespeare with such authority. He tells me that he is an out-of-work actor who substitute teaches between commercials. Before he moved to Los Angeles to pursue an acting career, he says, smiling, he had a long run as Othello in a Detroit repertory theater.

Later in the day, Braxton attends a meeting with administrators to prepare a contingency plan for Little's AP class in case she does not return. He has heard a rumor that she might apply for disability, which leads him to believe that she will miss the rest of the year. But Little has not yet announced her intentions—she has merely called in sick for a few days. So for now, the administrators can only hire substitutes and wait.

After school, a few teachers mill about the Gifted Magnet office and speculate about Little.

"I don't think she's coming back," a teacher says.

"That would be *so* unfair to her AP kids," another teacher says. "I can't believe she pulls this shit a month away from the test."

"If this was some other school district, they would fire her ass," the first teacher says. "But here, with our union, you've got to be Jack the Ripper to lose your job."

"If this was some Westside school, the parents would have her head," the other teacher says. "They wouldn't stand for her spending half the class time on her own bullshit. They wouldn't put up with her antics."

Many parents in South-Central, teachers say, are less involved in their children's schools than parents in the Westside or San Fernando Valley. It is not that the parents care less than the other parents, but there are more single mothers who have other children and little time. A higher percentage of the mothers work full-time—and sometimes juggle two jobs. The majority have not attended college, and they are unfamiliar with college-preparatory classes. And those who are involved usually have less political clout than more affluent, white parents.

Late Friday afternoon, before Braxton's long commute home, he sits at his desk, massaging his temples. His eyes are bloodshot. He looks exhausted. He was up until three in the morning, worrying about how he will replace Little a month before the AP exam, how he will tell the students that their teacher bailed out on them.

He thinks back to his senior year in college, when all he wanted to do was return to South-Central and teach English. His goals and ambitions seemed so uncomplicated then. He never thought he would end up as an administrator, entangled in bureaucratic battles, scrapping with recalcitrant teachers, so far removed from the classroom.

When Scott Braxton's father, Frank, was growing up in South-Central, his mother wanted to ensure that he had an opportunity for a good education, an opportunity she had been denied. She grew up in an Atlanta orphanage and, after moving to Los Angeles, worked as a maid. A determined woman, she managed to obtain one of the handful of coveted school district permits that allowed Frank to leave his neighborhood and attend a junior high school and high school with a much stronger academic program. His mother attributed much of his later success to his solid academic foundation. Frank studied art in college and became the first black animator at Warner Bros.

When it was time for Frank's daughter to attend junior high school, Frank followed his mother's lead. He wanted his daughter and young son to attend a predominantly white junior high school near Hollywood that was considered a much better school than the junior high near their house. The school, however, only issued twenty-five permits a year to students who lived outside the neighborhood. The permits were handed out on a Monday morning—on a first-come-first-serve basis. Frank camped out in a sleeping bag outside the school on Friday, Saturday, and Sunday nights, and his wife relieved him and held his spot in line during the day. On Monday morning, Frank obtained the eighteenth permit for his daughter.

When it was time for Scott to attend junior high school, he was automatically accepted by the same school, because his older sister was enrolled there. He had attended an all-minority grammar school, and now he was one of only a few dozen black students at the junior high, which had an enrollment of more than 2,000. A good-looking, athletic youth, he had little difficulty adjusting socially. In class, however, he had problems, initially. In grammar school, he had always been one of the top students, but now he had to adjust to more demanding teachers, more homework, more motivated students.

During his first year at the junior high school, his parents divorced, and when his mother felt he was slacking off, she would send him to live with his father, who was a stern taskmaster with extremely high standards. Sometimes, Frank would return home late on a weeknight and, while Scott was sleeping, scrutinize his homework. If he spotted an incomplete assignment, he would wake Scott up—sometimes well after midnight—and force him to finish his homework right then.

The black students with permits were allowed to attend a Westside high school, along with their junior high school classmates. This is where Scott's sister was enrolled. But when Scott graduated from junior high, he decided he wanted to attend his neighborhood school—Dorsey High School, which is Crenshaw's archrival. Scott was swayed by the black power movement sweeping his neighborhood at the time. He felt insulted by the idea that he could only get a good education if he went to school with whites, that he could only prepare for college by leaving the neighborhood.

When he was in the eighth grade, his father died of Hodgkin's disease. Had he been alive, Scott knows he would have attended high school with his sister because his father would have simply ordered him to get his butt to the school with the highest academic ranking. His mother was more flexible, and he enrolled at Dorsey.

He was a solid student at Dorsey, but not an inspired one. His father was no longer around to push him. And during his sophomore year, his mother became the road manager for the singer Roberta Flack, and left for long stretches at a time. He and his sister were on their own. He often coasted in school and devoted most of his energy to football—he played defensive back—and student government. During his senior year he was student body president.

When it was time to apply to college, he took the path of least resistance. He only applied to one school—La Verne College, a small private institution about forty-five miles from Los Angeles that had been attempting to recruit more minority students. His college counselor escorted him and a few other Dorsey seniors to visit the school. He had been considering a local community college, but when he received enough loans, scholarships, and financial aid to afford La Verne, he enrolled.

At La Verne, Braxton wrote a lengthy paper on the controversy over "black English." The research he conducted had a profound impact on him. He then decided to return to South-Central to teach English. When he walked down the halls, the other students would call out, "Welcome back, Kotter."

"The thought of all these kids who were bright, but whose futures were limited because they could only speak in ebonics and couldn't communicate properly outside their neighborhoods . . . well, that's what spurred me to be a teacher," Braxton says. "I knew someone needed to approach them with sensitivity, to let them know the way they spoke was okay, but also to let them know that to make it in the outside world they had to learn to switch, to be able to speak in newscaster language, too, when they had to. I was very idealistic. I thought I could really influence lives. I wanted to return to the 'hood. I didn't want to teach anywhere else.''

He was hired to teach English at a South-Central junior high school, but after only one semester, he received a notice from the school district that he was being transferred to a San Fernando Valley school. The transfer was part of a ''staff integration'' program. The school district was shifting white teachers to inner-city schools and black and Latino teachers to all-white schools with all-white teaching staffs. Braxton was adamantly opposed to leaving South-Central, so he and his principal finagled a way for him to thwart the school district mandate. He had to give up all his English classes and, instead, teach in a federally funded program at the school that was designed to boost reading skills. He had enjoyed trying to instill a passion for literature in his students. Now the teaching was rudimentary, with little intellectual challenge. But he stuck it out for two years before his principal managed to reassign him to regular English classes.

After a few more years at the school, Braxton decided he wanted to teach high school literature. The principal at Palisades, a highly regarded Westside high school, tried to recruit him, but Braxton was reluctant to leave the neighborhood. Still, he was flattered by the offer. And he felt that he needed to prove himself, needed to show that he was a good enough teacher to reach affluent white kids accustomed to a high-powered academic program.

Braxton spent two years at Palisades and then returned to South-Central and headed the gifted magnet program at a junior high school. Three years later, the principal at Crenshaw, who had heard parents talk about how committed Braxton was to his students, recruited him to be the coordinator of the high school's gifted program. At Crenshaw, he was immediately inundated. In addition to all his administrative tasks, he had to spend even more time helping the students through multifarious personal crises. One student's brother was murdered by police, and another student's brother was murdered by gang members, and another student's brother was convicted of murder, and another student's mother, who was a crack addict, abandoned him, and another student, who lived with his grandmother, had to raise his younger brother when she died, and another student was about to be thrown out of her group home after she punched a girl, and another student was molested by her stepfather, and on and on. During all of these crises, as the students failed classes, or dropped out of school, or ran away from home, or joined the service, or broke down emotionally, they all came to Braxton for support.

During his first year at Crenshaw, he spent many hours counseling a promising student who lived in one of the most impoverished, gang-ridden sections of South-Central. The boy's father had been murdered in a gang shootout. His mother was a crack addict. The boy had been a gangbanger, but was extremely bright and was trying to leave the gang scene.

During his senior year he was named the outstanding literature student at Crenshaw and won a Bank of America scholarship. He received a full scholarship to a small black college in the Midwest. A few weeks before he was scheduled to begin college, however, he decided to give up the scholarship. He had been looking after his mother since he was a boy. He nursed her after days-long cocaine binges, made sure she ate, and tried to prevent her from roaming the streets late at night. If he left home, he did not know how his mother would survive.

Finally, a few days before school was scheduled to begin, Braxton told him, "It's not *your* responsibility to save your mother. But it *is* your responsibility to save yourself." Braxton then called a travel agent and charged the boy's plane ticket to his own credit card. He met him at the airport and ensured that he boarded the plane.

The boy thrived at the school, and at the end of his freshman year he was on the honor roll. He is scheduled to graduate in June.

When Braxton started teaching at Crenshaw, he owned a house a few miles east of the school. He often had to contend with the unruly gang-bangers and the teenage prostitute who lived next door. Sometimes, drug addicts gathered on his front lawn. Once, a delirious crackhead ran through his front door, stood beside his sleeping, five-month-old son, and began screaming. During the 1992 riots, Braxton stood on the roof of his house, mesmerized by the surreal, panoramic view of fires in every direction.

One Sunday morning, a crackhead tried to steal his car stereo and a neighbor chased him away. Later that night, the crackhead, still miffed about the confrontation, returned and fired several rounds at the neighbor's house. One of the shots missed, hit Braxton's house, and punched through a picture in his living room. Braxton found the slug on the floor. Just a few seconds earlier, he had been standing right in front of the picture, with his headphones on, listening to a new Mozart CD. This was the final provocation. He decided to move.

He decided to buy a house in a better neighborhood, just a few miles away. He handed the real estate agent a "good faith" deposit of $5,000. When he brought a friend over to see the house, the friend spotted a bullet hole in the back window. Braxton had to do some fast talking to persuade the real estate agent to refund his deposit. He eventually bought a house in a quiet suburb east of the city.

He enjoys the placid setting, but the commute is wearing him down. He spends almost two and a half hours a day fighting the freeways. At home, he and his wife are exhausted by the demands of a baby and a toddler. And at school, this has been his most difficult year.

He spent countless hours counseling Olivia and Toya and Claudia, who had flunked Little's class because she refused to turn in the writing assignments. And then there was Sabreen, the girl who, like Olivia, lived in a foster home and who dropped out of Crenshaw in November. Braxton recently spoke with Sabreen and discovered that she is living with her boyfriend and planning to get married next month. Sabreen is carrying a full load of classes at a community college, but she is overwhelmed. Her boyfriend has two jobs, and Sabreen is left with most of the household tasks. After working more than forty hours a week and then shopping, cleaning the house, doing the laundry, preparing dinner, and making her boyfriend's lunch for the next day, she does not have the energy to study.

"I didn't think it would be like this," Sabreen tells me during a recent conversation. "I've been trying my best to stay focused on school, but I'm just so tired all the time. I want to stay in school and stay on track for my degree. But I just don't know if I can keep up this kind of hectic schedule."

Sabreen, Olivia, Toya, and Claudia are just a few of the seniors Braxton has counseled extensively this year. There were also many freshmen, sophomores, and juniors with equally compelling stories, who demanded much of him.

In addition to the students, he has spent a stressful school year dealing with Toni Little and her multitudinous complaints and battles and schemes and threatened lawsuits. And now he discovers she might take a health-related leave for the rest of the year, leaving him scrambling for a substitute qualified to teach a college-level English course.

Braxton found out this morning that he passed the school district's assistant-principal exam. He plans to seek a position at another school in the fall. He does not think he can survive another year at Crenshaw.

TWENTY-EIGHT

YVONNE NOBLE

READING IS FUNDAMENTAL

None of the administrators have talked to Toni Little during the week following spring break. None of the students have any idea whether she is going to return.

The students, who have been worried about the upcoming AP exam, are even more anxious now that Little is gone. They know that they need her to prepare them. Many have repeatedly approached me at school and asked me when—or if—Little is returning. Finally, at the end of the week, I tell them that although I do not know, I will try to find out. I decide to talk to the principal, Yvonne Noble, and then visit Little at home during the weekend.

Noble is a commanding, intimidating figure at Crenshaw, who perpetually patrols the grounds during lunch and the nutrition break and seems to know the name of every student she encounters. Noble grew up dirt-poor in a Florida logging camp and was raised by her grandparents. She loved to read and felt that reading helped her to overcome segregated schools and substandard teaching. Now, every morning, on the school public address system, she concludes her short announcements with the refrain: "Remember, reading is fundamental."

Noble is one of those principals who engenders among the teachers diametrically opposed viewpoints about herself—without much middle ground. Some, such as Little, resent her and chafe under what they consider to be an autocratic reign. Others, such as Braxton and the AP government, AP science, and AP art teachers, appreciate her no-nonsense manner and how she can cut through bureaucratic double-talk and get things done. They also respect her because she is well read, a true intellectual, and she appreciates good teaching. She has a master's degree in English and still teaches a class every semester at a community college.

Noble tells me she has no idea if Little is planning to return and she speculates that Little probably has no idea herself. Noble still is working with Braxton on contingency plans. When I ask her about Little's various complaints about Crenshaw, she answers my question with a question. She asks if I know the meaning of the word "solipsistic." Then she nods, reluctant to elaborate.

During their conference before spring break, Noble gave Little a supreme compliment. She told her that she was the second best English teacher she had seen in her thirty years as an educator. "The best," she told her, "is me."

But she told Little that she is only a great teacher when she is focused on the literature and the students. When Little began at Crenshaw, Noble told her, she spent 95 percent of the time focusing on the literature and the students. Each year, the percentage has dropped. And each year her AP passage rate has dropped. This year, Noble told Little, the percentage of time she spends digressing on personal matters is at an all-time high.

"And who loses because of this?" Noble asks me, pointing to Little's third-floor classroom. "The students."

Little has been so dissatisfied with the school that she has attempted to persuade the parents of a number of her tenth graders to send their children to other high schools, Crenshaw administrators say. Two tenth graders have already transferred and several others are considering leaving the school at the end of the year.

Some of the parents have been influenced by Little's denunciations of the school. Others are simply put off by the contentiousness permeating Little's class, and feel their children have been caught in the middle of a battle that does not concern them. Noble has asked some students to write statements, buttressing her claim that Little has made comments in class that were "injurious to the community." Little has enlisted other students to write statements in support of her.

After Braxton talks on the telephone to a mother who was outraged that her daughter became ensnared in Little's dispute with school administrators, he slams down the phone and mutters, "This program is coming apart at the seams. Two kids have already left because of Little's influence. All these other kids are talking about leaving. This is like a virus that's spreading. She's hurt and offended virtually everyone involved with this program." He sighs, looking defeated. "I wish I could have found some way to have used her brilliance to make this a better program. The fact that, ultimately, I couldn't will haunt me until the day I retire."

Braxton now has to process the paperwork on the two students who have transferred. He knows that the next dropout slip he has to contend with may be Little's.

On Saturday morning, I stop by Little's one-bedroom duplex. It has a galley kitchen, a computer in the living room, and a strip of brick for a backyard. On the walls, she has two posters of Marilyn Monroe and a poster with a quote from Jesus:

"IF YOU BRING FORTH THAT WHICH IS WITHIN YOU, WHAT YOU BRING FORTH WILL SAVE YOU. IF YOU DO NOT BRING FORTH WHAT IS WITHIN YOU, WHAT YOU DO NOT BRING FORTH WILL DESTROY YOU."

Although her moods might be cyclonic in class, she still projects an aura of authority. Today, however, as she huddles on her sofa, clutching her three Papillons for security, she seems diminished, a frail and frightened woman. Her face is speckled with stress-induced rashes and blotches. Glassy-eyed and jumpy, she smokes one Marlboro Light after another. She is taking an antianxiety medication that her doctor prescribed for her a few days ago.

The stress has been building all year, Little tells me, and finally reached a peak and overwhelmed her during the meeting with Noble. After school that day, she returned home and collapsed.

Little takes a few drags of her cigarette, fanning away the smoke. She has thought about the students every single day, she says, fighting back tears. She feels terrible leaving them in the lurch, just a month from the AP exam. She would like to rent a hotel room and teach the students there. Anything, she says, anything to avoid returning to Crenshaw. She takes another nervous drag and leans forward. She cannot return to Crenshaw right now, she says in a confidential tone. She is too frightened.

"Right before spring break this administrator came up to me at Crenshaw and threatened my life. She said to me, 'I saw you on the freeway all crashed up. I'm amazed that you're still alive.' " Little lights another cigarette, her hands trembling. "I told her that my car was *not* crashed up. 'Oh, well,' she told me. 'I thought it was you.' Then she laughed and walked away.

"I consider that a threat. These people are gangsters. I think that if I go back, I'm putting myself in harm's way. I'm really scared that they'll hurt me. I'm freaked out to the fucking bone."

Little smokes a cigarette without saying a word. When she stubs it out she launches into a long screed, encompassing her hatred for the school, her love for the students, how her discrimination complaint against the school is going nowhere, how the school district investigator is incompetent, how her district union representative does not like her because she is white, how the administrators who oppose her are liars and racists, how everyone conspires against her.

Someone strolls by the duplex and Little's three little dogs—Tara, Duluca, and Hannah—leap off the sofa and race about in a frenzy, yapping and pawing the door and jumping at the window. Little attempts to calm the dogs down, speaking to them in soothing tones. She strokes their necks, and coaxes them back onto her lap.

"I've cried every day about this because I feel so bad about the students," she says. "That's why I'm taking that antianxiety medication.

The kids don't deserve this. I was supposed to do a poetry section. They need that to prepare for their AP test. But I didn't do it. Too much was going on. I feel bad about that.

"They deserve to get the rest of their education. I consider it a privilege to teach these kids. They're so bright. They're the match of kids anywhere. They've been my comrades. But I can't die for them.

"I've really enjoyed the journey with them. We've been through so much this year together." She stares off into the middle distance, looking wistful as she reminisces about the year. "It was amazing how *Portrait of the Artist* made such an impact on Latisha's life . . . I'll never forget the way Miesha read the part of the preacher in *Inherit the Wind* . . . I was moved by how Curt got so into *Wuthering Heights* . . . The kids were so into it when Tommie Smith came to class."

She hugs her dogs and says, "I miss Danielle. I'd like to ensure that she gets what she needs so she can make it to Stanford. I miss Miesha and Latisha because they love me. I miss Venola because she cares so much about the literature." Tears stream down her face, and she wipes her eyes with a tissue. "I even miss that little shit Curt, who can be so arrogant sometimes. I wonder what Willie is thinking about all this. He used to call me sometimes when he had questions about the literature. I wonder why he hasn't called me. In fact, no one in the AP class has called me. A number of tenth graders called me, though. A few of them said, 'Please come back. Why did you leave? Is it something *we* did?' "

She lights another cigarette and emits a cloud of smoke, a deep sigh mingling with her exhalation. For a few minutes she watches her dogs frolic in the living room. Finally, I broach the question all the students have been pestering me to ask her: "Are you coming back?"

She stubs out her cigarette and stares at the ashtray for a moment. "It's a real possibility that I could miss the rest of the year," she says. "But right now, I just don't know."

TWENTY-NINE

MAMA MOULTRIE

CAN I GET AN AMEN?

If Little does not return, Braxton is considering drafting Anita Moultrie to step in and take over the AP class, although Moultrie already is overwhelmed. She owns her own business and teaches full-time, is chairman of the English Department and has five children—including an infant. But she knows these seniors and she cares about them. She taught many of them last year in her eleventh-grade English class. Moultrie does not want to see them stuck with an apathetic substitute a month before the AP exam. She tells Braxton she will teach the class if he needs her.

As Little was increasingly distracted as the year progressed, Moultrie—despite her manifold responsibilities—seemed to have gained momentum. As she interweaves African American history with the assigned literature, her outrage at black subjugation keeps her at an intense pitch and sustains a taut classroom ambience. During the first semester, her lectures on the history of slavery in the American colonies were a counterpoint to *The Scarlet Letter*. She discussed the Civil War and Reconstruction through the prism of *Jubilee*. Now, during the second semester, the students are reading *Native Son,* which enables Moultrie to tie in black migration from the rural South to the Northern cities and the new kind of racism this engendered.

"I call this making connections," she tells the students on a warm, crackly, desert-dry Monday morning. "I want us to read the literature with a knowledge of where we, as people of color, fit into the historical perspective. When we read *The Scarlet Letter,* we learned about America as a place founded with the promise of freedom. Yet at the same time, they were enslaving African Americans and killing off a third of the Native Americans. In *Jubilee,* when the Civil War was over, they still burned down the sista's house three times. Today, the Klu Klux Klan's still burning crosses on people's lawns.

"In this class, we're progressing from the slave era to the 1940s with *Native Son.* In the book, Bigger's bad. He's a gangbanger. That's right. There were gangs in the 1940s, too. He's so bad he'll cut you or kill you. He'll curse his own mama."

Moultrie tells the class that she will be screening a documentary this morning, one of a series of films she will show in class that traces twentieth-century black history in America. The students will then have to write an essay based on the documentary.

"You're going to be learning about the Black Panthers in today's film," Moultrie says. "You're going to see all their black berets and black leather jackets and guns. You're going to hear their slogan: 'By any means necessary.' They've been portrayed as crazed black men. But there was a reason that they came about. They saw a need in the black community. If there wasn't police brutality or we had control of our schools, we wouldn't have needed the Black Panthers.

"I've been to dozens of schools all over this district. I've seen what goes on. We still don't have control of our schools. We can't even get rid of teachers who aren't doing right," she says, a veiled reference, perhaps, to Little.

"I learned the hard way that nice don't get you anywhere. You got to fight. You think I got to be the owner of the largest black-owned party business in Southern California by just sitting around? Hel-*lo*?

"After you see this film today, and you write your essays, I don't want any of this namby-pamby stuff in your paper. I don't want any of this: 'Well, the Black Panthers did this and that,' " she says in a simpering voice. "I want you to challenge established notions.

"Y'all better wake up because times are changing. All this gimme, gimme, gimme just ended. They're takin' it all away. Affirmative action's going by the wayside. Government programs are being cut. Look at food stamps. You're in line at the market and they're sorting out the milk and the meat items and everyone in line's lookin' at you like you're a dog."

Several students nod. A girl calls out, "It takes sooo long."

"That's demoralizing," Moultrie says. "There's nothing wrong with food stamps. There's no reason they have to make you feel like you're less than nothin'. Well, all this is coming to an end. We got to get ourselves together as a people. We got to make things happen for ourselves. That's what the Black Panthers were trying to do. The way we do it in *this* classroom is through education. Education is how you help yourself and help your people."

Moultrie leans against her desk, breathes deeply, and exhales theatrically. "I'm done preaching for the day," she says. "Let's watch the film."

Moultrie starts almost every class now by writing an African proverb on the blackboard. The students then spend a half hour interpreting the proverb and writing a short essay. On this Wednesday morning, the proverb for the day is:

HE WHO IS UNABLE TO DANCE, SAYS THAT THE YARD IS STONE.
—Kenya.

After the students finish their essays, they begin reading the first assigned play of the second semester, *A Streetcar Named Desire*, which is part of the required curriculum for Crenshaw eleventh graders. Moultrie immediately interrupts the girl who is playing Blanche.

"Go on with your *bad* self," Moultrie says. "Put some feeling into your part, girlfriend."

A minute later she interrupts the boy who is playing Stanley.

"Don't be so wishy-washy," she tells him. "Play the part low down and mean. You Mack Daddy now."

The boy reads the passage in which Stanley is sifting through Blanche's wardrobe trunk. He examines a few of her furs and says to his wife, Stella: "I got an acquaintance who deals in this sort of merchandise. I'll have him in here to appraise it . . ." He checks out her jewelry and says, "I have an acquaintance that works in a jewelry store. I'll have him in here to make an appraisal of this . . ."

Moultrie places her book face down on her desk and says, "This brutha is plugged into the neighborhood. He knows everyone."

A boy named Che raises his hand. "It's like in the 'hood. Everybody's got a cousin to do this or that."

When Stella heads off to the porch and Blanche returns, she flirts with Stanley and asks him to help her button up the back of her dress.

Moultrie puts a hand on her hip and says, "Students, now why is Blanche acting like this? Don't you all know girls like this? They act like the bomb, but they're really insecure. Blanche is flirting like that and putting it out there because of the emptiness in her own life. When she's flirting like this, I can guarantee something's going to happen. You best listen to me. Y'all *know* Mama Moultrie's got the *vision*."

She puts her book down and asks, "What do you think of Stanley?"

A student named Shayla cups her hands around her mouth and barks. "He's a dog."

"It's interesting," Moultrie says, "that Stanley is very offended when he's called a Polack. But he'll make racist comments to Pablo and calls him a greaseball. You notice that?

"When the play begins, Blanche acts all hotsy-totsy and looks down on her sister for marrying some ol' Polack. She acts like her sister's living in a big dump. Now, when she's alone with Stanley, her attitude is like: My sister got herself a *maaaan*," she says, giving the word a throaty, bluesy inflection. "She layin' up with some fine, buff, good lookin' *maaaan*.

"Come on, men, when a girl comes on like that don't you think: Wha's up with *this* girl?"

A boy named Marcel says, "I'd think that I can have it if I want it."

"Come on, girls," Moultrie says. "Watch how you carry yourself.

Don't wear your dresses up to here and then get mad when a brutha says you have a nice A-S-S. Girls, when you use your sexuality—like Blanche—to get something, it can lead to trouble. It can lead to something like date rape. So be careful. Don't play like that.

"Bruthas, when a girl says no, she means NO! She could be prancing around in a red kimono like Blanche, but if she says no, it means NO! You got it?"

She wags a forefinger at the girls in the front row. "Sistas, respect yourself. People will respect you back. That's some free advice from Mama Moultrie."

When the students finish reading the next scene, Moultrie says, "Remember, a writer doesn't put anything in by accident. So why does Blanche buy the colored paper lantern and put it over the lightbulb when she talks to Mitch? It's so Mitch can't get a real good look at her face.

"Anglo women don't age as well as us women of color. The sun causes them a lot of wrinkles. Blanche doesn't want him to know how old she really is. Blanche deceives Mitch in some other ways, too. She tells him she's visiting New Orleans because Stella hasn't been well. That's not true. She doesn't want Mitch to know that she's destitute. You know how it is. You don't want to get wit' a brutha or sista if they have lots of problems. You afraid they'll bring you down with them. You know what I'm saying? You got it?"

A student reads the stage directions in which Blanche "turns the knobs on the radio and it begins to play 'Wien, Wien, nur du allein.' Blanche waltzes to the music . . ."

"What's that song mean?" a student asks Moultrie.

Moultrie studies it for a moment, looking confused. Finally, she says, "It means, wang, wang, do your thang."

She smiles and the class bursts out laughing.

The next Monday, before class, Moultrie writes on the blackboard: "East Coast rapper Notorious B.I.G. was recently gunned down. Tupac Shakur, a West Coast rapper, was killed last year. Share your feelings." Moultrie decides to use the murder as a segue to discussing *Native Son*.

"Why are two prominent rappers dead?" Moultrie asks the class.

"Why are we fighting among ourselves? What's the real issue here? It's not really about East Coast rap versus West Coast, is it? What are the economic, social, and political issues here? It's something bigger than the death of two bruthas."

"Black people who prosper seem to get killed," Shayla says.

"When black people get too big, white people want to bring 'em down," Clinton says.

"I agree with Clinton," Che says. "It's like with Johnnie Cochran. People always trying to bring him down. They always bringing up bad stuff about him."

"But Notorious wasn't killed by white people," Moultrie says. "He was killed by another brutha. The Bible says that if you live by the sword, you die by the sword. This is Mama Moultrie talkin' now. The good you give is going to come back to you. And so is the bad.

"Look at Tupac. He wanted to live the thug life. Did you really think that wasn't going to come back to him? We've got two rappers, two bruthas, two talented young men lying flat on their back, dead in the street. And for what?

"There's a lot of anger out there on the street. There's a lot of rage. You can see that rage very clearly in *Native Son* with Bigger. His rage builds and builds. Remember when he was sitting between those two white people in the restaurant. They were telling him, 'Oh, Bigger, we just *love* you folks,' " Moultrie says in a sugary, patronizing voice. " 'We just want to *relate* to you. Why don't you take us to one of your restaurants and eat—what do you call it—soul food. Why don't you sing one of those spirituals you all love to sing.' " Moultrie sings a few bars of "Amazing Grace" and abruptly stops.

"They thought Bigger was happy being with them. But he was getting angrier and angrier. They didn't have a clue. There was rage there, but they couldn't see it. Look at the rage that leads so many young African American men to jails and prisons. Look at the rage that sparked the Watts riots in '65 and the 1992 riots after the Rodney King verdict." In a mock-white voice she says, " 'This is Channel 7 News. Why are those people down there rioting and tearing up their own communities?' Here we are in the 1990s, and these people still don't have a clue.

"When Bigger's working for his white boss he's real timid." She casts her eyes down and mimics Bigger. " 'Yes, sah. No, sah.' But all the while his rage builds. Can't we get beyond the slave mentality today? My bruthas, you were kings at one time. You were building pyramids."

She draws a circle on the blackboard. Inside the circle she carves out a tiny sliver. "This is all we have out of the piece of pie. Yet you bruthas are fighting over this sliver of the 'hood. And it's not even yours. You don't even own any of it.

"And what's society doing about it? Well, there's plenty of black men wearing orange jumpsuits in jail." She says angrily, "They're all being told when to shit, when to piss, when to eat, when to sleep. I talked to a lady yesterday and she waited five hours at the jail to see her son for ten minutes. We all know someone in jail or in prison or on probation. We're becoming a demoralized people in a wealthy society." She claps an eraser on the blackboard. "That's some of the anger that Bigger has.

"All of you, listen to me. Nobody's gonna hand you nothin'—excuse the double negative. Y'all have the chance to be our doctors and lawyers and accountants. Don't just take these jobs to enrich yourselves. You need to be leaders in your community. You need to have a conscience. You need to give back to your community. You need to recycle your dollars in your community. After the '92 riots, my husband and I opened our business on Florence and Van Ness. People said, 'Oh, nobody's going to come to a business down there on Florence in South-Central.' Well, we're still there, still a black-owned business, still hiring neighborhood kids so they can be a part of our business."

She surveys the class. "Can I get an amen?"

"Amen!" the students shout in unison.

"When I see you come back and own businesses here and begin your professions, I'm rewarded. So I want y'all to be more politically and socially oriented—as people of color. Contribute something. Be like Thurgood Marshall, a man who worked for his people. Not like my brutha Clarence Thomas. The less said about him, the better. I'm talking to y'all from the heart. I'm telling it like a sister would."

"All right, now," a student says.

"Tell it," another student calls out.

Moultrie has returned to Sunday school now, teaching and preaching, bellowing to attract the students' attention and then whispering, confiding in them, pacing and waving her hands, challenging them, imploring them, leavening her literature lecture with street talk and Afrocentric ideals.

"Here at Crenshaw, all of you are in a comfort zone. But when you get out into the world, the whole world's going to be judging you, not just by the content of your character, but by the color of your skin. You'll be working under a veil of media misconceptions. You'll be looked at as gangbanging, undisciplined lowlifes. Some people may not be calling you a nigga, but a lot of them will be treating you like one. You know when it's going on. Let's get real. Do you hear what I'm saying? Hel-*lo*."

"We hear you," several students shout.

"People look at me and say, 'Anita, you're militant.' I'm not militant. I'm socially aware. Are you with me? Literature helps you take off the rose-colored glasses and helps you see reality. In *Native Son,* it helps you see Bigger's anger. It helps you see that the anger is still here today."

"Yeah, there's anger," Marcel says. "But that's the way it is. So we might as well move on."

Moultrie is furious. "You can be a stronger brutha than *that,*" she says with disgust. "I teach because I don't want you students to be complacent. But what I hear you saying, Marcel, is, 'Oh, well, That's how it is. That's how it's gonna be.' I hear you saying that we *can't* make a difference. That's a lie from the pit of hell. I hear you saying that we might as well give up. That's a slave mentality. And from a brutha who I thought had a *con*science." She looks Marcel up and down and shakes her head in disappointment. He is embarrassed, afraid to meet her gaze.

She pats him on the shoulder and says, "I still love you, Marcel. I love all you kids. I love you with the blood of Christ. Why? Because I do. It's a great honor for me to be a part of your lives. I don't teach for the money. I teach because I want to touch lives. I teach because I have a passion for making a difference."

Moultrie traces her social conscience to her high school years in Oakland, where the Black Panthers were founded, during the late 1960s, when the Panthers were capturing headlines. Others in her neighborhood were enthralled by the Panthers' swagger, their ultra-cool black leather jackets and black berets, their uncompromising "by any mean necessary" attitude. Moultrie, however, was impressed by the Panthers' concern for their community and their willingness to fight injustice and racism; by their free lunch and child-care programs, their community school for inner-city students, their "Panther patrols" to prevent police brutality.

Moultrie and her three brothers and sisters grew up in an all-black area of East Oakland. Her father, a graduate of the University of Arkansas at Pine Bluff, was an FBI agent who attended law school at night. Although he worked for an agency that was virtually at war with the Panthers, Moultrie held the organization—not the man—responsible. She still greatly respected her father for his community activism. He was a leader at their church—one of the most prominent black Baptist churches in Oakland— and after he passed the bar he volunteered to handle all of the church's legal services. He was still active in the black fraternity he had joined in college, which supported many programs for inner-city teenagers. And he frequently mentored and tutored black students in Oakland and helped raise money for scholarships.

He eventually left the FBI, established a law practice, and the family moved to an upper-middle-class neighborhood in the Oakland Hills. Moultrie encountered discrimination for the first time at her grammar school. One of her closest friends at the new school was having a slumber party and she gave her mother a list of all the fifth-graders she wanted to attend. The next day, the girl told Moultrie that she could not invite her because her mother did not want any black children at their house.

A few months later, the students vied for roles in the class Christmas pageant. Moultrie wanted to play Mary, but the teacher told her that a black Mary would be inappropriate. Again, Moultrie returned home from school devastated. But this time her mother, an elementary school teacher, could take action. She complained to the principal with such vehemence that he ordered the teacher to give Moultrie the role.

Moultrie attended a high school that was predominantly white and about one-fifth black. She was an excellent student, but during her senior year, her counselor offered the same advice she dispensed to all black girls: Forget about college and attend secretarial school in the fall. Moultrie's mother, who eventually earned a Ph.D. in education when her children were grown, was outraged. She visited the school and informed the counselor that both she and her husband were college graduates, and they expected all four of their children to also graduate from college. Furthermore, she told him, she planned to inform the principal about his racist assumptions and bigoted notions.

Moultrie and her three brothers and sisters all fulfilled their parents' expectations and earned college degrees. Moultrie majored in child development and graduated from the University of California at Davis. She then moved to Southern California and enrolled in a teaching-credential program—for both English and special education—at a state college, where she encountered a number of teachers whom she regarded as racists.

One of her teachers told the students during a lecture that "black children have smaller brain capacities than white children." Moultrie slammed her pen down, crossed her arms, and stared at the teacher. The rest of the students in the class were furiously jotting notes.

"Do you have a problem with what I said?" the teacher asked her.

Moultrie delivered a resounding malediction and concluded by demanding to see his research. He hemmed and hawed, and eventually acknowledged that he may have been relying more on speculation than fact.

Later that year, another teacher chartered a bus and transported the class on a tour of inner-city neighborhoods, where many of the students would soon start their teaching careers. As the bus rumbled through South-Central, the teacher, who narrated the tour, told the students: "See how the old men sit in front of the liquor stores all day . . . Look at how they write on the walls of their own neighborhood . . . Pay attention to how *these* people live because many of you are going to be dealing with *them* on your first teaching jobs."

The tour concluded at Locke High School in Watts, and the teacher asked the group: "Do you know who this school was named after?" No one raised his hand. He then pointed to Moultrie—the only black student in the class—and said: "Anita, *you* should know."

Moultrie did not know that the school was named after the first black Rhodes scholar. And she was insulted by his tone.

"Why should *I* know?" she growled through clenched teeth.

"Because he's black and you're black."

Again, Moultrie exploded in anger, berating the teacher for his condescending tone during the tour and his ethnic stereotyping. He, too, backed down. He had not imagined anyone would find his comments offensive, he told Moultrie. All he wanted to do, he insisted, was orient the students to the ghetto neighborhoods where many would soon be teaching.

Moultrie's first job was in Pacoima, an impoverished section of the San Fernando Valley, at a high school that was half Latino and half black. The school district was attempting to integrate the teaching staffs at the city's schools during this time. Moultrie frequently overheard some of the new white teachers denigrate their students, saying: "Those black kids can't learn *any*thing . . ." "*All* of 'em are probably on welfare . . ." "*None* of the parents give a damn about their kids' education."

This experience radicalized Moultrie. She realized she had to be a strong advocate for her students, that she had to stand up for them, look out for them because they faced discrimination, not just in society at large, but, sometimes, at their own neighborhood schools. After a few years in Pacoima, she transferred to a South-Central high school, where she taught English for five years. She was then picked for a federally funded school-district program that trained teachers to provide other English teachers with techniques for instructing black students. The program analyzed why some black children have difficulty with standard English and traced their distinctive speech patterns to West African languages. The program also emphasized incorporating black culture and history into English instruction, an emphasis that greatly influenced Moultrie when she later taught at Crenshaw.

Moultrie has been with the gifted magnet program for four years, and she never had the opportunity to teach an AP class. But because the pass rate in Little's AP classes has been slipping and because she has been so distracted this year, school administrators have discussed with Moultrie the possibility of teaching the AP class, perhaps as early as next year.

Moultrie has mixed feelings about teaching AP English. She believes the test is culturally biased and, along with many other academic achievement tests, is used as a way to hinder minority students. But she also knows that the exam would be the ultimate challenge for her as a teacher.

If Moultrie teaches AP English next year, she will include ethnic litera-ture in the reading list. She also plans to incorporate black history and culture into the AP curriculum. This will help students understand and appreciate traditional works of literature that she believes many find—initially, at least—alienating.

THIRTY

THE FOURTH SUBSTITUTE

IT'S HARDER THAN IT LOOKS

On Monday morning—the second week of Little's absence—a third substitute arrives. Like the first two substitutes she has not been prepped about the class, so she asks me what the students should be doing today. While I fill her in, the students complain about the timing of Little's absence.

"Miss Little is letting us down," says a girl named Brandi, the senior class president.

"What's the point of coming?" another girl asks, when she spots the substitute. She pivots around and walks out the door.

A boy glances around the room, sees only a third of the class in their seats and says, "This class is getting smaller and smaller every day."

The few remaining students start to read the last act of *Hamlet,* but only Venola and two other students seem interested in the play. The others clown around during the reading. One boy asks to play the part of the queen and he shows off for the girls by speaking in a falsetto. Other students read their lines in mock ebonics. One boy in the corner falls asleep, snoring loudly.

The final scene of the play, one of the most rousing in all of drama, is fraught with several climactic plot twists. In a rapid-fire concatenation of tragic events: Gertrude accidentally drinks the poisoned cup of wine that Claudius had meant for Hamlet; Hamlet and Laertes are mortally wounded in a duel; before he dies, Hamlet kills Claudius.

I feel bad that the few students interested in the play have to hear the final, dramatic scenes butchered and parodied. Their teacher is gone. Their substitute has been thrown into the breach, unprepared. Their AP exam is only a few weeks away. Their understanding of the play may prove a factor in whether they pass the exam or not. In their college English classes, they will be expected to have read—and understood—Shakespeare. Most of them are good students. Even the ones who are fooling around are acting out of character, a temporary lapse because of Little's absence. It is not fair that they are caught in the middle of Little's dispute with the school. Yet they are the ones who are paying the penalty. They all deserve better than this.

I do not feel comfortable usurping the substitute's authority and simply taking over the class. And I do not feel qualified. So I lean over and, in a whisper, ask if she wants to say something about the play in order to get the students back on track.

She shakes her head and says, "It's been a long time since I read *Hamlet*."

Exasperated, Venola and the few other students still interested in the play look as if they are ready to bolt the room. I feel I have to say something, anything, in order to salvage the class before there is not a single student left.

I clear my throat, tap my hand on my desk, and tell them I want to make a few points. The students initially quiet down and pay attention. They are amused at the novelty of seeing me in a teaching role. Drawing on a memory of a college Shakespeare class, a production of *Hamlet* I saw in England about fifteen years ago, and various snippets from magazine articles and books I have read over the years, I launch into a rambling, disjointed monologue about the play. I tell them why Hamlet is regarded as the first modern, introspective protagonist; why his ambivalence came at a great cost and led to the death of six other characters; why *Hamlet* is my favorite Shakespeare play; why they should care about the play; why some critics think there is an Oedipal theme in the play; why Hamlet's soliloquies are so compelling; why the play's themes are timeless.

Midway through my lecture, I watch as the students, one by one, lose interest. They fidget and gaze out the window and pass notes to each other. Still, I continue to barrel along. Finally, when it is clear that not a single student is paying attention—not even Venola—I talk more slowly, more softly, more slowly, steadily losing energy like a windup toy sputtering to a halt, until I finally stop, midsentence, discouraged and defeated.

At this moment I appreciate Little's skills as a teacher. I recall how she never simply unloaded information on the students—as I just did—and how she had a gift for drawing critical insights out of them. By asking the right questions or briefly highlighting a salient point, she enabled the students to make their own discoveries about the literature. This, I realize, is the art of teaching. So many times, I watched her engage virtually every student in the class into a passionate discussion and inspire in them a real enthusiasm for the literature and its themes. It seemed so effortless, so easy. I realize now it is not.

I decide to emulate Little's approach and ask the students questions about the play. But my first few questions do not interest them. Several students answer me, just to be polite. But they, too, soon lose interest. I feel stymied. I do not know what I can ask them that will spark their interest. There are thirty minutes left in class. I ask the substitute if she has any ideas. She shakes her head. I tell the class to spend the remaining time working on their Act 5 study questions.

On Wednesday morning, Latisha wanders into class eating a fast-food taco for breakfast. When she sees the substitute, she walks out. When Brandi sees that I am going to try to teach the class again, she says to me, "No offense, but nobody does it like Miss Little." She, too, walks out. Even Danielle, the most conscientious student in AP English, cuts class when she sees that Little is gone again.

Still, there are fourteen students left in class, a few of whom want to study *Hamlet*. And although my teaching debut on Monday was hardly a success, I feel I should, at least, try to help these students appreciate and understand *Hamlet*. So I decide to have another go at sparking a class discussion. If I can do this, then I figure they will be in the right frame of mind to read the last few acts of the play. I guess you could call this a lesson plan, of sorts.

I know the students live in one of the most murderous neighborhoods in the country—if South-Central were a separate city it would rank among the nation's top ten for homicides. They all know about Crenshaw classmates who have been killed for wearing the wrong colored shirt, or for standing on the wrong street corner, or for giving the wrong answer to the traditional gang challenge: "Where are you from?" These students are more intimately familiar with murder than any students in America.

I want them to think about why so many homicides in their neighborhood are committed without premeditation, with so little motivation, for such inconsequential reasons. How some of their gangbanging Crenshaw classmates could nonchalantly gun down a rival in a drive-by. And then I want them to contrast this to Hamlet's view of murder, how the taking of a single life was such a momentous decision for him, how he was almost driven to madness because of his tormented ambivalence, his interminable delays. Maybe this will generate some discussion. So I introduce the topic.

"I don't think people around here take murder so casually," says a girl defensively.

"Some people do," Sadi says. "People murder other people all the time around here for nothin'. They smoke a few sherms [marijuana laced with angel dust] and get all doped up and they don't even remember it. I know people who've shot people and they think it's cool. They say, 'I watched him drop—It was just like TV.' It's like they're bragging. They say, 'I'd do it again.' They don't even know it's bad. Like when a lion kills his prey and eats it. He doesn't feel bad. It's all about survival. And for some of these dudes, it's about recognition, too. It's like, 'Now I'm hard core.' It's like a trophy."

A boy raises his hand and waves it, until I realize that he is waiting for me to call on him.

I nod and he says, "They be shootin' people on the street here like they dogs. The fool who pulls the trigger don't even think that boy he kills is gonna have a grieving mama. He don't even think of the boy as human. He just an object to him. But Hamlet is different. He realizes that he gonna be killing a human being. He knows the taking of a human life is some serious shit. There's a real humanity to Hamlet, you know what I'm sayin'?"

Playing devil's advocate, I ask the class how Hamlet could approach one murder—his uncle's—with such gravity and then be so blasé when he discovers that he stabbed the wrong man behind the curtain—Polonius, not Claudius.

A girl nods and says, "It was an accident. It wasn't premeditated. After Hamlet did him, he figured: 'What's done is done. I can't change it, so I better move on and take care of my business.' "

Another girl shakes her head in disagreement. "Hamlet was like a gangbanger who shoots into some house during a drive-by. Then he kills an innocent bystander and says, 'Who cares.' I don't think Hamlet delays killing his uncle because he was such a great humanitarian. He delays 'cause he's not sure if the ghost was telling the truth about his uncle capping his daddy. He has to find out for sure. When he's sure, then he's ready to do his uncle."

I am relieved when I see the students probe the issue with some enthusiasm. When their interest flags, I introduce the topic of revenge— in the play and on the street.

"Hamlet lived for revenge," Sadi says. "Just like a lot of gangbangers. They waste their lives—all for revenge. A guy I know joined a gang 'cause his brother was killed. So he wanted to kill as many as he could for revenge."

"My dad's cousin was murdered," a boy says. "For the longest time all he could think about was catching that murderer."

"My dad's brother was murdered," a girl says. "The police didn't care. They didn't do shit. My dad was like Hamlet. He tried to find out the truth. But he could never catch the motherfucker. Because he never got revenge, he never got over the murder. Revenge would have been good for him. It would have been like a cleansing."

"The Bible says: 'Thou shall not kill,' " another girl adds. "I don't believe in murder. You should put someone in prison for the rest of their life.''

"The Bible also says an eye for an eye," a boy says. "Anyone who kills, should be killed.''

"It's not just Hamlet, who is looking for revenge in the play," Larrin says. "Laertes's father was murdered, too. He's looking to avenge the death of his father, too. So while Hamlet's seeking to avenge his father, by killing his uncle, Laertes is seeking to avenge his own father, by killing Hamlet.''

"That was Ophelia's father, too," says Robert, who, like Larrin, plays on the baseball team and writes for the school newspaper. "Look how different Hamlet and Ophelia respond to the death of their fathers. Hamlet wants revenge. But Ophelia doesn't. She just breaks down.''

The students nod, intrigued by Larrin's and Robert's comments. After a quiet, reflective moment, I ask them why Hamlet treated Ophelia so brutishly? Why didn't he confide in her? Did he distrust her, or was he trying to protect her?

"Hamlet didn't have to do Ophelia like that, but it's typical of the way these macho dudes treat their girlfriends," a girl says. "Somethin' comes up and all they say is: 'I can handle it.' They never want to tell you what's really happening.''

"If the dude did tell you, you'd probably cry: 'boo, hoo,' and go all hysterical and what good would that do?" a boy asks, smiling slyly.

When the discussion devolves into a screaming match between the boys and the girls, I ask them if there are any parallels between the political climate of seventeenth-century Denmark and twentieth-century America, between any characters in the play and twentieth-century political figures.

"The play shows that telling the truth is dangerous," a boy says. "Once Hamlet started to tell the truth, he was doomed. You tell the truth, you die. Look at Malcolm X.''

"And JFK and RFK," a girl says.

"And Martin Luther King," a boy adds. "The FBI tried to set him up and make him look bad and then lied about it. That's the kind of thing Claudius did.''

"The government of Denmark was corrupt, just like our government is corrupt," Larrin says. "Look how the CIA sent cocaine into South-Central during the Contra war."

The discussion proceeds for ten more minutes before I halt it. The students seem sufficiently engaged and interested in the play. Now is the time, I feel, to read the last two scenes of *Hamlet*. The students pick parts and resume reading. There is no miraculous transformation; the students do not suddenly read with insight and passion. They still struggle with the lines and some still read in a monotone. But at least they appear to be trying, and most of the class seems to understand the story line. When Gertrude sips the poisoned wine, a few students gasp. When Hamlet is mortally wounded, everyone is following along intently.

At the play's conclusion, Venola raises her hand. "I'm sad," she says. "I really got to like Hamlet. Why did he have to die?"

I explain that Hamlet is a tragedy, and that Shakespeare's plays are divided into comedies, histories, and tragedies. The class discusses the meaning of tragedy for a few minutes, and then the bell rings.

"What are we going to do Friday?" Larrin asks me, as he walks out. I shake my head. "I have no idea."

On Friday morning, I bring to class the movie version of *Hamlet*, starring Mel Gibson. But I cannot find a VCR in the neighboring classrooms. One teacher just had his second VCR stolen—including one he had brought from home—and there is currently a VCR shortage at the school. A few students volunteer to wander through the halls in search of one. They bring back what looks like the first VCR ever made, and we watch the movie for a few minutes, but the picture is so dim and faint the actors are mere shadows. I call a teacher I know, tell him my predicament, and he promises to secure a newer model for me in a few minutes. I send a student to pick it up, and we watch the movie.

During previous classes, when students realized Little was gone again, they simply cut class. But this morning, when they see that a movie will be shown, they stick around. Most of them are interested in the movie, but a few talk and giggle, distracting the other students. The substitute is unable to keep order, so I, reluctantly, try to quiet them down. As a reporter, I do not feel it is appropriate for me to discipline students; this is not a role I am comfortable with. But by attempting to teach the class, I have already crossed some sort of line. And I figure the students who are trying to watch the movie are counting on me. So I walk over to the obstreperous students, kneel beside their desks, and attempt to reason with them. I return to my desk. When I see my approach has not worked, I simply point at them whenever they begin to chatter. For some reason, this is effective. They smile shyly and look embarrassed—almost as embarrassed as me—that a reporter has to resort to this kind of inane tactic to keep order.

Because of the VCR snafu, we had a late start this morning and will not be able to finish the movie. So, with about fifteen minutes left in the class, I shut off the VCR and turn on the lights. The students are excited about the movie and eagerly discuss how it changed their perception of the play.

"The play seemed a lot more contemplative," Danielle says. "In the movie, Hamlet's rage and anger were more apparent."

"Oh, you *know* the brutha was angry," Latisha says. "He was out of control. The brutha was out there killin' folks. But I couldn't really see that Oedipal thang when I was reading it. But the movie played it out. Moms was scandalous. What a slut!"

"I thought it was going to be boring," a girl says. "But it was cool. I'm definitely coming to class Monday. I want to see the rest of it."

As I watch the students file out after class, I feel somewhat uncomfortable because my role has shifted so quickly. I had been accustomed to sitting in the back of the class and scribbling notes. Now I wonder if the dynamic of my relationship with the students will be inalterably changed because of my new role as a teacher and disciplinarian. I wonder if they will resent me, if it will now be difficult for me to return to the role of a reporter and resume interviewing the students and their families.

When Latisha lingers after class and thanks me for quieting the students down during the play, I am reassured. "That was sweet the way you've tried to show some leadership in class," she says. "All of us appreciate it, even the loudmouths who wouldn't shut up. We're grateful that you care enough about us to try and help out."

THIRTY-ONE

AFFIRMATIVE ACTION

EQUALITY AS A RESULT

Little still has not announced whether she is returning, and Braxton is increasingly distressed by the uncertainty of the situation. If Little is not coming back to Crenshaw this year, he would like to hire a replacement as soon as possible so the students are not subjected to a steady diet of substitute du jour. But he is at the mercy of Little, and since she has not yet declared her intentions, he has to accept this maddening, tenuous situation.

For Braxton, the saving grace of a difficult year occurs when the seniors march into his office, smiling proudly, and hand over their college acceptance letters—the culmination of their four years together. Braxton congratulates the students and then Xeroxes the letters and tapes them to a wall in his office. Now, mid-April, the wall is about half full. Braxton is particularly proud of the letter Danielle just handed him, which reads:

Dear Danielle,

It's with great pleasure that I write to offer you admission to Stanford

*University . . . I invite you to become a part of Stanford, not because
you fit a mold, but because you convinced us that you will bring something
original and extraordinary to the intellectual life of the university . . .*

Danielle—like Chelsea Clinton—was accepted to Stanford's class of
2000. But, unlike Chelsea, Danielle cannot afford to attend Stanford. The
University offered her about half of the approximately $30,000 a year she
needs for room, board, and tuition. But her family cannot pay the difference. The shortfall is such an unfathomable sum to her that she is not
particularly distressed when she realizes she will have to turn Stanford
down. She simply cannot afford to attend the school. That is an incontro-
vertible truth, so she has spent little time worrying about it.

"It's strictly a matter of money," she says with a philosophical shrug.

Fortunately, Pitzer College offered her almost a full scholarship and
financial-aid package, and she is enthusiastic about the school. She plans
to commit to Pitzer this week.

Curt just found out he was rejected from Stanford. He had attended
the university during the summer before his junior year, and the experience
transformed him. Unfortunately, it transformed him a year too late. The
session at Stanford inspired in Curt a newfound seriousness toward school.
At the end of the summer, he dreamed of returning there for college.
That is all he has talked about during the past two years.

Curt and Danielle were the best students at Crenshaw during their
junior and senior years. But during Curt's sophomore year, his grades
were not up to Stanford's standards. And these were the grades that
doomed him. Curt has been accepted by UCLA, but Braxton senses Curt's
deep disappointment. Braxton plans to keep close tabs on him during the
next month.

Every year several Crenshaw students have the grades for Ivy League
colleges, but they rarely apply. Most think the schools are too far away
from home, or too expensive, or have too few minority students. The top
Crenshaw students usually aim for Stanford or a University of California
campus or the schools that aggressively recruit them and offer them full
scholarships. For many students at Crenshaw, applying to Harvard would
be like applying to the Sorbonne. They would never even consider it.

Sheila is the only student in AP English who applied to an Ivy League college. She was accepted by Cornell, but as with Danielle, the financial-aid and scholarship package was insufficient. She is now planning to attend Xavier, a black college in New Orleans.

Miesha was accepted by UC Berkeley. Latisha, who decided she wanted to attend a college in Alabama, near her mother and brother, was accepted by Alabama A&M. Willie was accepted by Morehouse. Brandi, another student in Little's class, was accepted to Pitzer. Venola was accepted by Colby College in Maine. They all received enough scholarships and financial-aid grants to be able to afford the schools.

After Venola received the news from Colby College, her mother was ecstatic. The school sent Venola a Colby College decal, and her mother immediately affixed it to the back window of her dusty Ford Escort. She called about half of her thirteen brothers and sisters, most of whom live on the East Coast and in the South. The other half she wrote. She then notified friends and neighbors and other relatives. At the convalescent hospital where she works, she informed all of her coworkers and most of the patients. That night, she treated Venola and her sister to a dinner at Sizzler. And the next Saturday, she invited all of Venola's friends to a celebratory backyard barbecue.

Sadi was accepted by Clark College in Atlanta. This was his first choice, a school he had picked because of its excellent speech team and communications department. Sadi's mother, Thelma, who needs a liver transplant and cannot work, survives on welfare. So the only way Sadi can attend college is if all of the costs are covered. But because his grades the past year and a half were mediocre, the school only offered him a partial scholarship and a limited financial-aid package. Still, his mother is a determined, persistent woman. She has been calling the school repeatedly in an effort to see if she can rustle up more grants and loans.

Thelma, who is sitting in the living room of her small apartment, jerks a thumb at Sadi and rolls her eyes. "I've been very flustrated by this boy. If he had done what he should have done, we wouldn't be in this fix now. As smart as he is, his grades should have been a lot better. Then he'd have all the scholarships he needed, and I wouldn't have to be doing all this scrambling. I've called back to Atlanta so many times, my phone bill was sixty dollars last month.''

Sadi looks sheepish as he tries to explain why he did not put more effort into his studies this year. In the tenth grade, he began the year as a gangbanger. He ended the year a scholar. He changed his friends. He changed his style of clothes. He changed the way he spent his evenings and weekends. He changed his relationship with his mother. He changed his aspirations and he changed his inclinations. By his senior year, the momentum from this monumental effort dissipated, and he felt as if he were a balloon whirring around a room, rapidly losing air.

Little was so impressed with Sadi when he was a sophomore because he had such passion for the literature and his comments in class were so insightful. She also was impressed by how he constantly strived to improve. His writing showed flashes of brilliance, but it was raw and undisciplined. Almost every day after school, he stopped by her classroom and she worked with him, editing his copy, improving his grammar, teaching him essay structure. During his senior year, Little expected great things from him. Sadi, however, was content with Bs on his papers, and he showed little of the passion and creativity that had impressed Little so much during his sophomore year.

Sadi works after school for an accounting office, and he has spending money for the first time in his life. This year, he has been more interested in making money—and spending it—than in school.

''My main objective this year was material stuff,'' he says. ''I've been into buying clothes and CDs. In the tenth grade I had no distractions. I was just a kid. When I got out of school, I would come home and study. This year I saw money for the first time in my life. It got me off track.

''Also, Miss Little was a different teacher than when I was in the tenth grade. She didn't spend all this time in class talking about her own problems. She was more inspirational. I can't use that as an excuse, 'cause I know it's all on me. But it's still real.

''I guess this year I was just happy to make it through high school,'' Sadi says with a shrug. ''So many of my friends are dead and in jail. That's where I was coming from. I would have been satisfied going to junior college. That seemed like an accomplishment to me.''

Thelma wags a forefinger at him. "You ain't going to no junior college next year. I'm getting you to Clark, one way or another. I want you out of this neighborhood. No one's doin' nothin' here."

"Unless it's illegal," he says with a grin.

"You need to get out of L.A., out of my house. You need to be on your own. That'll make a man out of you." She faces me and says, "From the time he was a baby, I told him he had to go to a university, that I'd accept nothing else. That's still my attitude."

Braxton tapes Sadi's letter from Clark University to his wall and then studies some of the other letters for a moment. This has been a good year. In Little's class, alone, eight students were admitted to UCLA and UC Berkeley—the most selective schools in the UC system—and about a dozen students were accepted to other campuses in the UC system, which accepts the top eighth of the state's high school graduates.

Braxton believes that future classes at Crenshaw probably will have much lower admittance rates to UC schools, in particular to UCLA and UC Berkeley. Because of Proposition 209, which goes into effect next year for undergraduate admissions, this will be the last class at Crenshaw to benefit from affirmative action. Braxton has mixed feelings about affirmative action, but, in the end, he voted against Proposition 209. There are elements of race-based preferences that trouble him, but he realizes that, after more than three decades, the advantages greatly outweigh the disadvantages, and affirmative action continues to tremendously benefit blacks in America.

The first time the word "affirmative" was conjoined with the word "action" was in 1961, during a presidential inaugural ball for John F. Kennedy. While shaking hands in the receiving line, Vice President Lyndon Johnson spotted a young black attorney, Hobard Taylor Jr., and asked him to help presidential advisors write an executive order barring federal contractors from racial discrimination in hiring.

"I put the word 'affirmative' in there at that time," Taylor recalled in an interview for the Lyndon Baines Johnson Library. "I was searching for something that would give a sense of positiveness to performance under that executive order, and I was torn between the words 'positive action' and the words 'affirmative action.' And I took 'affirmative action' because it was alliterative.''

Taylor and the presidential advisors drafted Executive Order 10924, which was signed by President Kennedy in March 1961, and stated: "The contractor agrees not to discriminate . . . the contractor will take affirmative action to ensure that applicants are employed, and that employees are treated during employment without regard to their race, creed, color, or national origin.''

This initial interpretation of affirmative action, which was created to aid impoverished blacks, simply meant banning discrimination. And the Civil Rights Act of 1964 specifically prohibited racial quotas. Still, many believed at the time that merely outlawing legal segregation in the South did not go far enough in resolving America's racial divide. But because those who were most vociferous in decrying the dangers of reverse discrimination and quotas were Southern segregationists, few predicted how unpopular race-based preferences would later prove to be among middle-class and working-class whites.

In 1965, President Johnson delivered a commencement speech at Howard University that is regarded as the founding document of affirmative action. Johnson, in a speech drafted by Assistant Secretary of Labor Daniel Patrick Moynihan, told the graduates: "You do not take a person who, for years, has been hobbled by chains and liberate him, bring him up to the starting line in a race and then say, 'You are free to compete with all the others' and still justly believe that you have been completely fair . . . We seek . . . not just equality as a right and a theory, but equality as a fact and equality as a result.'' The phrase "equality as a result" departed sharply from the simple nondiscrimination assurances of the past. Equality of result shifted the debate on affirmative action from the protective to the proactive, an interpretation that later would ignite so much controversy.

In higher education, the civil rights movement prompted a number of universities to reevaluate their admissions policies and begin to recruit and admit black students. This was seen as necessary to increase black enrollment and to improve the economic conditions of blacks in America. In

1965, less than 5 percent of all U.S. colleges students were black. Only 1 percent attended elite New England colleges. Only 1 percent attended law school, and only 2 percent attended medical schools, more than three-quarters of whom were enrolled at all-black colleges.

The dean of Harvard Law School, Erwin Griswold, was troubled that the law had played such a critical role in the lives of blacks during the civil rights movement, but no black students were enrolled at Harvard Law School. In 1966, the law school started to admit black students, although their test scores were substantially lower than those of their white classmates. Soon admissions officers at other law schools, medical schools, and undergraduate institutions initiated similar recruiting programs, and the percentages of black students increased substantially.

By the late 1960s, civil rights lawyers, both inside and outside government, clamored for decisive action. Eliminating bias was no longer enough. Minorities, they believed, should be guaranteed a proportional share of jobs, promotions, and college slots. This change in focus was considered essential because blacks still were excluded from a number of professions. Construction unions in New York, Cleveland, Philadelphia, and a number of other cities refused to hire black workers. And inner-city riots during the mid- and late 1960s forced Americans to confront the great chasm between white and black America as well as the abysmal conditions of the nation's ghettos.

It was during the administration of President Richard Nixon, who had campaigned against quotas, that the government instituted its most explicit quota plan, one that introduced into the American workplace the concept of proportional representation by race. George P. Schultz, Nixon's labor secretary, issued in 1969 what was known as the Philadelphia Plan, which forced federal construction contractors in Philadelphia to submit "affirmative action compliance programs" that set goals for hiring minorities and to make a "good faith effort" to meet the goals—or face sanctions.

Nixon endorsed the Philadelphia Plan, partly because of a Machiavellian political strategy that was vintage Nixon. He saw the plan as a highly effective way to pit blacks and labor against each other, a way to divide and conquer a traditional Democratic base. In 1970, Nixon's labor department expanded the Philadelphia Plan to include federal construction contractors across the country. These aggressive interpretations of affirmative action were eventually challenged in court and vilified by politicians, but for the next twenty-five years, affirmative action remained largely intact.

In academia, integrating student bodies during the 1960s had been voluntary. But by the early 1970s, affirmative action at universities—many of which received federal funds—was no longer simply encouraged by federal officials. It now seemed mandatory. In the affirmative action plans federal officials now required from universities, they wanted a racial breakdown included in the enrollment data.

During the 1980s, affirmative action had been transformed by the umbrella concept of diversity, and blacks had to compete for financial-aid funds with many other deserving students. Blacks faced much greater competition for places at top universities from the burgeoning Latino population, in addition to an increasing number of highly qualified Asian Americans and whites. Still, the educational gains made by blacks were impressive. The percentage of blacks aged twenty-five to twenty-nine who had graduated from college tripled from about 5 percent in 1960 to about 15 percent in 1995. Blacks represented only about 1 percent of the nation's law school students in 1960, but the number increased to more than 7 percent by 1995.

During the affirmative action years, the number of blacks in technical and managerial jobs doubled, and the number of black police officers and electricians tripled. Affirmative action clearly played a major role in enabling a significant number of blacks to enter the middle class and share in the American dream.

During three Republican administrations, from 1980 to 1992, there was much posturing about eliminating affirmative action. Both Presidents Ronald Reagan and George Bush campaigned against quotas. When their administrations began gearing up to eliminate affirmative action programs, however, they backed down after the public outcry.

But during the 1990s, momentum against race-based preferences intensified. Affirmative action has been eliminated in California's and Texas's public institutions, and is under serious challenge in a number of other states.

Yes, affirmative action is an imperfect solution to an intractable problem. Yes, some affirmative action programs are deeply flawed. But critics, who pontificate about the many reasons why affirmative action should be dismantled, offer few practical alternatives. The one alternative that *is* frequently offered—a major reclamation of America's inner-cities schools—is a worthy and necessary objective. The chances of actually accomplishing this objective, however, is negligible, given federal budget constraints and antitax sentiment in America.

Those who argue that affirmative action is no longer needed should look closely at the lives of inner-city students, and the neighborhoods where they live, and the conditions of the schools they attend, and their lack of SAT preparation, and the many crises they are routinely confronted with, and their work schedules, and their families.

Nathan Glazer, who has been one of academia's most prominent affirmative action critics during the past few decades, who denounced race-based preferences in his influential 1975 book, *Affirmative Discrimination,* recently changed his position on the issue. He still opposes numerical quotas for black admissions, but he also opposes legislative bans on the use of race in making decisions on admissions.

". . . We cannot," Glazer wrote, "be quite so cavalier about the impact . . . of a radical reduction in the number of black students at the Harvards, the Berkeleys, and the Amhersts. These institutions have become, for better or worse, the gateways to prominence, privilege, wealth, and power in American society. Higher education's governing principle is qualification—merit. Should it make room for another and quite different principle, equal participation? . . . Basically the answer is yes—the principle of equal participation can and should be given some role. The decision has costs. But the alternative is too grim to contemplate."

THIRTY-TWO

TONI LITTLE

I COULD USE A LITTLE MORE TIME

The AP exam is three weeks away and Danielle decides that whether Little returns or not, the students desperately need her help to prepare for the test. She calls Little at home and asks if she will come to a Sunday afternoon study session and tutor the students. Little agrees.

Khaliah volunteers her house for the study session. Khaliah, whose father is a bank examiner for the state, lives near Curt in Los Angeles's wealthiest black neighborhood, in a spacious, Spanish-style house. Many of the students in Little's class have to work on weekends and others have to attend afternoon church services with their families, so only nine students—including Sadi, Curt, Venola, and Danielle—show up. The study session was supposed to begin at 3 P.M., but by 3:45, Little still has not arrived. The students decide to proceed without her. They gather around the living room table, pull out their *Hamlet* study questions, and discuss the play among themselves. At four o'clock, Little still has not arrived. The students spend a few minutes speculating if she will return to school this year, or miss the rest of the year.

At 4:15, Little rings the doorbell and makes a theatrical, emotional entrance. She sweeps through the room, shouting students' names, hugging them, fighting back tears. "Even Sadi's here," she cries, skittering across the room and embracing him.

She spots Curt. "Did you hear from Stanford?"

He stares at his shoes. "Yeah. Didn't get in."

"I can't believe it. Are you freaked?"

"Naw. I'm okay. I'm going to UCLA."

"Did you get in?" she asks Danielle.

"Yeah. But I'm not going. Costs too much. I'm going to Pitzer."

"Thanks so much for calling me," she says to Danielle. "That meant a lot to me."

She points to Khaliah and asks, "Where are you going?"

"Berkeley."

Venola hugs Little and says, "I'm going to Colby College." Venola kisses her on the cheek and says, "I'm so glad you're back." She pauses and then asks, "You are back, aren't you? You'll be in class tomorrow, won't you?"

Little nods. "I'll be there." She heads into the kitchen to get a soda and whispers to me, so the students cannot hear, "I have to go back. I've got no alternative. I used up all my sick days, and I've been on temporary disability. My lawyer recommended that I go back. He told me, 'You're broke and you need money to fight this thing.' "

She returns to the living room and pulls up a chair and says, "Let's discuss *Hamlet*." For the next hour Little effortlessly leads the students in a spirited discussion about the play. After my own abortive teaching attempt, I appreciate the way she asks just the right question to spur debate, how she deftly makes a point—briefly and incisively—without boring them, as I had. She leads the students through a discussion about Hamlet's relationship with Ophelia; the meaning of "true love"; the similarities and differences between Heathcliff and Hamlet; the characteristics in Hamlet that "you recognize in yourselves"; the meaning of tragedy.

One of the students quotes something I had said about tragedy—when I had taught the class—and I have a disturbing premonition about how they will do on their AP exam. If they are relying on an unqualified and overmatched teacher like me for literary interpretation, they are in trouble.

After about an hour of discussion, the study group breaks up because several of the students have to go to work. As Venola stuffs her book and notebook into her backpack, she tells Little, "You'd be so great in college. You seem so much happier teaching a small group like this. You're so much more relaxed." Venola waves to her, as she walks out the door, and says, "See you tomorrow."

Little waves back and says, "See you tomorrow."

On Monday morning, Little, wearing an orange- and yellow-streaked silk blazer and slacks, strides down the hall toward her classroom. When a group of students clustered by the door see her, they clap and call out:

"Welcome back, Miss Little."

"We missed you, Miss Little."

"So glad you're back, Miss Little."

She hugs several of the students and opens the classroom door with her key. As she organizes her desk, students wander in and greet her. When Latisha walks in and sees Little, she frames her face with her hands and freezes for a moment, wide-eyed. "I'm filled with joy," Latisha says. Miesha wanders into class—for the first time in weeks—and hugs Little.

Little dabs her eyes with a Kleenex and says, "I missed you guys."

When the bell rings, Little sifts through a thick pile of yellow absence slips. "How come so many students were absent while I was gone?"

"We went on strike," Miesha says.

"You were being bad," Latisha says, "so we were being bad. Even Danielle missed some classes."

"You ditched, Danielle?" Little asks, incredulous.

Danielle says sheepishly, "Yeah."

"So what's going on?" Miesha asks. "Why, exactly, did you miss so much class? We heard some things, but give us the real deal?"

Little shakes her head. "At the end of the year we'll have a barbecue and I'll tell everyone the whole story. But, for now, we better get to it. We've got so little time before the AP test and so much to do. We've got to close out *Hamlet* before we can roll out the other stuff."

I brought the movie again and I tell Little the students only saw the first half on Friday. She scrounges up a VCR, flips in the movie, and dims the lights. Now that Little is back, the students watch *Hamlet* without any clowning around. But occasionally they shout out exhortations or warnings to the characters, not to disrupt the class, but because they are engrossed in the play.

When Ophelia starts to babble, a girl calls out, "She done lost it!"

When Hamlet denounces Claudius, a boy shouts, "Right on, brutha!"

Before the sword fight between Laertes and Hamlet, Curt calls out, "Let's get ready to rumble."

Before the queen reaches for the cup of poisoned wine, Latisha shouts, "Don't drink it, sista."

While the students watch the movie, Little tells me she feels terrible about missing so much class right before the AP exam. "I'm like Hamlet," she whispers. "I'm obsessed and other people have been harmed. I was self-indulgent, like Hamlet was self-indulgent. I know it's a flaw. I've had to reevaluate some things in my life." She stares into a corner of the darkened room, lost in thought for a moment. "But I also have a burden, like Hamlet. I have to try and right a wrong."

After the movie, Little leads the class in a discussion, summing up the major elements of the play, the motivations of the various characters, and themes the students might need to know for the AP exam. She assigns the students their last essay of the year and tells them it will be due in mid-May. She writes it on the blackboard: ". . . Consider whether distaste for revenge might be one reason for Hamlet's hesitation to kill Claudius. The crown, to which Hamlet has been heir, was responsible for upholding injustice and was now being worn by a murderer. Was Hamlet's mission one of personal revenge or public justice?"

After class, more students tell Little how glad they are that she is back. A few, however, shuffle out the door, whispering among themselves about how they are miffed at Little for missing so much class, during such a crucial juncture, for such cryptic reasons.

After the class empties, Little hunches over her desk and thinks about how much material she still has to cover before the AP exam. She chews her lower lip and, with an anguished expression on her face, sketches out a lesson plan for the next few weeks.

The Monday when Little returns is a wild, frenzied day that throws Braxton and the other school administrators into a panic.

In the morning, Gwen Roberts, who teaches math in the gifted magnet program, is walking back to her classroom, after making copies of an exam. She spots about fifteen students hanging around behind the quad who are cutting class. None look familiar; they are not in the gifted program. She smells marijuana, but Roberts does not want to confront the students. There are too many, and a few of the boys, who are dressed like gangbangers, look menacing.

She stands there for a moment, clutching the stack of math exams with both hands. The students stare at her defiantly, blocking the entrance to the annex where her classroom is located. She has to pass them to get inside. Finally she says, "I smell marijuana." There are no other teachers or school policemen around. Roberts is fifty-four years old and she feels alone and vulnerable. She has no intention of busting the students. She just wants them to disperse. "Nobody has a pass," she tells them. "So you need to go to class."

A moment later, she is sprawled out on the pavement with an intense, searing pain shooting along the side of her head. She wonders if she was shot. She is barely conscious. All she can see are little flecks of light around the periphery of her vision. Blood pours from her ear.

She raises her head for a moment. A teenage boy with a clenched fist is staring down at her, shouting, "Bitch!" She has never seen such an intense look of pure hatred. She will never forget his eyes. They smolder with fury, a murderous expression that chills her to the bone. She is terrified that the boy, whom she has never seen before, is going to punch her again.

The other students just stand around and watch. Not a single one had warned her the punch was coming. Not a single one offers to help her now.

"Give me a hand," she calls out weakly, as she tries to stand up.

They all turn their backs on her and casually saunter off. The boy who had punched her begins running, but when he is about fifteen feet away, he stops, turns around, shouts, "Bitch!" and flashes her that same murderous look. Then he runs off.

After a few minutes on the ground, Roberts finally summons the strength to stand up. She staggers toward the security office. One of her gifted math students spots her, sees the blood streaming down her face and shouts, "Oh, my God, Miss Roberts!" He helps her to the security office. She tells the security officers what happened to her, and they search the campus. A nurse then ices the side of her head.

A few minutes later, two boys run when they spot the officers. The officers chase them down and bring them back to the office.

"Did one of these guys do it?" the guards ask Roberts.

She points to one of them and says, "He did it."

"Do you want him arrested?"

"Yes," she says.

Braxton drives Roberts to a hospital emergency room. She has a black eye and one side of her face is completely discolored. She has a concussion and torn ligaments in her elbow, which she injured trying to break the fall. Her neck is severely sprained and so sore she cannot move it. The doctor gives her a prescription for pain pills and anti-inflammatory medication and tells her she should not return to work for at least a month.

Shortly after Braxton drives Roberts home from the doctor, Lisa Lippa, who is teaching twelfth-grade physiology to a class of gifted magnet students, is lecturing on the vestibule of the inner ear. She suddenly hears a cracking sound. Lippa turns toward the window of her third-floor classroom and she sees a girl frantically picking glass out of her hair. A few other girls scream and dive for the floor. Lippa studies the hole in the window and tells the class that she thinks someone threw a rock.

A boy, who has seen a few bullet holes in his time, raises his hand and says, "Mrs. Lippa, no rock makes a hole like that."

Curt and another boy, Akindeji, who also is in Little's AP English class, trace the trajectory and search for the bullet. They study the shattered window and then find a hole in the wall the size of a quarter. Akindeji, like a good detective, notices that the class parakeet is squawking frantically. He figures the bullet whizzed by the bird, so he looks beside the cage. He finds the flattened slug, which had ricocheted around the room, inside a sink. The slug is still warm.

Lippa calls the school dean. He evacuates the class to the library. She continues lecturing about the inner ear, but a few students are too upset to concentrate and are allowed to go home. The other students, however, are blasé about the shot.

"No big deal," Venola says, shrugging, after the incident.

Latisha, however, is angry. "I hear gunshots all the time at home. But you don't figure to get them on the campus. And not this close. School is supposed to be your sanctuary."

Lippa, who is eight months pregnant, has long, light brown hair, freckles, big green eyes, and does not look much older than her students. She is from Indiana, attended college in Western Kentucky, and had little experience with black students when she began teaching in South-Central about seven years ago. She has found the work rewarding and has particularly enjoyed teaching Crenshaw's gifted students. But this is the second bullet that has ripped through one of her classrooms. A few years ago, when she was teaching at another South-Central high school, a bullet struck her classroom wall. Fortunately, she had been out of the room at the time. Later, she traced the bullet's trajectory and figured that if she had been lecturing in the front of the class, the bullet would have hit her in the chest.

This time, she had been lecturing in the front of the class. Had she been sitting at her desk, she figures, the bullet would have struck her in the head. She does not want to risk any more close calls, especially now that she and her husband are expecting their first child. Lippa, along with every other teacher in Los Angeles, is familiar with what happened to Alfredo Perez, a South-Central elementary school teacher. Last year, Perez was teaching when a bullet meant for a rival gang member smashed through his classroom window and into his brain. He survived, but is seriously impaired. After Lippa has her baby, and her pregnancy leave runs out, she decides, she will look for a teaching job away from inner-city Los Angeles.

The shot into Lippa's classroom and the attack on Roberts culminate a tumultuous week. A few days ago, two students were beaten up on campus in gang-related attacks. Another student, who was walking home from school, was beaten so badly he was hospitalized. There also have been a number of shootings near the campus. And during the weekend, a group of Bloods covered an outside wall of the high school with the kind of gang graffiti that usually presages a shooting.

Crenshaw's principal sends a memo to all of the teachers:

". . . We have had some extremely serious incidents connected with gang activity. Most of these occurred off campus, but several have occurred on campus. Consequently, to get the situation back under control, we are locking the campus down for the remainder of the week . . . As you can see, our 'safe haven' is beginning to show early signs of crumbling, but we are determined to hold 'the barbarians at the gates.' "

On Monday afternoon, Little discovers that two students from her class will not be taking the AP exam, or any other exam at Crenshaw. They have been expelled from school. The two girls, best friends who had always dressed in slinky outfits that violated the school dress code, had frequently disrupted Little's class with their giggling and chattering. They both worked for the school's college counselor and stole several scholarship checks. They handed the checks over to a cohort, who cashed them and split the money with them. When police tracked him down, he snitched on the two girls. The bank did not press charges, so the only punishment the girls faced was expulsion. They will soon enroll at a nearby high school.

"These girls are out on the street," Little tells me after school. "They'll graduate in June. But look at Olivia. She did the same thing. And who knows when she's getting out of jail."

Olivia recently has suffered a few setbacks. County juvenile authorities, unfortunately, will not give her permission to take the AP exams at Crenshaw. So several times Olivia called the Crenshaw college counselor who is in charge of administering the Advanced Placement exams and attempted— unsuccessfully—to convince her to mail the exam to the juvenile jail.

Babson College, where Olivia had dreamed of going, offered her a substantial scholarship. But when a school official called Braxton, and he reluctantly informed them where she was, they rescinded the offer. Fortunately, Olivia also has been accepted by a few state colleges in California, and she is still hoping she will be released from custody in time for the fall semester.

During the final few weeks of April, Little gives the class a crash course in poetry. A handful of poetry lectures, however, will not adequately prepare the students for the AP exam, Little realizes.

During these final classes before the exam, Little is so harried, feels so behind schedule, that she is extremely focused and has no time to digress. The students read some poems, and they interpret them in class. Little hands out study sheets listing various types of poetry, such as lyric, narrative, blank verse, free verse; she hands out study sheets, listing various terms the students can use when analyzing poetry, such as alliteration, allusion, personification, onomatopoeia, imagery, denotation, and connotation. The students spend a few hours in class discussing the terms.

On the first Friday in May—the last class before the AP exam—the students chatter among themselves before the bell rings. Most are jittery and do not feel prepared. The poetry section was rushed and superficial, a cram session, they feel. They are insecure about their ability to analyze poems. They do not express much confidence about other elements of the exam, either.

On Fridays, classes at Crenshaw are abbreviated—less than an hour. So on this final class before the exam, Little does not have much time for in-depth suggestions. In a hurried, discursive lecture, she briefly touches on numerous topics.

''Remember, your job as the writer is to persuade . . . It's not just content that's important. You have to rely on presentation and construction, too . . . You have to know that a comma follows a subordinate clause . . . In your essays, you can ask a rhetorical question . . . The first hour there are about sixty questions. Don't let that burn you out . . . Read the essay questions carefully. Find the verbs, verbs like 'define,' 'diagram,' 'interpret,' 'contrast.' The verbs will tell you what to do . . . Remember, 'analyze' is *not* the same as 'describe' . . . And 'a lot' is two words. Some of you still have it as one word. If you do that, they won't take your essays seriously . . . From this year, you have Shakespeare, Brontë, Joyce. When I had you as tenth graders we had Fitzgerald and

Faulkner and a lot of other great writers. Make them your friends . . .
You've been on this journey for three years. Remember what you
learned . . ."

She hands out passages from previous exams. "Over the weekend,"
she tells them, "study these. And review your literary terms. If you don't
know what figurative language is, you're sunk!"

When the class ends, she flashes me a worried look and says, "Those
weeks I was off killed us in poetry." She stares out the window and
nervously rakes her fingers through her hair. "What do you think?"

I shrug.

She drums her fingers on her desk and says, "I could use a little
more time."

THIRTY-THREE

THE EXAM

WHERE THE RUBBER MEETS THE ROAD

On Monday morning, as the students file into the classroom, Little paces nervously, looking like a coach before the big game. She asks the students, "Did you spend the entire weekend studying, going over the literary terms?"

Most shake their heads.

Little looks dismayed. "Why not?"

"We had to work," several students say in unison.

"I had to work twenty-four hours this weekend," a girl says.

"I worked until midnight last night," a boy calls out.

Little holds up her palms. "Okay, okay."

Before Little can rally the class with a final pep talk, the college counselor arrives and marches the students down to the library, where they will take the exam under her supervision. After the class empties, Little walks over to the window and studies the quad for a few minutes. This is the first Monday in May, a radiant spring morning. A warm breeze ruffles the blinds in Little's classroom, carrying the scent of freshly cut grass. The jacaranda trees are blossoming, a scattering of lavender amid the profusion of fronds, and the bottlebrush trees are in full bloom, ringing the campus with garlands of scarlet, vivid splashes of color in a drab, institutional setting.

Little returns to her desk and attempts to handicap how the students will do on the exam, which is about three hours and composed of both multiple choice and essay questions. If students pass with a score of three or better—out of a possible five—they will earn college credit. Little figures Danielle—who earned a five last year on the AP Art History exam—and Curt are the only students who have a chance for fives. Another dozen students, Little believes, have a good chance to pass the exam. Miesha, Venola, and a boy named Robert are the most likely candidates, Little believes.

Robert lives with his mother and younger brother in a down-at-the-heels South-Central neighborhood, east of the Harbor Freeway, in a small house behind a house, next door to an abandoned, boarded-up bungalow. His mother, a sign-language interpreter for the deaf, grew up in the house, which is still owned by her parents. When she and Robert's father split up eight years ago, she moved back. Robert is uncomfortable when asked about his father and is reluctant to discuss him. All he will say is: "He's not part of my life."

Robert always has tested well. In the fifth grade, when he was classified as gifted by the school district, he scored well above the 90th percentile in several categories. Last year, he passed the AP American History exam, with a three. Robert, who is soft-spoken and slender and wears a silver hoop earring, is one of the best writers in the class, but he has a poor attendance record, and when he does show up, he rarely participates in class discussions. On the rare occasions when he proffers an opinion, the other students take notice. Like Sadi, he is an independent thinker who will challenge Little's point of view and the orthodoxy of the class.

This has been a busy year for Robert. He writes for the student newspaper, works for Moultrie's party business, and plays center field on the Crenshaw baseball team. He will attend UCLA next year on a combination academic scholarship, financial-aid, and part-time work package.

During his high school years, Robert has not been a particularly conscientious student. He crams for his exams and frequently writes his papers at the last minute. Somehow he manages to get maximum results with a minimum of effort. Little hopes that on the AP exam, he can pull it off one more time.

At the midway point of the AP English exam, Little is too nervous to sit still, so she walks down to the library. A pink sign covers the window: THE LIBRARY IS CLOSED FOR TESTING. Little pulls back the sign and peeks inside.

"They're writing away," she tells me. "They must be on the essay. Look at Andriana. She's jamming. All of them are concentrating so hard."

She returns to her classroom and says, "This is where the rubber meets the road. This is where they have to compete against kids from throughout the country. My kids are smart kids, as smart as any kids, anywhere. But their biggest disadvantage is that they don't read."

This is not simply excuse-making by Little; it is an obvious handicap. A number of students in Little's class have told me the only books they have ever read are the ones assigned in class, and they have never read a single novel for pleasure. Many Crenshaw students grow up in households without a tradition of reading. Their parents do not read. There are no books in the house. Other students have full-time jobs and do not have time for outside reading. In other neighborhoods, AP Literature students have had the guidance, the inclination, and the time to read extensively since they were in elementary school. As a result, their vocabulary, their use of language, their writing skills are often much more advanced than those of the Crenshaw gifted students. That is one reason why the average score of Crenshaw gifted students is always higher on the math sections than the verbal sections of standardized tests.

Shortly before noon, the students complete their AP exams and file out of the library, dazed and discouraged. This is not a good sign.

"How'd you do?" one girl asks another, as they stroll across campus.

"I'm shooting for a three," she says with a half smile.

Her friend nods knowingly, and they exchange high fives.

*   *   *

On Wednesday morning, Little interrogates the students about the exam.

A girl shakes her head and says, "I could see the level I've got to get to for college. I'm not there yet."

"I didn't really understand the prompt," another girl says. "I didn't understand what they wanted."

"I was way too slow," a boy says. "I needed more time."

Robert is the only student who expresses confidence. "I didn't feel prepared the night before the test, but during the test I felt good. I didn't feel overwhelmed at all."

Most of the students, however, grumble about the exam and are pessimistic about their results. They tell Little that they had the option of choosing a literary work for one of their essay questions. About a third of the students picked *Hamlet*, which is a bad sign, because Little was gone or distracted during most of the *Hamlet* instruction. Much of the teaching was done by me and a collection of unprepared substitutes.

Sadi announces that he picked *The Great Gatsby*, which he studied in Little's tenth-grade English class. He tells Little, "That's the book that taught me that it's not about race. It's where I learned that there's a universality to human beings and that everyone has the same dreams."

Although Sadi knows he did not do well on the exam, he is in an ebullient mood this morning. He just discovered that Clark College will offer him a scholarship and financial-aid package totaling $13,000. He still is $5,000 short, but his mother continues to call the college almost every day. She is optimistic she can rustle up a few more thousand dollars in financial aid or—at the very least—loans.

Several students tell Little they were distracted during the exam by a long argument two girls had in the hallway, right outside the library.

"They were fighting and screaming," Miesha says. "It got louder and louder."

Miesha, the class actress, stands up, puts a hand on her hip and, impersonating one of the girls says, " 'Bitch, I'm gonna *whup yo ass.*' "

" 'You *wish* you could whup my ass,' " she says, impersonating the other girl.

" 'Fuck you, bitch!' "

" 'Fuck you, too . . .' "

She concludes her reenactment and says, "It went on and on. I wanted to go out there and push the two of 'em together and get the fight over with. When the girls weren't yelling, people were pounding on the library door every ten minutes. And all during the test, there were constant announcements over the PA system. That was another distraction. And some student library worker—a football player—was walking around videotaping us while we were taking the test. It was irritating."

Little was growing increasingly discouraged by the students' bleak self-evaluations, slumping in her chair, looking tired, and disconsolate. But when they talk about the distractions, she perks up.

"This is an *outrage!*" she announces, leaping out of her chair. "This school can't even provide you with a proper test environment."

She scurries over to her phone and calls the organization in New York that administers the Advanced Placement exam. She barks into the phone, "I'm an AP literature teacher and my students took the exam on Friday. I have a complaint. The test environment was outrageous. Who do I talk to?"

She jots down a few names and numbers and hangs up the phone. She tells the class, "If you failed miserably, it wasn't because you weren't prepared."

"Now *that's* a great excuse," Miesha says, laughing.

Little ignores her. "If the pass rate is real low, maybe the environment has something to do with it. Wouldn't you say?"

A few students offer half-hearted nods. Others mumble, "I guess so."

"There's a form we can fill out, listing irregularities surrounding this exam," Little says. "But if you pursue this, I'm sure everyone will say *I'm* the one who is at fault." She breathes deeply and extends her palms, a pose of martyrdom. "If there's an investigation, of course *I'll* get blamed for stirring it up. Oh, yes," she says sarcastically, "I'm a little Hitler."

She rests her head against the blackboard for a moment. Then she jabs a forefinger at the students, like a prosecutor hammering home a salient point to a dubious jury. "Did I *force* you to come up with all these distractions? Didn't you tell me about them on your own volition?"

She waves a hand airily and says, "I can't bring home scores that accurately reflect my ability to teach. This class was way too big—double the size of what it should have been. We didn't even have enough chairs. We had no AP progression. I taught you in the tenth and twelfth grades. And someone *else* was doing something entirely different with you in the ninth and eleventh grades."

She sinks into her chair and drops her chin to her chest and mutters, "I couldn't even get a literature textbook for this class."

About a week after the AP exam, I visit Olivia again at the Dorothy Kirby Center. She is more discouraged than the last time I saw her, more downcast and pessimistic about the future. She slumps in her chair, speaks with little animation, and gestures languidly.

The past few weeks have been a distressing time for her. She was very disappointed when she discovered she could not take her AP exams. And when she learned that Babson College would not accept her because of her arrest, she was devastated.

"After I heard about Babson, I felt like my life was over," she says, staring at her shoes. "Basically, it meant that all my dreams went down the tubes. I was in my room, crying and hitting the walls. When some of the other girls found out how upset I was they started teasing me, calling out: 'Ha, ha. She doesn't get to go to college.' "

She looks up and says, "What kind of evil shit is that? They didn't like it that I wasn't like them. They didn't like it that I had a future. They were happy when my plans were ruined."

I ask Olivia what are the chances that she will be able to attend college in the fall. Her eyes fill with tears. "I don't know if I'll *ever* be able to go to college. My counselor says she doesn't know when I'll be ready to leave here. When I finally *do* get out of here, I don't know how I'll swing college. How can I afford it? I'll have to work full-time, buy a car, get an apartment, and support myself. I remember how hard that was when I had my own apartment and supported myself in *high* school. I was going to quit school then, but Mr. Braxton talked me out of it."

Olivia wipes her eyes with a fist and says, "I'm afraid I'll get out of here, get a job, and wake up when I'm forty years old with nothing." She sets her jaw and says angrily, "I don't even care anymore."

Olivia will earn her high school diploma while in custody. In August, if the judge determines that Olivia has made satisfactory progress at the center, she will be released and can attend one of the California state colleges where she has recently been admitted.

After Olivia is led away, I talk with her counselor, Susanne Dunne. During Olivia's first month at the center, Dunne says, her approach to the daily group-therapy sessions was somewhat superficial. The other girls thought she acted aloof and superior, like a prima donna. Recently, however, Olivia has made progress. She has attempted to be more frank, to be more introspective, but some of the self-awareness she is gaining is painful for her.

"For the first time, she's talked about how totally alone she feels, how hard it's been for her to have no family, no one really close to her. It's been difficult for her to express that because she's so blocked emotionally . . . And that goes hand in hand with ripping someone off and saying, 'It's no big deal. It's just a bank, not a person.' It's also connected to that feeling of omnipotence—that she'd never get caught.

"Olivia's also talked about the [taxi] dancing that she's done. Again, her attitude was that it was no big deal. But the other girls in group confronted her on it. They helped her see that she was, in a way, prostituting herself, selling herself, not respecting herself as a woman. They made her see the reality of it."

Dunne holds her thumb and forefinger about an inch apart and says, "She's starting to acknowledge a little remorse for her crime. She's starting to get in touch, a little bit, with how her actions affect others."

I ask Dunne if Olivia has progressed sufficiently to attend college in the fall. I ask her what she will recommend to the judge.

She shrugs. "I don't know if she'll be ready—emotionally. She needs at least eight to ten months here. She needs the *full* program. In August, it will only be six months. I'll have to see how she progresses. So at this point, I don't really know what's going to happen with Olivia."

THIRTY-FOUR

SCOTT ALLEN

A DIFFERENT APPROACH

A week after the AP exam, about a dozen students from Little's class take the AP U.S. Government and Politics test, and they feel much more prepared and confident. Scott Allen, the government teacher, has shoulder-length hair and dresses as casually as the students. Initially, many of his students view him as a pushover, a hippie with little interest in rules and regulations. Instead, they discover he is a strict disciplinarian and a demanding teacher.

Allen's teaching style is diametrically opposed to Little's. He is a martinet, meticulous, and obsessively organized. Every morning, before the students arrive, he writes on the blackboard a detailed lesson plan for the day, including the subjects he will lecture about, the chapters in the textbook he will refer to, historical citations that are relevant. He gives frequent tests, quizzes, and daily homework assignments. He covers the material in a systematic fashion, does most of the talking in class, asks students brief, pointed questions, and rarely allows class discussion to meander off point.

Although his approach is antithetical to Little's, many seniors count the two of them as their favorite teachers. They enjoy Allen's sense of humor, the way he leavens the material with comic asides and one-liners. Despite initial resistance, they also appreciate his exacting standards, the way he pushes them. They know his class will prepare them for college.

Claudia, who flunked out of Little's class after the first semester because she refused to turn in her writing assignments, has succeeded in Allen's class. She still refuses to submit many of her writing assignments, but on Allen's multiple-choice exams, she invariably receives the highest grade, so she has managed to pass the class. Claudia still does not study, but she pays close attention during Allen's lectures and has a gift for synthesizing and quickly understanding complex material. On the economics final, she received the highest grade in the class, without cracking open the book. Venola received the second highest.

After Claudia flunked Little's class, Braxton was afraid she would drop out of school. But Claudia made up the F at night school, kept her grades up in her other classes, and is on schedule to graduate in June. She has been accepted by California State University, Long Beach. Claudia is so bright that at the beginning of the year Braxton had hoped she would attend an elite university like Stanford or Berkeley. Now he is simply grateful that she will graduate from high school and plans to attend college in the fall.

Allen believes that even though Claudia has not studied, she has a good chance to pass the AP exam. He also feels confident about a number of others, although they start the year on an unequal footing with suburban students.

"I was at a debating conference a few weeks ago, and I saw kids talking knowledgeably about all kinds of issues in the news," Allen says. "Their parents are doctors and lawyers and teachers. These kids read the newspaper every morning; they read *Time* or *Newsweek*; they watch the national news. They discuss current events at the dinner table every night. They're just better prepared, and they get a lot of this preparation at home."

Students are encouraged to use current events on the AP Government and Politics exam to draw connections between theory and reality. They can use events in the news to illustrate points and list examples. But the vast majority of the students in Allen's class are at a distinct disadvantage: The parents of only two students subscribe to a newspaper.

The AP program offers a total of thirty-one different tests in eighteen disciplines, from micro economics to Latin literature. Crenshaw students, however, do not take as many AP exams as students from schools in wealthier neighborhoods mainly because they simply do not have access to as many AP courses. Crenshaw offers eight AP courses—many more than most inner city schools because it houses the gifted magnet program. Still, the other Los Angeles high school for gifted students, which is located in the San Fernando Valley, schedules three times as many AP courses.

About 130 California public high schools, which serve predominantly black and Latino students, do not offer any AP classes, and more than 300 high schools offer four or fewer AP classes. The fact that inner city students do not have access to as many AP courses as students at affluent schools is a clear inequity. Many schools use weighted grading systems that award extra points for AP or honors course grades. As a result, at these schools, students can load up on AP and honors courses and inflate their grade point averages. When they apply for college, they will have a distinct advantage over Crenshaw students. (Two years after the Crenshaw students graduated, the American Civil Liberties Union filed a class-action lawsuit charging that because of the disparity in AP courses, blacks and Latinos are disproportionately rejected from elite public universities in California, such as UC Berkeley and UCLA.)

A month after math teacher Gwen Roberts was punched by a student and suffered a concussion, torn ligaments in her elbow, and a severely sprained neck, she still has pounding headaches and can barely move her neck. Her elbow is sore and swollen, she continues to take anti-inflammatory medication and has difficulty sleeping. Her doctor tells her not to return to school this year and she follows his recommendation.

An expulsion hearing for the student accused of punching Roberts is held at the school district office. The boy shows up forty-five minutes late with his stepfather, gives his version of the incident to a panel of three school district officials, while Roberts waits outside the conference room. Roberts is then called into the room, and she discovers that the boy denied punching her. She tells the school district officials about the attack, and they pepper her with questions and ask her to repeat the story about five times. She feels as if she is on trial.

They then bring the boy and his stepfather into the room. She is not allowed to ask the boy any questions, but his stepfather is allowed to question Roberts.

"When he hit you, did you turn around?" the stepfather asks.

"No," she says. "I was on the ground."

"Then how do you know it was him?" he asks.

"Because he just knocked the shit out of me, and he jumped in front of me, and taunted me," she says angrily. "He was the only student near enough to me to have hit me."

After the hearing, the school district officials can either expel the student or determine that there is insufficient evidence against him and allow him to return to school.

They allow him to return to school.

Each year, a bank awards a scholarship to the outstanding senior English literature student at Crenshaw and Little picks the winner. This year she selects Miesha. Danielle is the scholar of the class, but Miesha, Little believes, is the best all-around student. She is a talented actress whose readings frequently enliven the class. Her thoughtful comments often animate class discussions.

Danielle is in a league of her own, academically, Little believes, but she is shy and rarely raises her hand or participates in class discussions. A student like Miesha, Little believes, makes a class work.

Miesha credits her brother Raymond for her academic success. While her mother was working long hours as a bus driver, it was Raymond who always made sure she did her homework, who attended parent-teacher conferences, who baked cookies for her to bring to school bake sales. Now Raymond is in a bittersweet mood. He had hoped Miesha would attend a Southern California college, so he could continue to see her frequently, but now he discovers that next year she will be attending UC

Berkeley and living almost 400 miles from Los Angeles. Still, Raymond is proud that Miesha will be attending such a prestigious university, and he feels great satisfaction knowing that he has contributed so much to her success.

On Friday, May 16, there is no class for the seniors because few of the girls would bother showing up. Most are spending the day primping for the prom.

At many suburban high schools in Southern California, the senior prom and high school graduation merely serve as the prelude to college, where a more significant graduation and a plethora of social events await them. At inner-city schools, however, high school graduation is a momentous event, the final academic achievement of many students' lives. Some will join the service after graduation, or go to work, or start trade school. The prom is a valediction to their youth, the major social event of the year. At Crenshaw, *everyone*—from the gangbangers to the gifted magnet students—attends.

The girls save all year for their prom dresses. And instead of buying dresses off the rack at department stores, many visit neighborhood seamstresses and design their own custom-made gowns.

A few weeks ago, a senior approached Moultrie and confided that she could not afford to buy a dress or pay for the prom ticket. Her date did not have enough money to rent a tuxedo. The girl's mother had died of a drug overdose and her father is in prison. She lives with her grandmother, who had just suffered a mild stroke. The grandmother told the girl that she was proud of her for finishing high school and had planned to help her pay for the prom, but her medical bills had eaten up all of her savings. The girl was devastated.

The next week, however, the girl bounds into Moultrie's classroom during the lunch period and announces that all her problems have been solved. She and her boyfriend can now afford the prom. She just bought a new dress, she tells Moultrie, her boyfriend rented a tuxedo, and they will hire a limousine.

"My uncle's slingin'," the girl tells Moultrie. "He's a big-time baller.

When he heard about my problem, he just pulled a big wad of hundreds out and threw twelve of 'em down on the table. Isn't that great?"

The girl sees the angry expression on Moultrie's face and asks her what is wrong. "This guy's dealing drugs, he's pumping poison into our community, into the veins of our children," Moultrie tells her. "Your mother died from drugs. Now your uncle's selling the same thing that killed her. You don't see anything wrong with that?"

The girl shrugs and says, "Yeah, I know it's wrong. But he's got a record and can never get a job that'll pay enough for him to survive on. So if slingin' is the only way he can make his money, then he's got to go out and do it to survive."

Moultrie fails to alter the girl's perspective, and on Friday night, at the Intercontinental Hotel in downtown Los Angeles, the girl arrives at the prom and marches right up to Moultrie, who is a chaperone. She hugs Moultrie and introduces her to her date.

Later, Princess, the queen of the prom, arrives, and several girls in Little's class surround her and tell her how glamorous she looks. Three months ago, Princess was planning to drop out of high school because her mother was in such dire financial straits. Princess's mother finally landed a job in late February, after a long stretch out of work. With her first paycheck, her mother brought Princess a beautiful, white, floor-length gown, trimmed in beads and sequins, which she is wearing tonight, along with her prom-queen tiara.

The other girls in Little's class also have been transformed. In class they usually wear jeans and T-shirts. Now they are all in evening gowns, with necklaces and corsages and sophisticated hairdos: Danielle is wearing a pale blue satin gown, trimmed in white lace and pearls. Latisha dons a taupe spaghetti-strap gown with white beaded panels in the front and back. Venola is wearing a white, crushed-velvet gown with matching elbow-length gloves. Even Naila, the class jock, looks elegant in a brown satin gown with halter straps.

Six months ago, Toya was a high school dropout, living in a shabby Watts apartment with her baby. Now Toya, who is wearing a black, form-fitting gown with rhinestone spaghetti straps and matching necklace, is back in school and reveling in the ambience of the prom. "Everyone looks so beautiful," she says, her eyes welling up with tears.

The boys, too, are elaborately turned out. A popular rap star recently began carrying a cane, so this is a big year for tuxedos with matching canes. Of the boys in Little's class, Larrin, who will be attending UCLA next year, has the most eye-catching ensemble. He is wearing a white double-breasted suit, a bright red satin shirt—open at the throat—with an enormous collar, matching red bowler hat, red pocket handkerchief, and red leather boots. His date is wearing a matching red gown, red shoes, and red, baby-rose wrist corsage. Sadi, too, is looking dapper, but more subdued, in a black tuxedo with a cognac-colored checked vest and matching bow tie.

A sober counterpoint to the festivities are the school policemen, dressed in suits, who wander about the ballroom, on the lookout for gang skirmishes. Several teachers signed up to chaperone, including Little, but a number of students from her class search the hotel and cannot find her. They whisper to each other: "Why isn't Miss Little here?" When she finally arrives, after 10 P.M., several girls race across the ballroom, teetering on their high heels, hug and kiss her, and call out: "We're so glad you made it." Despite the difficulties of the year, the students genuinely want to be with Little and share this night with her.

On the Monday following the prom, after the eight o'clock bell rings, Latisha raises her hand and asks, "You gonna be teaching at Crenshaw next year, Miss Little?"

She tells the class she has been going on interviews and is still trying to land a job at another high school. "I don't want to be here next year; I don't want *those* students," she says, referring to the eleventh graders currently in Moultrie's class. "There. I've said it. And I don't care if you repeat it."

In her last rant of the year, she recounts the "fucking white bitch" incident and insists she is being persecuted at Crenshaw because she is white. "They're saying I can't teach black kids. That's a lie! . . .

"They're trying to run the white teachers out of here. They're trying to run *my* ass out of here. Why?" she asks, loudly banging her fist on her desk. She stares at the students for a moment, but no one calls out the answer she is waiting for. She sighs impatiently and shouts, "It's racism! It's racism! It's racism!"

There are only a few more AP English classes before graduation, and on this Wednesday morning, Little has vowed to maintain her composure and not get distracted by extraneous issues. After the students are seated, she reads them a quote from the writer Ursula Le Guin: "It's good to have an end to a journey; but it's the journey that matters in the end."

Little paces in front of the class for a moment and says, "Think back on this year and the journey you've taken and all the literature you've read. Think back to that hot day in early September, that first day of school, when this class was overflowing with kids and we began reading *The Crucible.* Now, let's look at the connections between everything we've read, from *The Crucible,* to *Streetcar Named Desire.* What are the connections between all these great works? Why would a teacher choose this collection of works?"

"Because these were written by the aces, the Columbians," Latisha says.

"It's more than that," Little says. "In *The Crucible,* Christian orthodoxy's threatened by the dancers in the beginning of the play . . . by the presence of other religious beliefs . . . In *Inherit the Wind,* what's questioned? Public education and the role of Christian orthodoxy in schools. In *Wuthering Heights,* what's questioned? Exalting love and negotiating honor and obedience. In *Portrait of the Artist,* what did we discover that we have in common? We all come from a family; we're all introduced to a religion; we're all identified by our nationalism. In *Hamlet* we revisited the theme of nationalism, as well as personal revenge and public justice, and a number of other themes. In *The Elephant Man* we saw the importance of seeing the humanity in everyone, in loving our fellow man."

Little holds out her arms and asks the students, "What will you take from this class?"

"The knowledge of how to think critically," a girl says.

"Intellectual growth," another girl says.

"That you can learn who you are through literature," a boy calls out.

Latisha nods. "I learned that I could relate the literature to my own life. The literature helped me understand and deal with the problems in my life."

Little asks the students what works had the greatest influence on them.

"Portrait of the Artist," Latisha says. "I really connected to that stream-of-consciousness thang. The way Stephen had to look back on his life in order to get a handle on his future was meaningful to me. I learned from that."

Miesha raises her hand. *"The Elephant Man* struck a chord with me. When that woman showed him some kindness, it made him look inside himself. That made me realize it's the inside part of you that really matters."

Princess, the prom queen, one of the prettiest girls in the school, says of all the characters, she most closely identified with the disfigured, grotesque-looking Elephant Man. "I had to get through a lot of trials and tribulations this year. So when I read about what the Elephant Man had to go through, I could relate. I was inspired by the way he found the courage to overcome his problems. That helped me."

Brandi, the senior-class president, calls out, *"Wuthering Heights.* I, too, had to choose between two people that I loved. And that's all I'll say about it."

Larrin, who wore the white suit and matching red hat, shirt, and shoes to the prom, says, *"Wuthering Heights* made me think about a lot of things. I realized that my existence, like Heathcliff's, has been shallow in a lot of ways. That book made me face up to it."

A painfully shy girl named Carol, who will be attending Berkeley next year, tentatively lifts her hand. "I could really relate to *Streetcar Named Desire.* I learned from Blanche. She put up so many illusions and messed up her own life by not facing up to reality. That's like me, when I don't want to think about things, and I turn on the radio and pretend everything's hunky-dory. The play made me realize I shouldn't put up illusions. I should face up to things and deal with them."

Little asks the students, "Can you continue to inhabit the characters we studied? Will the great truths you learned from the literature stay with you? Can reading great works alter who you are and shape your lives?"

The class shouts in unison: "Yes!"

THIRTY-FIVE

MAMA MOULTRIE

SOME FREE ADVICE

If Little lands a job at another high school, or if she returns to Crenshaw, but does not teach AP English next year, Moultrie will teach the class. She knows most of the students who will take AP English next year because they are now enrolled in her eleventh-grade class.

As the semester draws to a close, Moultrie's eleventh graders—and the students in another class she teaches—are reading *The Great Gatsby*, which is part of the Crenshaw curriculum. But she has been unable to obtain enough copies for both classes. So now, she hands out copies of *The Great Gatsby* to her eleventh graders and they spend the first half of the class reading at their desks. She then collects the books, so during another period, her other class also will have an opportunity to read the novel.

She ordered the books from the school district months ago, but she did not receive enough copies because of what she calls ''a typical bureaucratic delay.'' As a result, Moultrie can no longer give her eleventh graders a daily writing assignment because the students spend half of the class reading *The Great Gatsby*. She knows this is not the ideal way for the students to read a great American novel. She knows students in more affluent neighborhoods are not subjected to these kinds of snafus. But, at this point, she has no alternative. So she improvises.

Moultrie decides to devote the second hour of every class now to *Othello*. She teaches the play every year to show her students that a man of color can be a lead in a Shakespearean play. She introduces the play to the students by telling them, "Othello is a Moor. That means he comes from North Africa." She holds up her copy of the play, which has a drawing of Othello on the cover. "Notice the strong African nose and mouth. In giving the lead to a person of color, Shakespeare was reacting against the conventions of the period, which equated beauty to whiteness." She sets the book down and says, "Don't we still equate beauty with white skin and golden hair?"

The students nod.

"Last time we read *Othello,* I took my eleventh graders to a Shakespeare festival to see the play. Othello was played by a black man. This brutha was *fine*. Tall. Great ebony skin. Beautiful piano-line teeth. He had it to-geth-*or*. Anyone who saw him would know you don't have to be white to be *fine*-looking.

"Let me introduce a few of the characters. Desdemona is the woman Othello loves. She's the daughter of a senator. So y'all know *she's* not trash. Do you think her father, Brabantio, a senator, would have a problem with his daughter eloping with a brutha?"

A few students laugh and shout, "Oh, *yeah!*"

In addition to trying to read *Othello* and *The Great Gatsby* before the end of the year, Moultrie's students are furiously completing a number of unorthodox assignments. They are sketching a newspaper front page, depicting the murder in *Native Son*. They are creating a children's book for impoverished South African students. They are compiling "character graphs" for the main characters in *A Streetcar Named Desire,* charting on graph paper the various traits that make up their personas. They are rehearsing their roles for the *Native Son* murder trial, which they will act out in class.

These are the types of assignments that infuriate Little. She feels they are frivolous and do not prepare the students for AP English. The eleventh graders, Little insists, need to spend the year writing traditional essays about literary works that will develop their interpretative and analytical skills. But Moultrie contends that assignments such as these—and her assignments that reflect black history and culture—pique the students' interest and enable them to immerse themselves in the literature. A steady diet of traditional essays, she feels, would not be as effective.

Moultrie knows she might be called upon to teach the AP English class next year, so she has been attempting to hone her teaching skills and recently has attended a number of workshops and conferences. She spent three days in Sacramento at a conference that explored innovative ways to teach gifted children. She has attended several conferences for teachers at UCLA. She also plans to enroll in a one-week seminar at Stanford this summer that prepares high school English teachers for Advanced Placement instruction.

At 11:30, on a warm June morning, after the students spend an hour reading *The Great Gatsby* at their desks, Moultrie discusses the end of the first act of *Othello*. The Santa Anas are blowing, most of the students are wearing shorts, and many are mopping their brows. Moultrie, however, who wears a flowing skirt, African bracelets, a top with a colorful African pattern, seems unaffected by the heat. She discusses the play with her customary verve.

"Desdemona is saying to Othello: 'Give me a brutha, like *you*.' " Moultrie rolls her shoulders and gives the class a sultry look. "Whoo-ee!"

She reads a few lines in which Desdemona's father admonishes her:

> . . . *Do you perceive in all this noble company*
> *Where most you owe obedience?*

"He's telling her: 'Don't you go up there and embarrass yo' daddy,' " Moultrie says. "And know who yo' mama is, too. And don't let me hear that you didn't act right."

She reads a passage in which Othello tells Desdemona:

Come Desdemona. I have but an hour.
Of love, of worldly matter, and direction
To spend with thee. We must obey the time.

"What's Othello saying?" she asks.

Che raises his hand. "He's sayin': 'Let's get busy.' "

"That's right," Moultrie says. "He's trying to get his groove on. He's telling her: 'I just have an hour for you, baby. So let's get it *onnnn!*' "

Moultrie reads a few lines from one of Iago's speeches:

. . . Our bodies are our gardens, to the which our wills are gardeners . . .
why, the power and corrigible authority of this lies in our wills . . .

"Listen to what he's saying," Moultrie tells the students. "He's saying: *We* control our own destiny. You guys talk about being doctors, lawyers, and accountants. It's your will, drive, and determination that'll make it possible. Keep negativity out of your life. Can I get an amen?"

"Amen!" the students shout.

"All those raggedy people who're giving you a hard time for being serious students, for caring about your future, don't let them into your gardens. All those people who tell you: 'Don't study, come hang out with me and we'll do yang, yang, yang' . . . Leave it be. Negativity is like weeds. It'll ruin your gardens."

She surveys the room, nodding at the students, and says, "That's some free advice from Mama Moultrie."

THIRTY-SIX

GRADUATION

STILL WE RISE

On a cool, foggy Monday morning in mid-June, Toni Little is preparing for her final AP English class of the year. This is typical June gloom weather in Los Angeles: The mornings, which are dank and misty, feel more like November than the cusp of summer. The fog often does not burn off until midafternoon. The sweltering summer days, days when dawn breaks clear and bright, without a hint of morning haze, do not begin until July.

The jacaranda trees that frame the quad are in full bloom and clusters of lavender, trumpet-shaped blossoms look lustrous against the backdrop of Kelly-green fronds—anomalous daubs of color against the wash of gray sky. Beneath the trees, there is a carpet of fallen blossoms, and the sidewalks are stained purple where legions of students have walked.

Before class, Little's students are busy exchanging yearbooks and writing inscriptions. When the bell rings, Little raps her knuckles on her desk and tells the class that before they begin the final exam, she wants to read them a farewell letter she wrote on Sunday night.

In the past, on the last day of AP English class, she has given spontaneous farewell addresses, sometimes going through her roll book and imparting brief comments to each student. She feels there was something special about this class, however, so she wants to give them a special farewell.

What made this class so different was its diversity. Past AP classes of Little's were more homogeneous, with many serious, soft-spoken students who were more interested in garnering As than in the dialectics of literary discussion. Although perhaps not as academically oriented, there was a serendipitous mix of students in this year's class. These students willingly drew from their own experiences, sharing the difficulties of their own lives, and they brought a rare visceral honesty, a passion and profundity to class discussions. Because Little feels a strong bond with these students, and because this has been such an emotional year for her, she wanted to leave the class with a valediction, a formal gesture of farewell.

She hands out copies of the letter to the students so they can read along with her.

"Today marks the culmination of a year of studying some of the greatest works in literary history," Little reads. "It has been my privilege to facilitate you in the process of growing and learning . . . learning that is based on a journey rather than in collecting facts . . .

"At the heart of my curriculum choices for you was a desire to impart that 'in each of us is a little of all of us.' I believe that you have entered into the worlds created by Shakespeare, Emily Brontë, James Joyce, Tennessee Williams, Arthur Miller . . . I would wager to think that . . . you have concluded that all of the above writers in some way or another altered your life.

"Each one of you has made a contribution to my life and has, in some way, altered it. I would be remiss if I didn't share with you some of the things I learned about you that wouldn't be found on an objective test. So here's to your lives:"

She asks each student to read what she has written about them:

Latisha reads: "There is Latisha, always willing to enter into an inquiry, always willing to express her point of view . . . savvy as ever in taking the stage. Her generosity of spirit and desire to advance her life, despite difficult circumstances, is a demonstration that we can overcome when we are dealt a lousy hand of cards. Her wisdom was presented with a style all of her own and will stay with me throughout the many years I have ahead of me to teach.''

Latisha waves the copy of Little's letter and shouts, ''That's *it*! Miss Little, you *feel* me, sista. That's the *whole* truth.''

Miesha reads, ''I think my relationship with Miesha has been obvious from the beginning. Here was this little tenth-grader, as smart as the day is long, trying to give her English teacher a run for her money. I knew then that it was going to be a struggle for the two of us to figure out who was in charge, but we did . . . and in the end we learned that a mutual respect would benefit us both in the long run. I love Miesha with all my heart and think that we are sisters from another lifetime.'' Miesha pauses, swallows hard, and reads, ''I have so enjoyed Miesha's willingness to work with the literature, to find the truths that are so befitting her high intelligence . . .''

As other students read what Little has written about them, a few girls sniffle. Little dabs at her eyes with a palm.

Venola reads: ''My Venola, God, I love her, too.'' Venola flashes Little a sweet smile. ''Venola is another sister who finds roots in relationships. She has from the tenth grade been there for me. She offered support and guidance and organization to a busy classroom environment. Her sense of humor and intelligent insights carried me through some rainy weather. Venola has the capacity to look at the whole picture and bring balance. Her big heart and mature wisdom are unquestionably valuable . . . Venola is special and a true friend to all the things that are ultimately important in life—love, wisdom, and communication.''

Now more students are crying and tears are streaming down Little's face. ''Don't cry, Miss Little,'' Venola calls out.

Naila reads: ''I came to know Naila a little bit this year and have learned firsthand what a scholar-athlete she is. Naila was always on time, rarely absent, offered insight, and worked hard for her grade. She was a positive asset to the class and allowed us to integrate the competitive nature she has on the basketball court into the academic search for truth in literature . . . You are bound for glory at Stanford and I will be rooting for your success.''

Half the class is crying now. Little shields her eyes and a student grabs a box of Kleenex and hands it to her.

Sadi reads: ''Sadi was a bit of a disappointment this year. His light was shining very brightly in the tenth grade and it seemed to dim this year . . ." Sadi looks a bit sheepish, but he brightens when he reads, "Nonetheless, I have the greatest respect for his academic insights and am hopeful that he will again let his light shine brightly in a world that so needs his point of view. I will never forget his oratorical delivery when Tommie Smith was here. Sadi, please . . . bring the same zest that you brought to us two years ago to your college studies. We missed the contribution you bring to the study of fiction. That contribution more accurately represents who you really are."

Danielle reads: "This leads me to a . . . scholar, Danielle. What can I say? You're awesome." Danielle looks down and smiles shyly. "Danielle has been, from the first day I met her, exemplary . . . I, like many, am honored to have been a part of Danielle's life and respect every single word she has ever written. She exemplifies excellence. In addition, she is a quality human being . . . She always provides a caring heart to situations. That, mixed with her intelligence, will make for a very fulfilling life."

When the students finish reading, Little dabs at her eyes again with a tissue and reads, "There you have it. That is a little insight into what was going on in my head while I was delivering lectures, grading essays, testing objectively, and trying to stay afloat among some of the brightest young people I have ever encountered. I will never forget this year . . .

"So, we're at the end of this journey." Little's voice breaks and she pauses, drying her eyes, until she regains her composure. "I hope that in some small way I have made a difference. At best, I hope that I was able to shed some light on how awesome it is to take the literary journey. I hope that the authors were good teachers to you. They have been to me. As you carry on in life, remember the lessons you learned from them. Use those lessons . . . Use the wisdom . . .

"I, like Holden Caulfield, am a kind of 'catcher in the rye' . . . I hope that your journey into *my* world, aided by the authors whose works are unparalleled, has illuminated *your* world. Thanks for the opportunity. I will miss you. Do try to keep in touch. If I don't hear from you, know that I am in the stands rooting for you. Get on the court and play this game of life out . . . and let your gifts shine. This world will be a better place because you're in it.

"Your friend, Toni."

For several minutes, the class is silent. The only sounds are sniffles and muffled sobs. A few students walk up to the front of the class and embrace her. The fog, the mist that beads against the windows, and the gray overcast skies add to the bittersweet mood in the classroom.

Finally, Miesha wipes her eyes, stands up and says, "I want to thank you for making us read all those books. I used to think it was all about money, but through the literature and our class discussions, you made me look deeper and examine more important values. You're the best teacher I ever had."

Miesha's comments rouse the class and, one after another, the students stand up and offer testimonials to Little.

"You've been like a mentor to me," Latisha says. "When I had problems this year, you listened to me—behind the scenes. Thank you."

Lena, who will attend UC Santa Barbara, is ranked second in the senior class. She sat in the back row and rarely participated in class discussions, but now she stands and says, "One reason I always liked to come to class was because you were always so animated, so crazy. It was never boring. This is the first year I ever learned anything in English. I used to write superficially, but you pushed me to write in depth."

Larrin, who will attend UCLA, is another student who sat in the back of the class and rarely spoke. Now he walks to the front of the class, hugs Little, and says, "I don't want to be remembered as the boy who never said anything. A million things are going through my head right now." He begins crying. "I just want to say: Thank you, Miss Little."

Sheila, who will attend Xavier University next year, says, "I've never had a class that had such interesting discussions. They were always based in reality, and they helped me understand the literature. So whenever the faculty asked me about you, I always had your back." Sheila sobs, "I love you, Miss Little."

Curt stands up and says, "I can say on behalf of everyone, we all have respect for you. We admire you because of your passion, even your passion about O.J.—although we don't agree with you." The class laughs and pounds their desks. "You taught me what I needed to learn. When I went to summer school at Stanford, I got As and Bs on all my papers. That's because you taught me to write in the tenth grade and prepared me to compete. You've given me the path to leave high school."

Little sits on the edge of her desk, her face flushed, her eyes watery, lips trembling.

Brandi, the senior-class president, is not in the gifted program, and this was her first class with Little. She stands up and says, "You're the first *real* English teacher I ever had. Thanks to you, I now have the confidence to go on to Pitzer next year."

Robert waves his hand and says, "I remember you as a teacher who taught me to write. But I appreciate your class more than for the writing and reading. You made me see that these books are not just words on paper; you made me see that they're about life. You helped me look deeper, not just at the literature, but at my own character."

Miesha walks over to Little, hugs her and says in a quavering voice, "There were times when the only people who were there for me were you and my brother. I look at you as more than a teacher. You really are Toni Little, my home girl."

There have been so many testimonials, there is not enough time left for the final exam. Little stands up and says, "I guess we won't have a test today. The AP exam was really your final, anyway. And, ultimately, this is more valuable. This is what you'll remember ten years from now."

Little takes a deep breath and says, "I want to tell all of you that it was a privilege teaching you. Do well with your lives. Read on your own. Don't wait for someone to assign books. Teach yourselves. Make people proud of you."

She pauses, tears streaming down her face, and says, "Congratulations, you guys. It's all over."

The bell rings, but the students are reluctant to leave the classroom. Most gather around Little and wait to hug her. She wishes them well in college and urges them to keep in touch. The students hug each other and talk excitedly about graduation. When the last student finally files out, and the classroom is empty, Little sits at her desk, sniffling and wiping her eyes with Kleenex.

After this class, it is clear that, despite her shortcomings, Little has had a tremendous impact on the students. She may have digressed too often in class; she may have been too consumed with her own demons; she may have been too distracted by her battles with the administration; she may have missed a few crucial weeks of school during a critical juncture; she may not have thoroughly prepared the students for the AP exam. But this outpouring of emotion by the students is a rare, authentic testimony to the power of her presence in the classroom. In the end, the students were moved by the way she linked the literature to life; the way she galvanized class discussions; the way she generated enthusiasm for literary themes and analysis; the way she inspired students from South-Central Los Angeles to care deeply about Joyce and Shakespeare and Brontë.

Years after they graduate, the students may forget their AP score, or their grades in the class, or her tirades, but the way she sparked their appreciation for the world of ideas and their love of literature will stay with many forever.

Three days later, the students' families stroll across campus in the late afternoon, on their way to the football field for graduation. There is something sad about an empty campus at the end of the school year, a place where there was once so much frenetic activity, but now is eerily quiet. Notebook paper and candy wrappers skitter in the wind across the desolate quad, like tumbleweeds across a barren plain, as the families traverse the campus and filter into stands flanking the football field.

It is a glorious, sparkling afternoon with a great sweep of powder blue sky. The fog has burned off, a soft, salty breeze blows in from the ocean and, in the distance, the towering palms sway in the wind, the fronds dappled with sunlight. While the families wait for the graduates to march onto the field, they listen to a jazz guitar CD playing from the public address system.

At 4:30, the more than 400 graduates—about 40 of whom are in the gifted magnet program—march onto the field to the evocative strains of "Pomp and Circumstance." The students wear royal blue caps and gowns and many have, over their shoulders, Ghanaian kente cloths, decorated with bright geometric patterns that symbolize the students' African heritage.

The stands, which are packed, erupt in cheers when the students emerge onto the field. On the elevated stage, in front of the rows of folding chairs for the graduates, Little and Moultrie, wearing black gowns, sit a few feet from each other, but avoid each other's eyes. They head different honors societies and will hand out awards.

The students' reactions to Little and Moultrie indicate that, despite the animosity between the two teachers, they are both admired by the students. One of the first student speakers begins his address by saying, as the graduates cheer: "I want to thank Mrs. Moultrie . . . for showing us it's our right and our duty to make a difference in our community."

When Little is introduced, the graduates give her a standing ovation and students shout at her: "We love you, Miss Little," and "We'll miss you, Miss Little."

Danielle is the class valedictorian, and as she strides to the podium to give her speech, the crowd grows silent. In Little's class, Danielle rarely participated in class discussions, and when she did make a comment or answer a question, it was always haltingly, shyly, with eyes cast down.

But this afternoon, as Danielle delivers her speech, she is transfigured. She is poised, confident, and commanding. "Good afternoon, family, friends, and fellow graduates," she says, her voice strong and clear. "This day represents the pinnacle of all of our efforts as high school students. It is at this time that we have a chance to stop, reflect on our past, before we progress into the future . . .

"We are a class of survivors. We survived the loss of affirmative action. We survived the loss of Tupac and Biggie. We survived the O.J. Simpson trials that have been going on since we were *ninth* graders . . . But most importantly, we survived the scrutiny of our potential by this society that labeled us failures. We learned to place less importance on what this society thinks of us, and more what we think of ourselves . . .

"As Eleanor Roosevelt said, 'No one can make you inferior without your consent.' Well, we did not give our permission *or* our submission," she says, pausing, and nodding at the students. "I am reminded of a poem I was once taught by my kindergarten teacher, Mrs. Hunt, a poem by Maya Angelou entitled, 'Still I Rise,' only, in this instance, the more appropriate title would be, *Still WE Rise*. Not only did we survive, but we *succeeded*.

"How do we know we succeeded? What is a measurement of our success? Is it *solely* the grades that we received, or all the As on our report cards? Not quite. It is also the pride that we detect in our parents' eyes. The smiles that we see in the faces of all those who were instrumental in passing the knowledge on to us . . . Most of all, it is what *we* know we've accomplished, and how we apply what we know . . .

"Now we are at a crossroads in our lives. This is the point where we all go our separate ways. As seniors, we all have our ambitions, our own dreams to pursue . . . That brings me to where we are today. The past is behind us, the present is upon us and the future is before us. So what should we do?" she asks, extending her arms.

"I leave you with these words:

"Remember the past.

"Cherish the present.

"Conquer the future."

The parents in the stands and the students on the field rise and clap and cheer and stamp their feet. There are a few more speeches, more awards are presented, and then the students form a long, serpentine line and the principal, whom Little feuded with all year, gives each student a diploma and a handshake.

Finally, the students march across the field and gather in the school parking lot, as LAPD and school police officers patrol the perimeter. A few of the students seek out Little, hug her, and introduce their parents to her, some of whom have been estranged from their children, or who live across the country.

When Latisha was growing up in an Alabama housing project, her mother, a cocaine addict, battered her. Latisha's relatives decided she would be safer in Los Angeles, where her father lived, and she moved in with him when she was thirteen. Her mother is off drugs now and has flown in from Alabama to attend graduation. Latisha is beaming and, with her arm around her mother's shoulder, introduces her to Little.

When Willie was a child, his mother became addicted to cocaine and he moved in with his father. Willie's mother lives in Northern California now, is off drugs, and she, too, is here today.

When Sadi was five, his father walked out on the family. He disappeared for long periods of time and drifted in and out of his son's life. Even though Sadi professes not to care, his mother can tell he is secretly pleased that his father showed up for graduation.

Miesha brings her brother Raymond to say hello to Little. Raymond, who was a surrogate parent to his younger sister because their mother worked such long hours as a bus driver, had mixed emotions about Miesha attending UC Berkeley and living so far away. But now Miesha tells Little she was just awarded a full scholarship to USC. Berkeley offered a partial scholarship and the remainder of the financial-aid package consisted of loans and a part-time job.

"I've got to go where the money is," Miesha tells Little, hugging her. "Now I'll be able to stop by and see you next year because I'll only be a few miles away."

"Yessss!" Raymond shouts, smiling and pumping a fist.

Another student introduces his mother to Little and then asks her, "You coming back next year?"

"I've got a few interviews at other high schools lined up," Little says. "If I get a decent offer, I'm gone. That's why our last class was so wonderful. It gave me closure. I feel my work here is done."

Scott Braxton watches the students line up to embrace Little and introduce their parents to her. Braxton recently passed the school district's vice principal exam, and he expects to be transferred next year to another school. Graduations always put him in a melancholy, reflective mood. And now, these feelings are accentuated because he knows he probably will not return to Crenshaw and because this has been such a draining and demanding year.

There was Little and her many moods and the long stretch when she refused to speak to him, and her weeks off shortly before the AP exam, and her threatened lawsuits, and her battles with the principal, and her feud with Moultrie.

There was Olivia, whom he counseled while she was AWOL, while she was miserable at her foster home, while she lurched from court appearance to court appearance, until she was finally incarcerated—a dismal conclusion to their four-year relationship. Braxton thinks of her now, locked up, while her classmates are graduating, and he sighs and stares into the distance.

There was Sabreen, who also lived in a foster home and who dropped out of school in November. During the first two months of school, Braxton often counseled Sabreen every day, sometimes hours at a time, while she fretted—and sometimes sobbed uncontrollably in his office—about balancing a full-time job, a full load of honors classes, and a fiancé. She dropped out of school in November, married her boyfriend a few weeks ago, and now is considering dropping out of community college because she has so little time to devote to her studies.

There was Claudia, a girl for whom he had such great hopes. He spent so much time talking to her in his office, trying to discover why she would not turn in her exams in Little's class. She eventually flunked AP English and had to leave the class, leaving Braxton feeling bitterly disappointed. But at least Claudia's high school years ended on a propitious note because she made up the F in night school and graduated today.

There was Toya, who had been accepted for Cornell's summer program last year—which feels like a lifetime ago to Braxton. He had admired Toya so much, had such great expectations for her future, had tried so hard to keep her in school after she had her baby. He was so despondent when she dropped out, and so elated when she returned. But, it turns out, Toya returned too late. She did not have enough credits to graduate. If she attends summer school, she can graduate in August. But she was so disappointed that she could not graduate with her classmates, and is so overwhelmed by the exigencies of motherhood, Braxton is uncertain whether Toya will make the effort to attend summer school.

Braxton's mournful musing is interrupted when he sees Venola bounding across the parking lot with her mother. He reflects on students such as Venola and Miesha and Danielle and Latisha and Willie and Princess and Robert and Curt, and he realizes he has spent so much time dealing with students in crisis—putting out fires, as he thinks of it—that he had little time left to spend with the other students, the students who breezed along this year, or the students who never sought him out.

But now, as the sun dips past the campus buildings, and the light drains from the sky, and the wind dies down to a whisper, and the crickets thrum in the bushes, and the students give their classmates and teachers a final hug and stroll across the parking lot with their parents, and drive off to graduation parties or celebratory dinners or backyard barbecues, Braxton realizes that while there have been a handful of casualties this year, the vast majority of the gifted seniors—despite myriad obstacles and steep odds—have thrived and excelled. And he is proud of them.

EPILOGUE

A few months after the students in Toni Little's class graduated from high school, they received their scores from the Advanced Placement English Literature and Composition exam.

The results were a disaster. Only Danielle and Robert passed.

A grade of three, four, or five on an AP exam is a passing mark—and earns the student college credit. Both Danielle and Robert received threes.

It is clear that Little bears much of the responsibility for the students' showing because a number of the same students who performed poorly on the exam passed the AP Government and Politics test taught by Scott Allen. More than a third of his students passed, seven of whom were also in Little's class, including Venola and Curt. Claudia, the student who flunked Little's class the first semester and rarely cracked a book in Allen's class, received a four on the AP Government test. The others who passed received threes.

Allen was well organized, disciplined, and kept the students focused on the exam throughout the year. His students felt much better prepared and much more confident than the students in Little's class.

"I was too undisciplined," Little acknowledged, after she discovered the test results. "You have to have discipline to demand discipline. I didn't reinforce the basic skills like I should have. I didn't give them enough practice exams or vocabulary tests. I had barely enough energy to teach the literature."

At the end of the school year, Little applied to several other Los Angeles high schools, but none of the principals would hire her. She believes her battles at Crenshaw have crippled her search for another job in the school district.

Also, during the summer, Little filed a lawsuit against principal Yvonne Noble, Scott Braxton, a number of school district administrators, and the school district. The lawsuit stems from the incident during the second semester when a parent advisor referred to her as a "fucking white bitch." She claims Crenshaw administrators ignored the incident and retaliated against her when she complained. Little also alleges in the lawsuit, which is pending, that she has been discriminated against at Crenshaw because she is white and is forced to work in a "racially hostile work environment."

Noble took a leave of absence at Crenshaw for medical reasons and was briefly hospitalized. She believes her health problems were a result of stress, partly as a result of her battles with Little.

The ballot measure that ended affirmative action in California—Proposition 209—has had a profound impact on the fate of minority students in California.

The number of first-year black students enrolled at UC campuses in the fall of 1998—the first freshman class after the proposition went into effect—dropped by almost 20 percent from the previous year. The numbers of all other underrepresented minority students also decreased.

The declines were steepest at the most prestigious and competitive campuses, such as UC Berkeley and UCLA. The number of black freshmen enrolled at UC Berkeley plummeted by more than 50 percent compared to the previous year and by almost one-third at UCLA. The number of Latino students enrolled at UC Berkeley declined by 43 percent and at UCLA the number fell by 23 percent.

Black enrollment in 1998 at UC campuses was the lowest in eighteen years, despite tremendous growth in the overall student population.

In the second undergraduate class after Proposition 209 went into effect, however, recently released statistics indicate that the University of California admitted almost as many underrepresented minorities as it did before the affirmative action ban. Admissions directors attribute the gain to aggressive recruitment of talented minority students and more flexible selection criteria.

Still, the number of black undergraduates accepted at the eight UC campuses for the fall of 1999 was down about 8 percent, compared to 1997. And the number of minorities admitted at UC Berkeley and UCLA for the fall of 1999 were still well below the admissions figures prior to the affirmative action ban. The number of black undergraduates admitted to UC Berkeley for the fall of 1999 dropped by 51 percent compared to 1997, and at UCLA the number fell by 43 percent. The number of Latino students at UC Berkeley was down 41 percent and dropped by one-third at UCLA. Many of those minority students who would have been accepted by UCLA and UC Berkeley in the past were disseminated to less competitive campuses.

University of California graduate, law, and medical schools also have accepted fewer minorities since the affirmative action ban.

For example, at UC Berkeley's Boalt Hall Law School, which is the state's finest public law school, only one black student was enrolled in the fall of 1997—the first year the ban on affirmative action went into effect for graduate programs. The next year, nine black students were enrolled, but this number was still well below the previous two decades, when an average of 24 black students attended the law school.

At UCLA law school, only nine black students were enrolled in 1997, a more than 50 percent drop from the previous year. In 1998, the number of black students dropped again, to seven.

In a few years, many of the students who were in Little's English class will be applying to law and medical schools and other graduate programs. At that time, some of them will see their career choices greatly diminished because of the elimination of affirmative action in the state.

AFTERWORD

As of this writing, about three and a half years after the students graduated, Yvonne Noble is the principal at a Los Angeles middle school.

Scott Braxton was promoted and is now an assistant principal at a predominantly Latino high school on the East side.

Anita Moultrie, who was scheduled to take over Little's AP English class, was also promoted and left Crenshaw. She is a teacher advisor for about ten schools—and hundreds of teachers—in South Los Angeles. She is also the coordinator for a school district program that trains teachers.

After graduation, Toni Little taught two more years at Crenshaw. She then left teaching and headed a program—funded by the state—to integrate computer technology into the curriculum at Crenshaw. The next year she injured her back while at the school and is currently on disability.

Most of the students I profiled are now in the middle of their senior year in college. All of them have to work, from part- to full-time, depending on their scholarship and financial-aid packages. Many also volunteer for inner-city tutoring or mentoring programs. All of these students, some of whom were admitted because of affirmative action, are on track to graduate.

—Miesha is at University of Southern California, majoring in management consulting. She works about twenty-five hours a week as a bookkeeper. She also volunteers about fifteen hours a week for Rites of Sisterhood—a mentoring program for inner-city high school girls—and for several community service projects sponsored by her black sorority.

—After a lackluster senior year at Crenshaw, Sadi finally regained his motivation. The summer after graduation, he attended a program at a nearby state college that prepares minority students for college. Sadi was named the program's outstanding male student.

After countless phone calls to Clark College in Atlanta, Sadi's mother managed to insure that Sadi obtained enough financial aid, loans, and scholarships so he could attend the school. Sadi's mother died last year.

Sadi still has to work about thirty-five hours a week to pay for rent and food. He is a customer service representative for an express mail company.

Sadi still writes poetry, and he is attempting to compile his poems and short stories into a book. His major is speech communication and he is considering, after graduation, teaching African American history to inner-city students.

—Danielle is at Pitzer College in Southern California, majoring in sociology and black studies. She works about thirty hours a week for the Black Student Affairs department. She was the president of the Black Student Union during her sophomore and junior year. She also volunteers for a program that encourages minority students to attend college. She spent the first semester of her senior year attending college in Ghana.

—Toya needed to attend summer school in order to graduate from Crenshaw because of the classes she missed after the birth of her baby. But the demands of her infant overwhelmed her. She did not attend summer school, and she did not graduate from high school.

The next fall, however, she completed a church program that provided child care for teenage mothers so they could earn their high school equivalency certificates.

She is currently working as a teller for a credit union.

A chapter of this book that featured Toya recently ran in the *Los Angeles Times Magazine* and dozens of people responded, offering to help finance Toya's college education. Toya hopes to take advantage of this opportunity and return to college next year.

—Willie is at Morehouse College in Atlanta, majoring in business. He works more than thirty hours a week as a waiter. He attends school during the day and works at the restaurant from 5:00 P.M. to 11:00 P.M. He studies on weekends and between classes.

—Claudia is at California State University, Long Beach, and is majoring in psychology and anthropology. She works forty-five hours a week as a waitress and for the catering department at a film studio. Despite a hectic schedule—and a poor senior year in high school—she has excelled in college. Claudia has regained her enthusiasm for learning. She has a 3.7 grade point average and has been on the school's honor roll every semester except one.

—Venola is at Colby College and is majoring in Spanish. She works about thirty hours a week. She is the program coordinator for the African American Studies department, a research assistant for the Spanish department, and a peer mentor for freshmen.

She plans to attend graduate school in business. Her goal is to open a financial consulting firm that will promote investment in the inner city.

Venola wrote an article for the *Christian Science Monitor* about the adjustment of attending a predominantly white college after spending four years at an all-minority high school.

"As I get older, I understand that my world has been very confined," Venola wrote. "Being at Colby . . . has helped me realize that there is an entire world waiting for me to embrace it. I have grown tremendously since my departure from Los Angeles, and it hurts to see some people at home in the same place they were when I left.

"I owe it to myself and everyone who has helped me to reach out and try to help other poeple . . . I have great plans for my life . . . and I hope I can be an example to a lot of people who come from the same place I have."

—Latisha attended Alabama A&M, but dropped out during her sophomore year. She was bored with small-town life in Alabama and missed Southern California. She moved back to Los Angeles and obtained a job as a receptionist at a clothing company. She is now a customer service manager for the company and takes night business classes at a community college.

—Princess is at the University of California, Santa Barbara, majoring in communications. She works about twenty hours a week as a resident coordinator for university-owned housing. She volunteers about fifteen hours a week for philanthropic projects sponsored by her black sorority and for a campus organization that provides tutoring to minority high school students. She plans to attend graduate school in journalism and pursue a career as a television news reporter.

—After Sabreen dropped out of Crenshaw, she moved in with her boyfriend and they married a few months later. She never returned to high school. Instead, Sabreen passed the General Education Development (GED) test, and earned a high school equivalency degree.

During the next year, she worked full-time and took several classes at a community college. But her husband had two jobs, and Sabreen was left with most of the household tasks. At the end of the day she had no time or energy to study. She ended up dropping out of college.

After about a year of marriage, she left her husband. "He threw me around the apartment one night," she said, "so that was it for me." Sabreen had been abused by her mother as a girl, and she vowed she would never let anyone hurt her again. She moved to New York to live with relatives, "for a fresh start," she said. Sabreen hopes to attend college there.

—Curt is at UCLA, majoring in physiology. He had a difficult time during his freshman year at college. He has always been high-strung and short-tempered, and he found dorm living intolerable. He could not study or sleep amid the noise and tumult of the dorm, and his grades suffered. Also, he was devastated when his girlfriend of two years broke up with him.

During his sophomore and junior year, he lived alone in an apartment near South-Central and was completely self-supporting. Although both his parents are professionals, they believed it would benefit him to work his way through college. He worked almost forty hours a week—twenty-five hours for UCLA's parking service and twelve hours tutoring inner-city students for a federal program.

He now plans to transfer to Howard University next semester. Although this will delay Curt's graduation by a year, he believes he will be happier at a predominantly African American school with smaller classes and a more intimate classroom environment. He still wants to attend medical school and become an orthopedic surgeon.

—Naila is at Stanford and majors in medical administration. College basketball was an adjustment for her. She is almost six feet tall, and in high school she was an all-American power forward. But the forwards at Standord are well over six feet and the center is 6 feet 7. Naila was a reserve guard at Stanford and never adjusted to a new position.

Although she quit the team at the end of her junior year, she retained her scholarship. She now works about twenty hours a week at the student center restaurant. After graduation, she plans to work as a hospital administrator.

—Robert is at UCLA, majoring in African American Studies and history. He works about thirty hours a week at a campus office and at a nearby mall. He is also a leader of the campus organization for black students, volunteers for a program that invites black high school students to campus for workshops, and spends a few weeks during the summer at a camp for minority students. After graduation, he plans to return to the inner city as a community organizer.

—The summer after the students in Little's class graduated, Olivia was still locked up. At court, the judge announced that if she made satisfactory progress while in custody, she would be released in August, in time to attend college. The judge decided to rely on the assessment of Olivia's therapist at the center, Susanne Dunne.

At the end of the summer, Dunne felt Olivia needed at least another six months of therapy at the center. Dunne knew, however, how important it was to Olivia to attend colledge in the fall. And she was pleased at Olivia's progress. In August, Dunne made her decision.

Olivia was released.

She moved directly from county custody to the dormitory at California State University, Northridge. When I visited Olivia, shortly after she moved to the dorm, she did not even have enough money to buy a blanket or bedspread. All she had on the bed was a single frayed sheet. But she was happy.

At Northridge, Olivia worked more than forty hours a week as a supervisor on the overnight shift at two group homes, a world she knows well. She continued to hustle—but legally this time. She wanted to travel and used her education to see the world. She has spent a semester at the University of Hawaii on an exchange program, part of a summer studying in Cuba, and another summer in New York working for a Wall Street firm.

During her first two years of college, Olivia excelled, earning all As and only a single B.

When Olivia was in high school, she read a magazine article that rated Babson College in Massachusetts as the best business college in the nation. Since then, her dream was to enroll there. She was accepted to Babson, but then she was arrested. She reapplied during her sophomore year in college, was accepted again, and was given a full-tuition scholarship. She transferred to Babson for her junior year.

She is currently the vice president of public relations and webpage designer for the Babson Black Student Union. She is also attempting to launch her own company—while in college—which will provide a link between minority businesses and Fortune 1000 companies. After graduation, Olivia plans to obtain a job with a management consulting firm. After a few years, she hopes to return to school and earn an MBA from Harvard or the University of Pennsylvania's highly regarded Wharton School of Business.

Although Olivia is extremely busy, she spends every Saturday morning as a volunteer tutor to impoverished minority students in the Boston area.

Helping the students is important to her because she knows that, despite the myriad problems she faced as a child, it was school that ultimately saved her.

ACKNOWLEDGMENTS

I would like to express my thanks to all the teachers and administrators at Crenshaw High School. I am indebted, in particular, to four people who accepted the risk of my presence with great graciousness:

Principal Yvonne Noble approved my proposal to spend the school year at Crenshaw, and I am most appreciative of the free reign she granted me.

Scott Braxton could not have been more hospitable, treating me more like a colleague than a reporter.

Anita Moultrie was as enthusiastic about this book as she is about all of her many endeavors. She helped me understand the world—and the literary world—from a different perspective and always made me feel welcome in her classroom.

Toni Little was extremely generous with her time and spent countless afternoons with me, discussing the students and her teaching approach. Little was always open and forthright with me, despite our occasional disagreements and disputations. A year with Toni Little is never boring, and I enjoyed her dynamic classroom presence.

Additionally, I'd like to express my thanks to all the Crenshaw students in AP Literature—and their parents—who opened up their lives to me. I learned much from these students. They were, and continue to be, an inspiration to me. They are the true heroes of this book.

Barney Karpfinger is a brilliant agent and, more important, a valued friend. In the beginning, when I had grave doubts, he convinced me that this was a book worth writing. It is reassuring for me to know that I can always count on Barney and his unerring advice. He is a true mensch.

I am indebted to Jennifer Hershey at Morrow/Avon for her early enthusiasm, insight, and direction.

Kelly Notaras of Morrow/Avon was always efficient, enthusiastic, a pleasure to deal with, and, at all times, extremely helpful.

My editor Hamilton Cain was a marvel. He has a wonderful ear for language and his suggestions and emendations improved the manuscript immeasurably. I am thankful for his belief in the students—and the value of their stories—and the fervent manner in which he championed the book.

I received essential assistance from two longtime friends. Ruth D'Arcy's careful reading and excellent suggestions were very helpful. I am also grateful to Michael Shapiro for his many insights and thoughtful assessments.

Finally, I would like to thank most of all my wife, Diane. In the beginning, her belief in this book motivated me. During the research, her unflagging support encouraged me. During the writing, her often double-duty days of child-care sustained me. During the rewriting, her careful, energetic editing greatly assisted me. Because I shared every aspect of the book with her—from the initial spark of the idea to lunches with the students long after graduation—the research and writing was never a chore and most often a joy.

NOTES

This book is a work of nonfiction. No names have been changed, no pseudonyms have been used, no incidents have been altered.

Chapter 2

After about a week, Toya's mother could no longer afford: Bonnie Swindell, "Man arrested, charged with a strangulation death of wife," *The Coastal Courier,* January 16, 1990.

Chapter 8

One Southern California SAT preparation firm: Elaine Gale, "A 5-year Quest to Ace the SAT," *Los Angeles Times,* October 14, 1998.

For all ethnic groups, the higher a parent's educational background: Editorial, "SAT Shock," *Washington Post,* August 29, 1991.

Since World War I: Christopher Jencks and Meredith Phillips, *The Black-White Test Score Gap* (Brooking Institution Press, Washington D.C., 1998) p. vii.

Even when black and white students have the same family income: Pam Belluck, "Reason Is Sought For Lag By Blacks in School Effort," *New York Times,* July 4, 1999; Brent Staples, "How the Racial Literary Gap First Opened," *New York Times,* July 23, 1999.

The college environment often is a greater predictor: William G. Bowen and Derek Bok, *The Shape of the River* (Princeton University Press, Princeton, New Jersey, 1998) p. 259.

Chapter 9

In the years following the Bakke decision: Nicholas Lemann, "Taking Affirmative Action Apart," *New York Times Sunday Magazine,* June 11, 1995.

A mandate to ignore race: William G. Bowen and Derek Bok, "Affirmative Action: The Use of Race-Based Selection Has Opened Many Fields for Blacks, A New Study Shows," *Los Angeles Times,* September 23, 1998.

This policy, which is common in the top tier of law schools nationwide: Elaine Woo, "Boalt Hall Kills its Grade-Weighting Policy Admissions," *Los Angeles Times,* November 27, 1997; Susan Sturm and Lani Guinier, "Race-Based Remedies," *California Law Review,* July 1996.

I would tell black youngsters: Ethan Bronner, "Study Strongly Supports Affirmative Action in Admissions to Elite Colleges," *New York Times,* September 9, 1998.

The authors, however, did not have the political savvy: Peter Schrag, *Paradise Lost: California's Experience, America's Future* (The New Press, New York, 1998) p. 235.

Pete has been a strong supporter of the affirmative action efforts: R. Drummond Ayres Jr., "Wilson's Moderate Path Veered Quickly to Right," *New York Times,* August 9, 1995.

Later, as governor, Wilson signed: Dave Lesher, "Wilson Confronts Charges of Broken Pledges, Flip-Flops," *Los Angeles Times*, August 7, 1995.

Yet when Wilson was a United States senator: Paul Jacobs, "Wilson's Border Record—Success or Opportunism?" *Los Angeles Times*, May 15, 1995.

So when Wilson suddenly changed his position on affirmative action: Shrag, pp. 235–36.

The campaign manager for Proposition 209 acknowledged that trotting out Connerly: Barry Bearak, "Questions of Race Run Deep for Foes of Preferences," *New York Times*, July 27, 1997.

One angry regent, Ralph Carmona: Ralph Frammolino and Mark Gladstone, "UCLA Chief Admits Possible Favoritism," *Los Angeles Times*, March 17, 1996.

His father, however, was considered a prime target: Ralph Frammolino, Mark Gladstone and Henry Weinstein, "UCLA Eased Rules for the Rich, Well-Connected," *Los Angeles Times*, March 21, 1996.

The chancellor of UC Berkeley said Connerly: Mark Gladstone and Ralph Frammolino, "UC Berkeley Panel Handles Admission Requests by VIPs," *Los Angeles Times*, April 11, 1996.

Wilson recommended several dozen students: Ralph Frammolino and Mark Gladstone, "Politicians Sought Aid of UC Lobbyist," *Los Angeles Times*, March 3, 1996.

Regent Leo Kollogian, who voted to eliminate affirmative action: Ralph Frammolino, Mark Gladstone and Amy Wallace, "Some Regents Seek UCLA Admissions Priority for Friends," *Los Angeles Times*, March 16, 1996.

One, who had a 3.5 grade-point average: Frammolino, Gladstone and Wallace.

Right after the regents voted to end all racial preferences: Peter King, "The Curtain Pulled Back, For a Moment," *Los Angeles Times*, September 11, 1996.

While most Californians strongly opposed numerical quotas: Lydia Chavez, *The Color Bind: California's Battle to End Affirmative Action* (University of California Press; Berkeley, 1998), p. 245.

In 1988, 280 of 1,602 Harvard freshman: Jerome Karabel and David Karen, "Go to Harvard, Give Your Kid a Break," *New York Times,* December 8, 1990.

If legacies had been admitted to the 1988 freshman class at Harvard at the same rate: Karabel and Karen.

At Stanford, alumni children are admitted: Elaine Woo, "Belief in Meritocracy an Equal-Opportunity Myth," *Los Angeles Times,* April, 30, 1995.

In addition to children of alumni and athletes: Barbara R. Bergmann, *In Defense of Affirmative Action* (Basic Books, New York, 1996) p. 123.

Chapter 13

A few passages on the history of South-Central Los Angeles and the Los Angeles Police Department were taken from the author's book, *The Killing Season: A Summer Inside an LAPD Homicide Division* (Simon & Schuster, New York, 1997).

The boom in defense production in Southern California began as early as 1940: Arthur C. Verge, *Paradise Transformed: Los Angeles During the Second World War* (Kendall/Hunt Publishing Company, Dubuque, 1993), p. 45.

Before the war, Los Angeles' black population was relatively small: Lonnie G. Bunch III, *Black Angelenos: The Afro-American in Los Angeles, 1850–1950* (California Afro-American Museum Foundation, Los Angeles, 1988) p. 36.

Historian Lonnie Bunche wrote: "Talk with any Black Angeleno: Lonnie G. Bunch III, "A Past Not Necessarily Prologue: The Afro-American in Los Angeles," in Norman M. Klein and Martin J. Schiesl, eds., *20th Century Los Angeles: Power Promotion, and Social Conflict* (Regina Books, Claremont, Calif. 1990), p. 123.

From 1940 to 1960 the black population in Los Angeles increased 423 percent: U.S. Bureau of the Census statistics.

From 1963 to 1965, 60 black Los Angeles residents—25 of them unarmed—were killed by police: Robert Gottlieb and Irene Wolt, *Thinking Big: The Story of the Los Angeles Times, Its Publishers and Their Influence on Southern California* (G.P. Putnam's Sons, New York, 1977) p. 376.

By the mid-1950s, a moldering Central Avenue: Central Avenue Sounds (University of California Press; Berkeley, Los Angeles, London, 1998) p. 405.

Yet in other areas of the city there were many empty classrooms: Gerald Horne, *Fire This Time: The Watts Uprising and the 1960s,* (Da Capo Press, New York, 1997) p. 228.

Until 1965, Jordan High School in Watts was the only high school in the city without a chemistry laboratory: Horne, p. 228.

One California legislator interpreted Proposition 13 this way: Jonathan Kozol, *Savage Inequalities* (Crown Publishers, 1991, New York) p. 220.

But there has been a steady diminution in all facets of the public school system since 1978: Shrag, p. 66.

In La Jolla: Jay Mathews, *Class Struggle: What's Wrong (and Right) with America's Best Public High Schools* (Times Books, New York, 1998) p. 185.

A parents booster club at the Westwood Charter Elementary School: Doug Smith, "Funding and Fairness Clash in Public Schools," *Los Angeles Times,* February 15, 1999.

During the year of the Watts riots, California was ranked seventh in the nation in education spending: Editorial Notebook, "How California Betrayed Its Schools," *New York Times,* February, 10, 1997.

But all ethnic groups in California—including whites—scored near the bottom: Editorial Notebook, *New York Times.*

Because Proposition 13 capped government revenue, each decision about spending: Fox Butterfield, "Crime Keeps on Falling, but Prisons Keep on Filling," *New York Times,* September 28, 1997.

One union local, for example, which organized the predominantly black janitors: Mike Davis, "*Chinatown* Revisited? The 'Internationalization' of Downtown Los Angeles" in *Sex, Death and God in L.A.,* edited by David Reid (Pantheon Books, New York, 1992) p. 32.

Five years after the riots, the rebuilding efforts have, in essence, merely ensured that conditions in South-Central returned to pre-riot levels: Hector Tobar, "Riots' Scars Include 200 Still-Vacant Lots," *Los Angeles Times,* April 21, 1997.

On these sites, hundreds of vacant lots: Tobar, *Los Angeles Times.*

In Hollywood and the Wilshire district, for example, the 30 buildings: Tobar, *Los Angeles Times.*

Chapter 16

But several minority school board members intimated: 1997 author interview with Rita Walters.

"The middle class takes care of its own": Robin Pogrebin, "Gifted Programs: Necessary Elitism?" *New York Times,* February 25, 1996.

A landmark report by the U.S. Department of Education: National Excellence: A Case For Developing America's Talent (U.S. Department of Education, Office of Educational Research and Improvement, Washington D.C., 1993).

Chapter 20

At a high school with one of the richest traditions in boys' and girls' basketball: Eric Shepard, "Moseley Had Charted the Territory Ahead," *Los Angeles Times,* February 22, 1997.

Chapter 31

This initial interpretation of affirmative action: Andrew Kull, *The Color-Blind Constitution* (Harvard University Press, Cambridge, Mass., 1992) p. 200.

But because those who were most vociferous in decrying the dangers of reverse discrimination and quotas were Southern segregationists: Lemann, *New York Times Magazine;* Lemann, "Second Thoughts About Integration," *GQ,* December 1997.

Only one percent attended law school: Bowen and Bok, p. 5.

By the late 1960s, civil rights lawyers: David G. Savage, "Battle Against Bias Waged on Shifting Legal Ground," *Los Angeles Times,* February 20, 1995.

Construction unions in New York, Cleveland, Philadelphia and a number of other cities refused to hire black workers: Savage, *Los Angeles Times.*

It was during the administration of President Richard Nixon, who had campaigned against quotas: Kevin Merida, "The Firm Founder of Affirmative Action," *Washington Post,* June 13, 1995.

He saw the plan as a highly effective way to pit blacks and labor against each other: Lemann, *New York Times Sunday Magazine.*

It now seemed mandatory: Bok and Bowen, p. 8.

The number of blacks who graduated from law schools increased from about one percent in 1960: Bok and Bowen, p. 10.

During the affirmative action years, the number of blacks in technical and managerial jobs doubled: Lemann, *New York Times Sunday Magazine.*

When their administrations began gearing up to eliminate affirmative action programs: Lemann, *New York Times Sunday Magazine.*

"... *We cannot,*" *Glazer wrote, "be quite so cavalier about the impact* . . .": Nathan Glazer, "In Defense of Preferences," *The New Republic*, April 6, 1998.

Chapter 34

About 130 California public high schools, which serve predominantly black and Latino students: Louis Sahagun and Kenneth R. Weiss, "Bias Suit Targets Schools without Advanced Classes," *Los Angeles Times*, July 28, 1999.

Epilogue

The number of Latino students enrolled at UC Berkeley declined by 43 percent and at UCLA the number fell by 23 percent: Enrollment statistics provided to the author by the University of California Public Information Office. Enrollment statistics for Latinos was compiled by combining statistics for Chicano and Latino Students.

Admissions directors attribute the gain to aggressive recruitment of talented minority students: Kenneth R. Weiss, "Minority Admissions at UC Almost at 1997 Level," *Los Angeles Times*, April 3, 1999.